Substance Abuse Treatment for Persons With HIV/AIDS

Treatment Improvement Protocol (TIP) Series

37

U.S. DEPARTMENT OF HEALTH AND HUMAN SERVICES
Public Health Service
Substance Abuse and Mental Health Services Administration
Center for Substance Abuse Treatment

1 Choke Cherry Road
Rockville, MD 20857

Acknowledgments

This publication was written under contract number 270-95-0013 with The CDM Group, Inc. (CDM). Sandra Clunies, M.S., I.C.A.D.C., served as the CSAT government project officer. Warren W. Hewitt, Jr., M.S., served as CSAT content advisor. Rose M. Urban, M.S.W., J.D., LCSW, CCAC, CSAC served as the CDM TIPs project director. Other CDM TIPs personnel included Raquel Witkin, M.S., project manager; Jonathan Max Gilbert, M.A., managing editor; Susan Kimner, editor/writer; Cara Smith, production editor; Erica Flick, editorial assistant; and Y-Lang Nguyen, former production editor.

Electronic Access and Copies of Publication

This publication may be downloaded or ordered at http://www.samhsa.gov/shin. Or, please call SAMHSA's Health Information Network at 1-877-SAMHSA-7 (1-877-726-4727) (English and Español).

Recommended Citation

Center for Substance Abuse Treatment. *Substance Abuse Treatment for Persons With HIV/AIDS*. Treatment Improvement Protocol (TIP) Series, Number 37. HHS Publication No. (SMA) 08-4137. Rockville, MD: Substance Abuse and Mental Health Services Administration, 1998.

Originating Office

Quality Improvement and Workforce Development Branch, Division of Services Improvement, Center for Substance Abuse Treatment, Substance Abuse and Mental Health Services Administration, 1 Choke Cherry Road, Rockville, MD 20857.

DHHS Publication No. (SMA) 08-4137
Printed 2000
Reprinted 2002, 2003, 2006, 2008, and 2009

Contents

What Is a TIP?

Treatment Improvement Protocols (TIPs) are best practice guidelines for the treatment of substance abuse, provided as a service of the Substance Abuse and Mental Health Services Administration's Center for Substance Abuse Treatment (CSAT). CSAT's Office of Evaluation, Scientific Analysis and Synthesis draws on the experience and knowledge of clinical, research, and administrative experts to produce the TIPs, which are distributed to a growing number of facilities and individuals across the country. The audience for the TIPs is expanding beyond public and private substance abuse treatment facilities as alcoholism and other substance abuse disorders are increasingly recognized as major problems.

The TIPs Editorial Advisory Board, a distinguished group of substance abuse experts and professionals in such related fields as primary care, mental health, and social services, works with the State Alcohol and Drug Abuse Directors to generate topics for the TIPs based on the field's current needs for information and guidance.

After selecting a topic, CSAT invites staff from pertinent Federal agencies and national organizations to a Resource Panel that recommends specific areas of focus as well as resources that should be considered in developing the content of the TIP. Then recommendations are communicated to a Consensus Panel composed of non-Federal experts on the topic who have been nominated by their peers. This Panel participates in a series of discussions; the information and recommendations on which they reach consensus form the foundation of the TIP. The members of each Consensus Panel represent substance abuse treatment programs, hospitals, community health centers, counseling programs, criminal justice and child welfare agencies, and private practitioners. A Panel Chair (or Co-Chairs) ensures that the guidelines mirror the results of the group's collaboration.

A large and diverse group of experts closely reviews the draft document. Once the changes recommended by these field reviewers have been incorporated, the TIP is prepared for publication, in print and online. The TIPs can be accessed via the Internet on the National Library of Medicine's home page at the URL: http://text.nlm.nih.gov. The move to electronic media also means that the TIPs can be updated more easily so they continue to provide the field with state-of-the-art information.

Although each TIP strives to include an evidence base for the practices it recommends, CSAT recognizes that the field of substance abuse treatment is evolving and that research frequently lags behind the innovations pioneered in the field. A major goal of each TIP is to convey "front line" information quickly but responsibly. For this reason, recommendations proffered in the TIP are attributed to either Panelists' clinical experience or the literature. If there is research to support a particular approach, citations are provided.

This TIP, *Substance Abuse Treatment for Persons With HIV/AIDS*, is a revision of TIP 15, *Treatment for HIV-Infected Alcohol and Other Drug Abusers* (CSAT, 1995b). It is intended to help a wide range of providers become familiar with the various issues surrounding clients with both substance abuse and human immunodeficiency virus (HIV) and to foster a better understanding of the roles of other providers.

Chapter 1 provides a basic overview of HIV/AIDS, including the latest available epidemiological data from the Centers for Disease Control and Prevention. Chapter 2 discusses medical assessment and treatment of HIV/AIDS. Chapter 3 discusses the treatment of mental health disorders in substance abusers with HIV/AIDS. Chapter 4 explains HIV/AIDS prevention, and Chapter 5 provides information about how to integrate treatment services via collaboration, so that all the needs of HIV-infected clients with substance abuse disorders can be met. Chapter 6 discusses case management and how to access the services that clients need. Chapter 7 provides information about counseling clients with HIV/AIDS and

substance abuse disorders, including information on staff issues, screening, and cultural competency. Chapter 8 discusses ethical issues, and Chapter 9 presents legal issues, including confidentiality and clients' access to services and programs. Chapter 10 provides information about funding sources for programs treating clients with HIV/AIDS and substance abuse treatment. The appendixes in this TIP provide additional information on several topics and include the 1993 Revised Classification System for HIV and AIDS, Federal and State codes of ethics, AIDS-related Web sites, and a list of State and Territorial health agencies and AIDS hotlines.

This TIP represents another step by CSAT toward its goal of bringing national leaders together to improve substance abuse treatment in the United States.

Other TIPs may be ordered by contacting SAMHSA's National Clearinghouse for Alcohol and Drug Information (NCADI), (800) 729-6686 or (301) 468-2600; TDD (for hearing impaired), (800) 487-4889.

Editorial Advisory Board

Consensus Panel

Chair

Steven L. Batki, M.D.
   Professor
   Department of Psychiatry
   SUNY Upstate Medical University
   Syracuse, New York

Co-Chair

Peter A. Selwyn, M.D., M.P.H.
   Professor and Chairman
   Department of Family Medicine and
      Community Health
   Montefiore Medical Center
   Albert Einstein College of Medicine
   Bronx, New York

Panelists

Deborah Wright Bauer, M.P.H., M.L.S.
   Health Project Consultant
   Georgia Ryan White Title IV Project
   Epidemiology and Prevention Branch
   Department of Human Resources
   Atlanta, Georgia

Margaret K. Brooks, J.D., M.A.
   New Perspectives
   Montclair, New Jersey

Robert Paul Cabaj, M.D.
   Medical Director
   San Mateo County Mental Health Services
   Mental Health Services Administration
   San Mateo, California

Susan M. Gallego, M.S.S.W., L.M.S.W.-A.C.P.
   Trainer, Consultant, and Facilitator
   Austin, Texas

Larry M. Gant, Ph.D., C.S.W., M.S.W.
   Associate Professor
   School of Social Work
   University of Michigan
   Ann Arbor, Michigan

Brian C. Giddens, M.S.W., A.C.S.W.
   Associate Director
   Social Work Department
   University of Washington Medical Center
   Seattle, Washington

Gregory L. Greenwood, Ph.D., M.P.H.
   TAPS Fellow
   Center for AIDS Prevention Studies
   University of California at San Francisco
   San Francisco, California

Elizabeth F. Howell, M.D.
    Substance Abuse Program Chief
    Georgia Department of Human Resources
    Division of Mental Health, Mental
        Retardation and Substance Abuse
    Atlanta, Georgia

Martin Yoneo Iguchi, Ph.D.
    Co-Director
    Senior Behavioral Scientist
    Drug Policy Research Center
    RAND
    Santa Monica, California

Susan LeLacheur, M.P.H., P.A.-C.
    Assistant Professor of Health Care Sciences
        and Health Sciences
    The George Washington University
    Physician Assistant Program
    Washington, D.C.

Andrea Ronhovde, L.C.S.W.
    Director
    Alexandria Mental Health HIV/AIDS Project
    Alexandria Mental Health Center
    Alexandria, Virginia

Ronald D. Stall, Ph.D., M.P.H.
    Center for AIDS Prevention Studies
    University of California at San Francisco
    San Francisco, California

Michael D. Stein, M.D.
    Associate Professor
    Department of Medicine
    Brown University
    Providence, Rhode Island

Foreword

The Treatment Improvement Protocol (TIP) series fulfills SAMHSA's mission of building resilience and facilitating recovery by providing best practices guidance to clinicians, program administrators, and payors. TIPs are the result of careful consideration of all relevant clinical and health services research findings, demonstration experience, and implementation requirements. A panel of clinical researchers, clinicians, program administrators, and client advocates debates and discusses its particular areas of expertise until it reaches a consensus on best practices. This panel's work is then reviewed and critiqued by field reviewers.

The talent, dedication, and hard work that TIPs Panelists and reviewers bring to this highly participatory process have bridged the gap between the promise of research and the needs of practicing clinicians and administrators to serve people who abuse substances in the most current and effective ways. We are grateful to all who have joined with us to contribute to advances in the substance abuse treatment field.

Eric Broderick, D.D.S., M.P.H.
Acting Administrator
Substance Abuse and Mental Health
    Services Administration

H. Westley Clark, M.D., J.D., M.P.H., CAS, FASAM
Director
Center for Substance Abuse Treatment
Substance Abuse and Mental Health
    Services Administration

Executive Summary and Recommendations

Many significant changes have occurred in recent years in the treatment of human immunodeficiency virus (HIV)/acquired immunodeficiency syndrome (AIDS). In recognition of these advances and their impact on substance abuse treatment, the Center for Substance Abuse Treatment (CSAT) convened a Consensus Panel in 1998 to update and expand TIP 15, *Treatment for HIV-Infected Alcohol and Other Drug Abusers* (CSAT, 1995b).

Major research advances have substantially improved our understanding of the biology of HIV and the pathogenesis (i.e., origin and development) of AIDS. The pathogenesis of AIDS is now known to result from the ability of HIV to replicate at the rate of a billion new virions (viral particles) per day and nearly 10 trillion new virions over the course of HIV infection. This, countered by the ability of the body to produce CD4+ T cell lymphocytes (a primary target cell for HIV), sets the stage for the struggle between HIV and the immune system—a struggle that lasts from the first day of HIV infection to end-stage disease and death.

Early in the U.S. HIV/AIDS pandemic, the role of substance abuse in the transmission of HIV and AIDS became clear. HIV is most efficiently transmitted through exposure to contaminated blood. As a result, injection drug users represent the largest HIV-infected substance-abusing population in the United States. In addition to contracting HIV through contaminated injection equipment, sexual contact within relatively closed sexual networks is another route of HIV transmission among injection drug users. These networks are characterized by multiple sex partners, unprotected intercourse, and the exchange of sex for drugs. The use of alcohol and noninjection drugs within this environment only increases the HIV/AIDS caseload. Because substance abuse and the HIV/AIDS pandemic are so interrelated, substance abuse treatment can play an important role in helping substance abusers reduce risk-taking behavior, thus helping to reduce the incidence of HIV/AIDS.

The current trend in the HIV/AIDS pandemic shows that a disproportionate number of minorities who live in inner cities are affected by or at risk for contracting HIV. This population is poor, hard to reach through traditional public health methods, and in need of a wide range of health and human services.

The recommendations and guidelines in this TIP continue to reinforce the approach established in TIP 15, which was the creation of a comprehensive, integrated system of care for HIV-infected substance abusers. Collaborative, efficient networks must be developed among substance abuse treatment centers, medical personnel, mental health personnel, and public health officials to prevent further spread of the disease and to provide high-quality care to infected individuals. Bringing together these disciplines that traditionally work independently of each other is an enormous challenge. An additional important challenge is to overcome misunderstandings and a lack of communication based on differences in ethnicity, culture, economic status, sexual orientation, and lifestyle.

The HIV/AIDS pandemic has induced some substance abuse treatment centers in HIV epicenters (e.g., San Francisco, New York, Washington, D.C.) to increase the range of services they provide in order to attend to all the needs of their clients: substance abuse treatment; HIV/AIDS treatment; and other medical, behavioral, psychological, and social needs. As a result, these treatment centers are providing clients with comprehensive diagnosis, treatment, and management of all presenting problems. For those times when services are unavailable, these treatment centers may establish referral networks and resource links with other treatment providers in their communities.

There are various audiences for this TIP, and different chapters are targeted to some of them individually. Nevertheless, the entire TIP should be of interest to anyone who wants to improve care for HIV-infected substance abusers. Prevention and treatment of substance abuse and HIV/AIDS require a multidisciplinary approach that relies on the strengths of a variety of providers and treatment settings. It is unrealistic to expect any single provider to be competent in all areas of care; this TIP will help a wide range of providers become familiar with the various issues surrounding substance abuse and HIV/AIDS and should foster a better understanding of the roles of other providers.

The Consensus Panel for this TIP drew on its considerable experience in both the HIV/AIDS and the substance abuse treatment fields. The Panel was composed of representatives from all of the disciplines involved in HIV/AIDS and substance abuse treatment, including physicians, alcohol and drug counselors, mental health workers, State government representatives, and legal counsel.

The TIP is organized into ten chapters, the first of which provides an introduction to HIV/AIDS, including the origin, life cycle, and progression of the disease. The second part of Chapter 1 provides an overview of the changes in epidemiology since 1995 when the first edition of this TIP was published. Epidemiological data from the Centers for Disease Control and Prevention (CDC) are summarized, and readers are provided with an overview of the pandemic in the regions of the United States, the current trends and populations most affected by the disease, and a discussion of special populations.

Chapter 2, which is targeted to medical personnel, discusses the medical assessment and treatment of HIV/AIDS, including adherence to treatment, barriers to care, treatment and testing, pharmacology, and prophylaxis against opportunistic infections. Chapter 3, which is aimed at mental health workers, explores the mental health treatment of clients with substance abuse problems and HIV/AIDS and discusses common mental disorders, assessment and diagnosis, pharmacology, counseling, and staff issues. Chapter 4 presents issues concerning HIV prevention. These issues include assessing clients for risk, risk-reduction counseling, sexual risk reduction, prenatal and perinatal prevention, transmission of resistant strains of HIV, syringe sharing, rapid HIV testing, and infection control issues for programs.

Chapter 5 discusses integrating treatment services, as well as the importance of linkages between substance abuse treatment programs and other providers. Chapter 6 provides information about case management and finding resources for HIV-infected substance abusers, including resources for substance abuse treatment, mental health, medical care, and income and other financial concerns for clients. Chapter 7 examines counseling issues, including staff training and attitudes, screening, and issues specific to the substance-abusing client with HIV/AIDS. Chapter 8 explores ethical issues, and Chapter 9 discusses legal issues and provides basic information about Federal laws regarding discrimination and confidentiality. Chapter 10, geared toward program administrators, presents information about funding sources and grantwriting.

In light of the volumes of information available about HIV/AIDS, this TIP is not intended to be exhaustive. A wide array of resources is provided for those who wish to find more information on topics of interest. The appendixes in this TIP provide additional information on several topics and include the 1993 Revised Classification System for HIV and AIDS, Federal and State codes of ethics, AIDS-related Web sites, and a list of State and Territorial health agencies and AIDS hotlines.

In order to avoid awkward construction and sexism, this TIP alternates between "he" and "she" for generic examples.

Throughout this TIP, the term "substance abuse" has been used in a general sense to cover both substance abuse and substance dependence (as defined by the *Diagnostic and Statistical Manual of Mental Disorders,* 4th ed. [DSM-IV] [American Psychiatric Association, 1994]). Because the term "substance abuse" is commonly used by substance abuse treatment professionals to describe any excessive use of addictive substances, it will be used to denote both substance dependence and substance abuse. The term relates to the use of alcohol as well as other substances of abuse. Readers should attend to the context in which the term occurs in order to determine what possible range of meanings it covers; in most cases, however, the term will refer to all varieties of

substance abuse disorders as described by DSM-IV.

The recommendations that follow are grouped by chapter. Recommendations supported by research literature or legislation are followed by a (1); clinically based recommendations are marked (2).

Summary of Recommendations

Medical Treatment

- Treating HIV/AIDS is extremely complex. It is important that the medical care team have experience working with substance-abusing clients because the combination of substance abuse and HIV/AIDS poses special challenges. Integrated care is the best treatment option, and medical practitioners who work with substance abuse treatment centers should be experienced in treating HIV/AIDS patients. (2)
- Primary care staff serving HIV-infected patients with substance abuse disorders should understand and be responsive to patients' needs, potential for relapse, and cultural variations. Primary care models that are incorporated as part of substance abuse treatment programs should be evaluated to identify how they can be modified and expanded to address the special needs of the HIV-infected substance abuse disorder population. (2)
- Adherence to antiretroviral treatment means that the client must follow a prescribed and often complicated treatment regimen. Adherence should be maintained because nonadherence can lead to the rapid development of drug resistance. (1)
- One means to encourage adherence is to educate clients and their significant others about HIV/AIDS treatment. (2)

- Ideally, all treatment programs should be capable of conducting HIV risk assessments and providing basic HIV/AIDS education and counseling to clients. In addition, all programs should provide access to HIV testing and pre- and posttest counseling. If such services cannot be provided, linkages should be established with other agencies that can provide these services. When clients are sent from substance abuse treatment programs to referral sites for primary medical care, a communications system should be in place to ensure that appointments are kept, that information about clients' medical care is sent back to the program, and that the communications system complies with Federal and State confidentiality requirements. (2)

- Optimally, primary care should be multidisciplinary, with social workers, physicians, physicians-in-training, nurses, and counselors included among the treatment staff. A case manager may be helpful in facilitating communication among treatment personnel. Existing primary care models should be evaluated to identify how they can be modified and expanded to address the special needs of HIV-infected substance abusers. (2)

- Testing for HIV is a crucial first step in engaging the HIV-infected substance abuser. A low threshold for testing should exist when one assesses the client's level of risk for HIV. This can be determined by the following: if the client has engaged in risky behaviors; if the client has ever had a sexually transmitted disease (STD); if the client has a history of sharing drug injection equipment; or if the client is presenting with any of a number of symptoms that might indicate recent infection with HIV or early symptomatic infection. (2)

- Medical care for HIV-infected patients will vary, depending on the stage of infection, but all patients should receive a minimum level of evaluation and followup. An assessment of the behaviors associated with HIV transmission is an important part of the initial assessment. (2)

- A thorough medical history is an important step to help the clinician proceed to clinical evaluation and formulate a treatment plan. Although HIV/AIDS and its complications may involve nearly every organ, the HIV/AIDS-directed general physical exam should focus on the skin, the eyes, the mouth, the anogenital region, the nervous system, the lymphatic system, and patient weight and temperature. Knowledge of a patient's immune status may also direct the clinician toward screening other areas. (2)

- Before starting antiretroviral therapy in any patient, laboratory studies should be done and may include HIV ribonucleic acid (RNA) (or viral load), CD4+ T cell counts, blood counts, screening chemistries, syphilis, toxoplasmosis, purified protein derivative (PPD), hepatitis A, B, and C viruses, and chest x-ray. (2)

- The decision to begin antiretroviral therapy in the asymptomatic patient is difficult and often involves multiple visits to review treatment options. The factors that must be considered include patient willingness to begin therapy and remain adherent, the degree of immunodeficiency, the risk of disease progression as determined by plasma HIV RNA, the risks of side effects, the ongoing treatment of other medical conditions, and barriers to care, such as lack of insurance and unstable housing. (2)

- Criteria for changing therapy include
  - Suboptimal initial reduction in HIV RNA level
  - Reappearance of viremia after suppression to undetectable levels
  - Persistent and progressive decline in CD4+ T cells

♦ Development of intolerable side effects

♦ The client's inability to adhere to a treatment regimen. (In all cases, the clinician must determine whether the treatment failure is due to imperfect adherence [because of toxicity or patient disinterest], altered absorption or metabolism of one or more drugs in a multidrug pharmacokinetics, or viral resistance to one or more agents. When the decision to change therapy is based on HIV RNA, a second viral load test is needed before any decision can be made.) (1)

■ In general, it is preferable to change all of the drugs used in failing combination, except in those instances when viral loads are undetectable and a side effect can be traced to a specific medication. In some cases in which the viral load is not suppressed completely, it may be best to continue the present regimen if it has been partially effective and the patient's options are limited. (1)

■ Managing acute and chronic pain in HIV-infected patients with substance abuse disorders can be a challenging clinical problem. As with all patients in pain, the provider's primary goal is to maximize comfort while minimizing side effects. Local measures (rest, heat, ice, analgesic rubs) should be used as a first line of pain treatment when appropriate. If these measures fail to relieve pain, a systematic pharmacologic approach is recommended. Should these medications prove inadequate for pain relief, narcotic analgesia may be necessary. (1)

■ The treatment plan and the reason for using narcotics for pain control must be clear to both provider and patient. It is important not only that the patient knows that his pain is taken seriously but also that narcotic use will not be extended beyond a limited period

required for analgesia. Pain management specialists should be consulted as needed to examine alternative management strategies. Because HIV/AIDS patients often have pain problems similar to those of cancer patients, the World Health Organization's (WHO's) "cancer pain analgesic ladder" is useful as a starting point for managing pain in HIV-infected persons. (1)

■ Setting clear limits and devising a consistent treatment plan can help to reduce the risk of medication abuse by patients. The following strategies are recommended: designate one care provider to dispense prescriptions for controlled drugs, dispense limited amounts of controlled drugs (e.g., 1-week supply or less), and advise patients that lost or stolen prescriptions will not be replaced. (2)

■ Clients who are symptomatic with AIDS frequently are prescribed narcotic analgesics and may also have an indwelling intravenous line for infusion therapy. Injection drug users are at very high risk of using this indwelling intravenous line to administer heroin, cocaine, and other drugs of abuse. It is therefore essential that clients with such lines be cared for in residential settings where adequate monitoring and support can be provided. (2)

■ Ongoing efforts are needed to educate patients about the importance of clinical trials and to alleviate their long-standing suspicion of the medical profession. Specific efforts should be made to include more substance abuse clients, women, and minorities in HIV clinical trials. All of these groups currently are underrepresented. To avoid a conflict of interest, it is recommended that, as far as possible, the clinician responsible for the clinical trial not be the patient's primary care provider. (2)

■ Care providers must be aware that HIV-infected patients may be using alternative or complementary therapies; for example, acupuncture, meditation, and vitamin and herbal dietary supplements. However, patients need not be discouraged from trying a therapy unless it is known to be harmful. Clinicians have a responsibility to discover, in a nonjudgmental manner, what alternative or unapproved therapies patients are using and then to obtain as much information as possible about these therapies. Clinicians should specifically ask about unsupervised antibiotic use because it can complicate the diagnosis and treatment of bacterial infections in HIV-infected substance abuse clients. (1)

■ The Consensus Panel supports the CDC's recommendation that HIV infection be considered an indication for pneumococcal vaccination because of the markedly increased risk of pneumococcal pneumonia among HIV-infected clients. The effectiveness of this vaccine in clients with severely weakened immune systems is questionable, but it has been found to provide moderate immunity when administered in the earlier stages of HIV infection. Vaccination against *H. influenzae* type B should also be considered because HIV-infected individuals, particularly injection drug users, are at increased risk for *H. influenzae* pneumonia. Hepatitis A vaccine should be administered when necessary because most injection drug users are hepatitis C positive and the CDC recommends hepatitis A vaccine in all hepatitis C-positive individuals. (1)

■ Primary care providers should be aware that, in general, the incidence of gynecological disorders is likely to be higher among female substance abusers than among non-substance-abusing women. Some disorders such as STDs result indirectly from substance abuse, while others may result from lifestyle factors that influence the overall health status

of women, such as the lack of regular medical care. (1)

■ Treatment personnel must be aware of the special nutritional needs of HIV-infected substance abusers. Staff should be familiar with guidelines concerning nutritional supplements and with interventions to address the causes of inadequate food consumption. (2)

Mental Health Treatment

■ Individuals with substance abuse disorders, whether or not they are HIV infected, are subject to higher rates of mental disorders than the rest of the population. Counselors working with HIV-infected substance abusers should be aware of the variety of both HIV- and substance-induced psychiatric symptoms. It is also important to recognize that psychiatric symptoms may be caused by substance abuse, HIV/AIDS, or the medications used to treat HIV/AIDS, as well as by preexisting psychiatric disorders. (1)

■ Treatment programs that do not have the resources to adequately assess and treat mental illness should be closely linked to mental health services to which clients can be referred. Open lines of communication will enable personnel in both locations to be informed about a client's treatment program. Treatment staff should maintain contact with the client and continue treatment during and after the psychiatric referral. (2)

■ Communication between medical and counseling staffs is important to ensure that cognitively impaired clients are not perceived as deceitful or manipulative. Care providers must keep in mind that cognitively impaired clients' nonadherence to treatment may be a result of the impairment and not caused by denial, resistance, or unwillingness to accept care. (2)

- It is essential to set realistic treatment goals that correspond to the client's functional capacities. (2)

- Therapeutic interventions must be sensitive to the culture and ethnicity of the client population. Whenever possible, therapists and support group leaders should share the culture of their clients and should speak the same language. Cultural compatibility between therapists and clients is important in creating an atmosphere of trust where sensitive issues, such as family support and group mores, can be addressed. (2)

- Assessment and diagnosis of mental illness in HIV-infected substance-abusing clients is a daunting challenge because of these clients' complex problems. Therefore, it is important to evaluate clients' behavior in context (e.g., acute depression is common in people who have just learned they are HIV positive). (1)

- Standard pharmacologic approaches may be used to treat psychiatric disorders in HIV-infected substance abusers, with some specific considerations. Without exception, a medical and psychiatric diagnostic evaluation should always be carried out before medication is provided. (1)

- When prescribing medications for HIV-infected substance abusers, physicians should use a graduated approach that increases the level and type of medication slowly, one step at a time. Low doses of medications that are safer and less likely to be abused should be tried first, and higher doses or less safe agents used only if the initial approach is ineffective. (1)

- With highly active antiretroviral therapy (HAART) the physician must be aware of potential drug interactions that can increase the toxicity of medications or reduce their levels in the patient's blood, resulting in suboptimal therapy and the development of resistance. The mental health counselor should be familiar with the symptoms that could indicate that a client is experiencing a drug interaction. (1)

- HIV-infected individuals may be more sensitive to prescription medications as well as to drugs of abuse. When prescribing, clinicians should attempt to use the lowest effective dose to minimize side effects. With clients symptomatic with AIDS, it may be wise to begin with very low doses, of the magnitude generally associated with geriatric patients. (1)

- Substance abusers are at increased risk of suicide. HIV-infected individuals may also be at risk of suicide, especially if they are suffering from a mood disorder. Medication should be dispensed in small amounts until a client's level of responsibility can be fully assessed. Prescribers should be aware that some medications such as tricyclic antidepressants (TCAs) (like amitriptyline [Elavil]) are especially likely to be lethal in overdose. (2)

- Counseling is an important part of treatment for all substance abusers, including those with comorbid psychiatric disorders. The goal of counseling is to help the HIV-infected substance abuser maintain health, achieve recovery from the substance abuse, and attain the best possible level of psychological functioning. (2)

- If a client is not acutely suicidal but wants to talk about suicide, the counselor should maintain interest, allow the client to discuss his feelings, assess the severity of the client's suicidality, and obtain help if needed. The counselor should not minimize the client's experiences because talking openly about suicide decreases isolation, fear, and tension. (2)

- Support groups fulfill a wide range of needs. Substance abuse treatment programs should actively refer clients to appropriate outside support groups where their specific needs can be met. (2)

Primary and Secondary HIV Prevention

- For HIV-infected clients in substance abuse treatment, there must be a comprehensive approach to treatment that includes three goals: living substance free and sober, slowing or halting the progression of HIV/AIDS, and reducing HIV risk-taking behavior. (2)

- Numerous risk assessment protocols exist and may be used with a minimum of training and familiarity. The goal of the HIV/AIDS risk assessment should be to identify behaviors that may place the client at risk for HIV infection. (2)

- A comprehensive sexual practices history is important and should be taken early in counseling, although not necessarily at the first session. Clients must be reassured of the confidentiality of the information they provide. (2)

- Counselors should address the full range of potential risk behaviors in their history taking, including both syringe sharing and unsafe sex. They must take into account a wide range of sexual orientations, including those of homosexual, bisexual, heterosexual, and transgender clients. Condom use and safer sex practices must be a special focus of the assessment. Counselors need to know what the client believes about HIV/AIDS, including any information the client received from other treatment professionals. (2)

- In promoting risk reduction, the alcohol and drug counselor should help the client understand the need for change, provide psychological support for behavior change, and assist the client in developing the appropriate skills to sustain the behavior change. (2)

- Discussion of risk behaviors should take place in language that is culturally appropriate, clear, and understandable. (2)

- HIV sexual risk reduction programs should be integrated into substance abuse treatment programs. Sexual risk reduction programs should provide clients with basic information about safer sex practices, as well as an array of alternative strategies and choices that are client controlled. (2)

- IDU risk reduction is best approached in a step-wise fashion; for example, abstinence is the best step, no syringe use is the second best step, *not sharing* syringes is the third best step, using *only clean* syringes is the fourth best step, and so on. (2)

- Federal law currently prohibits using Federal funds for syringe exchange programs. (1)

- The AIDS pandemic poses a number of challenges for infection control policy and practice in substance abuse treatment programs. Treatment programs should apply the same universal precautions that exist in hospitals and other health care facilities. (1)

- The most important approach to reducing the risk of occupational HIV transmission is to prevent exposure. However, in the event of occupational exposure, substance abuse treatment programs should follow the CDC's recommendations for postexposure prophylaxis. (2)

- Rapid HIV tests are becoming readily available, and these tests will alter how and when HIV prevention counseling is delivered. Counselors must understand the technical aspects of these screening tests, as well as how to assess each client's risk for infection. Reactive rapid tests must still be confirmed by a supplemental test (either Western blot or immunofluorescence assay). (2)

Integrating Treatment Services

- Treatment for substance abuse and HIV/AIDS should reflect the interconnected relationship they share and be coordinated as much as possible to maximize care for persons with both HIV/AIDS and substance abuse disorders. (2)

■ Substance abuse treatment counselors and HIV/AIDS service providers should continue to develop their skills in establishing and maintaining treatment plans that support the "total" person. (2)

■ In any effort to develop integrated treatment for substance abuse and HIV/AIDS treatment, either within a single agency or through individual care plans, the following are essential: having a strong case management model, including social services as a core part of the treatment plan, cross-training all providers in the requirements of the other treatment centers, and facilitating eligibility determinations. (2)

■ Many HIV-infected substance abusers are unable to maintain abrupt and total discontinuation of substance use. In dealing with clients' ongoing substance abuse, treatment programs must find a balance between abstinence-oriented approaches, where clients must immediately stop substance use, or public health–oriented approaches, where clients who cannot abruptly abstain are encouraged to reduce substance use gradually. (2)

■ Counselors who work with HIV-positive substance abusers should familiarize themselves with the local AIDS Service Organizations (ASOs) and substance abuse treatment services. (2)

■ When establishing a network of care coordination, the provider must consider the issue of confidentiality. Providers must be aware of State and Federal laws and professional ethical codes, along with agency and community policies and agreements. The provider should understand the difference between "consent" and "informed consent." (2)

Accessing and Obtaining Needed Services

■ A case management approach recognizes that satisfying such basic needs as general health and adequate housing and food when an individual is actively abusing substances can be overwhelming and that substance-abusing behavior will impair a person's ability to gain access to a formalized system of services. (2)

■ The Panel recommends using case management in dealing with the multiple problems presented by HIV/AIDS in combination with substance abuse. Case management promotes teamwork among the various care providers. For example, linkages among the client's primary care provider, AIDS case manager, mental health provider, and substance abuse treatment provider can greatly benefit the client and improve care. (1)

■ There are several procedures in multidisciplinary planning: determine who the significant providers are within the client's system; determine the nature of the group (i.e., fixed or ad hoc); discuss the expectations, rules, and structure of the group; establish formalized linkages with other agencies to help build a group; if there are several case managers, designate one to act as "lead" case manager; and keep client confidentiality in mind. (2)

■ To enhance effective teamwork, the multidisciplinary group should periodically assess itself to determine if there are any concerns or frustrations among its members. There also should be a periodic formal evaluation to allow members to review more thoroughly what is and what is not working. (2)

■ It is sometimes difficult for the HIV-infected substance abuser to find and fund needed services. The case manager can play an important role in helping find specific services and navigate the plethora of public and private funding options. The counselor should be familiar with funding options for services such as substance abuse treatment, mental health treatment, medical and dental care, and HIV/AIDS drug therapy. (2)

- Counselors should be knowledgeable about the eligibility criteria, duration of service, and amount of assistance in their States for basic financial assistance programs, including welfare, unemployment insurance, disability income, food stamps, and vocational rehabilitation. (2)

- When faced with potential barriers to finding resources for clients, counselors should explore alternative resources, such as friends, significant others, and the community; other areas of the State; and client relocation to areas where services are available. (2)

Counseling Clients

- Before conducting any screening, assessment, or treatment planning, counselors should reassess their personal attitudes and experiences toward working with HIV-infected substance-abusing clients. It is important for a provider to reassess comfort level with each client because clients vary in demographic and cultural background. (2)

- Staff members must have the proper training to screen, assess, and counsel clients. The most important aspect of staff competency is that it is an ongoing process. (2)

- Providers should identify other programs and agencies with which to network in order to provide care for their clients. At a minimum, client services should include the following in order of priority: substance abuse treatment, medical care, housing, mental health care, nutritional care, dental care, ancillary services, and support systems. (2)

- Providers must take precautions when notifying clients of HIV test results, complying with regulations to ensure that their confidentiality is preserved. (2)

- Treatment providers and counselors must examine two essential factors when working with linguistically, culturally, racially, or ethnically different populations: the socioeconomic status of the client or group and the client's degree of acculturation. A distinction may need to be made between a population as a whole and a particular segment of that population. (2)

- Providers must work to develop culturally competent systems of care. One component of this involves making services accessible to and highly usable by the target risk populations. Effective systems also recognize the importance of culture, cross-cultural relationships, cultural differences, and the ability to meet culturally unique needs. (2)

- Clients facing progressive illness and disability need a variety of supportive services. The counseling of ill and dying clients should be supportive and nonconfrontational, addressing issues relevant to the client's illness at a pace determined by the client. (2)

- Providers should increase their proficiency at counseling clients who are at the end stages of AIDS by examining their own beliefs about death and dying. (2)

- Providers should discuss end-of-life health care options with clients, such as making a living will, appointing a health care proxy, and so on, and they should do this before clients become ill. (2)

- In preparing their children for the loss of parents, clients should be practically assisted in the following areas: legal guardianship, standby guardianship, leaving a legacy of living memories, and dealing with survivor guilt. (2)

Ethical Issues

■ Because providers routinely encounter emotionally charged issues when treating substance abusers, they should possess the tools to explore ethical dilemmas objectively. By doing so, and by examining their own reactions to the situation, providers can proceed with the most ethical course of action. (2)

■ All programs should have a consistent process for dealing with ethical concerns. While ethical issues are usually complex enough to require a case-by-case evaluation, agency practices should include a routine process for approaching an ethical issue. (2)

Legal Issues

■ Substance abuse treatment providers may encounter discrimination against their clients as they try to connect them with services. Counselors should be familiar with Federal and State laws that protect people with disabilities and how these laws apply to HIV-infected substance abusers. (2)

■ Although the Federal law protecting information about clients in substance abuse treatment and State laws protecting HIV/AIDS-related information both permit a client to consent to a disclosure, the consent requirements are likely to differ. Therefore, when a provider contemplates making a disclosure of information about a client in substance abuse treatment who is living with HIV/AIDS, she must consider both Federal and State laws. (2)

■ The rules regarding confidentiality in the provision of substance abuse treatment to persons with HIV/AIDS are very specific. Generally, no more than two sets of laws will apply in any given situation. If only substance abuse treatment information will

be disclosed, a program is generally safe following the Federal rules. If HIV/AIDS–treatment-related information will be disclosed, and the disclosure will reveal that the client is in substance abuse treatment, the program must comply with both sets of laws (Federal and State). When in doubt, the best practice is to follow the more restrictive rules. (2)

■ Any counselor or program considering warning someone of a client's HIV/AIDS status without the client's consent should carefully analyze whether there is, in fact, a duty to warn and whether it is possible to persuade the client to discharge this responsibility himself or consent to the program staff doing so. (2)

Funding and Policy Considerations

■ At a minimum, treatment programs receiving funding for women's services must also provide or arrange for the following services for pregnant women and women with dependent children, including women who are trying to regain custody of their children: primary medical care, primary pediatric care (including immunizations), gender-specific substance abuse treatment, therapeutic interventions for children in custody of women in treatment, and sufficient case management and transportation. (1)

■ States with a certain rate of AIDS cases must spend at least 5 percent of their total Substance Abuse Prevention and Treatment (SAPT) Block Grant funds on HIV/AIDS early intervention services for persons in substance abuse treatment. HIV/AIDS early intervention services are defined as appropriate pretest counseling for HIV/AIDS, testing services, and appropriate posttest counseling. All entities providing early intervention services for HIV disease to an individual must comply with payment provisions and restrictions on expenditure of grants. (1)

■ Any organization that receives SAPT Block Grant funding for treatment services for injection drug users must actively encourage individuals in need of such treatment to undergo it. States require organizations to use outreach models that are scientifically sound, or, if no applicable models are available, to use an approach that can reasonably be expected to be an effective outreach method. (1)

1 Introduction to HIV/AIDS

The first cases of acquired immunodeficiency syndrome (AIDS) were reported in the United States in the spring of 1981. By 1983 the human immunodeficiency virus (HIV), the virus that causes AIDS, had been isolated. Early in the U.S. HIV/AIDS pandemic, the role of substance abuse in the spread of AIDS was clearly established. Injection drug use (IDU) was identified as a direct route of HIV infection and transmission among injection drug users. The largest group of early AIDS cases comprised gay and bisexual men (referred to as men who have sex with men—or MSMs). Early cases of HIV infection that were sexually transmitted often were related to the use of alcohol and other substances, and the majority of these cases occurred in urban, educated, white MSMs.

Currently, injection drug users represent the largest HIV-infected substance-abusing population in the United States. HIV/AIDS prevalence rates among injection drug users vary by geographic region, with the highest rates in surveyed substance abuse treatment centers in the Northeast, the South, and Puerto Rico. From July 1998 through June 1999, 23 percent of all AIDS cases reported were among men and women who reported IDU (Centers for Disease Control and Prevention [CDC], 1999b).

IDU practices are quick and efficient vehicles for HIV transmission. The virus is transmitted primarily through the exchange of blood using needles, syringes, or other IDU equipment (e.g., cookers, rinse water, cotton) that were previously used by an HIV-infected person. Lack of knowledge about safer needle use techniques and the lack of alternatives to needle sharing (e.g., available supplies of clean, new needles) contribute to the rise of HIV/AIDS.

Another route of HIV transmission among injection drug users is through sexual contacts within relatively closed sexual networks, which are characterized by multiple sex partners, unprotected sexual intercourse, and exchange of sex for money (Friedman et al., 1995). The inclusion of alcohol and other noninjection substances to this lethal mixture only increases the HIV/AIDS caseload (Edlin et al., 1994; Grella et al., 1995). A major risk factor for HIV/AIDS among injection drug users is crack use; one study found that crack abusers reported more sexual partners in the last 12 months, more sexually transmitted diseases (STDs) in their lifetimes, and greater frequency of paying for sex, exchanging sex for drugs, and having sex with injection drug users (Word and Bowser, 1997).

Following are the key concepts about HIV/AIDS and substance abuse disorders that influenced the creation of this TIP:

■ **Substance abuse increases the risk of contracting HIV.** HIV infection is substantially associated with the use of contaminated or used needles to inject heroin. Also, substance abusers may put themselves at risk for HIV infection by engaging in risky sex behaviors in exchange for powder or crack cocaine. However, this fact does not minimize the impact of other substances that may be used (e.g., hallucinogens, inhalants, stimulants, prescription medications).

- **Substance abusers are at risk for HIV infection through sexual behaviors.** Both men and women may engage in risky sexual behaviors (e.g., unprotected anal, vaginal, or oral sex; sharing of sex toys; handling or consuming body fluids and body waste; sex with infected partners) for the purpose of obtaining substances, while under the influence of substances, or while under coercion.

- **Substance abuse treatment serves as HIV prevention.** Placing the client in substance abuse treatment along a continuum of care and treatment helps minimize continued risky substance-abusing practices. Reducing a client's involvement in substance-abusing practices reduces the probability of infection.

- **HIV/AIDS, substance abuse disorders, and mental disorders interact in a complex fashion.** Each acts as a potential catalyst or obstacle in the treatment of the other two—substance abuse can negatively affect adherence to HIV/AIDS treatment regimens; substance abuse disorders and HIV/AIDS are intertwining disorders; HIV/AIDS is changing the shape and face of substance abuse treatment; complex and legal issues arise when treating HIV/AIDS and substance abuse; HIV-infected women with substance abuse disorders have special needs.

- **Risk reduction allows for a comprehensive approach to HIV/AIDS prevention.** This strategy promotes changing substance-related and sex-related behaviors to reduce clients' risk of contracting or transmitting HIV.

The first part of this chapter provides a basic overview of the origin of HIV/AIDS and the transmission and progression of the disease. The second part of the chapter presents a summary of epidemiological data from the CDC. This second part discusses the impact of HIV/AIDS in regions of the United States and the populations that are at the greatest risk of contracting HIV.

Overview of HIV/AIDS

Origin of HIV/AIDS

Of the many theories and myths about the origin of HIV, the most likely explanation is that HIV was introduced to humans from monkeys. A recent study (Gao et al., 1999) identified a subspecies of chimpanzees native to west equatorial Africa as the original source of HIV-1, the virus responsible for the global AIDS pandemic. The researchers believe that the virus crossed over from monkeys to humans when hunters became exposed to infected blood. Monkeys can carry a virus similar to HIV, known as SIV (simian immunodeficiency virus), and there is strong evidence that HIV and SIV are closely related (Simon et al., 1998; Zhu et al., 1998).

AIDS is caused by HIV infection and is characterized by a severe reduction in CD4+ T cells, which means an infected person develops a very weak immune system and becomes vulnerable to contracting life-threatening infections (such as *Pneumocystis carinii* pneumonia). AIDS occurs late in HIV disease.

Tracking of the disease in the United States began early after the discovery of the pandemic, but even to date, tracking data reveal only how many individuals have AIDS, not how many have HIV. The counted AIDS cases are like the visible part of an iceberg, while the much larger portion, HIV, is submerged out of sight. Many States are counting HIV cases now that positive results are to be gained by treating the infection in the early stages and because counting only AIDS cases is no longer sufficient for projecting trends of the pandemic. However, because HIV-infected people generally are asymptomatic for years, they might not be tested or included in the count. The CDC estimates that between 650,000 and 900,000 people in the United States currently are living with HIV (CDC, 1997c).

In 1996, the number of new AIDS cases (not HIV cases) and deaths from AIDS began to decline in the United States for the first time since 1981. Deaths from AIDS have decreased since 1996 in all racial and ethnic groups and among both men and women (CDC, 1999a). However, the most recent CDC data show that the decline is slowing (CDC, 1999b). The decline can be attributed to advances in treating HIV with multiple medications, known as combination therapy; treatments to prevent secondary opportunistic infections; and a reduction in the HIV infection rate in the mid-1980s prior to the introduction of combination therapy. The latter can be attributed to improved services for people with HIV and access to health care. In general, those with the best access to good, ongoing HIV/AIDS care increase their chances of living longer.

HIV/AIDS is still largely a disease of MSMs and male injection drug users, but it is spreading most rapidly among women and adolescents, particularly in African American and Hispanic communities. HIV is a virus that thrives in certain ecological conditions. The following will lead to higher infection rates: a more potent virus, high viral load, high prevalence of STDs, substance abuse, high HIV seroprevalence within the community, high rate of unprotected sexual contact with multiple partners, and low access to health care. These ecological conditions exist to a large degree among urban, poor, and marginalized communities ofinjection drug users. Thus, MSMs and African American and Hispanic women, their children, and adolescents within these communities are at greatest risk.

HIV Transmission

HIV cannot survive outside of a human cell. HIV must be transmitted directly from one person to another through human body fluids that contain HIV-infected cells, such as blood, semen, vaginal secretions, or breast milk. The most effective means of transmitting HIV is by direct contact between the infected blood of one person and the blood supply of another. (See Figure 1-1 for an illustration of the structure of the virus.) This can occur in childbirth as well as through blood transfusions or organ transplants prior to 1985. (Testing of the blood supply began in 1985, and the chance of this has greatly decreased.) Using injection equipment that an infected person used is another direct way to transmit HIV.

Sexual contact is also an effective transmission route for HIV because the tissues of the anus, rectum, and vagina are mucosal surfaces that can contain infected human body fluids and because these surfaces can be easily injured, allowing the virus to enter the body. A person is about five times more likely to contract HIV through anal intercourse than through vaginal intercourse because the tissues of the anal region are more prone to breaks and bleeding during sexual activity (Royce et al., 1997).

A woman is eight times more likely to contract HIV through vaginal intercourse if the man is infected than in the reverse situation (Center for AIDS Prevention Studies, 1998). HIV can be passed from a woman to a man during intercourse, but this is less likely because the skin of the penis is not as easily damaged. Female-to-female transmission of HIV apparently is rare but should be considered a possible means of transmission because of the potential exposure of mucous membranes to vaginal secretions and menstrual blood (CDC, 1997a).

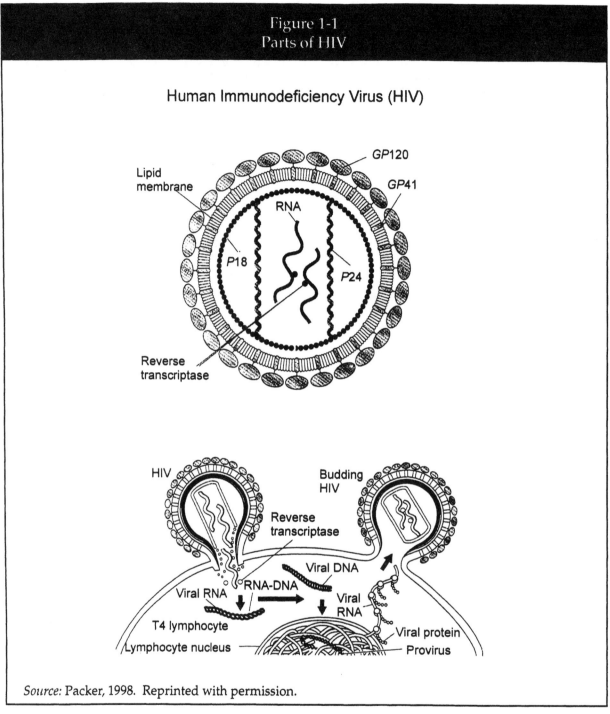

Figure 1-1
Parts of HIV

Human Immunodeficiency Virus (HIV)

GP120

GP41

Lipid membrane

RNA

P18

P24

Reverse transcriptase

HIV

Budding HIV

Reverse transcriptase

Viral DNA

Viral RNA

RNA-DNA

Viral RNA

T4 lymphocyte

Lymphocyte nucleus

Viral protein

Provirus

Source: Packer, 1998. Reprinted with permission.

Oral intercourse also is a potential risk but is less likely to transmit the disease than anal or vaginal intercourse. Saliva seems to have some effect in helping prevent transmission of HIV, and the oral tissues are less likely to be injured in sexual activity than those of the vagina or anus. However, if a person has infections or injuries in the mouth or gums, then the risk of contracting HIV through oral sex increases.

Role of circumcision in male infectivity

A possible link between male circumcision and HIV infectivity was first observed during studies conducted in Kenya in the late 1980s (Cameron et al., 1998; Greenblatt et al., 1988; Simonsen et al., 1988). Since then, numerous studies have been done on the possible relationship between male circumcision and

HIV infectivity. Data have not revealed a direct causal link between circumcision and HIV transmission, and scientific opinion has been divided on this topic. While some studies indicate that circumcision can play a protective role in preventing HIV infection (Kelly et al., 1999; Moses et al., 1998; Urassa et al., 1997), the bulk of recent scientific research has concluded that the reverse is true and that circumcision can actually increase the rate of HIV transmission (Van Howe, 1999). Clearly, further research and analysis of circumcision as a prophylactic against HIV transmission is needed.

Risks of transmission

Several factors can increase the risk of HIV transmission. One factor is the presence of another STD (e.g., genital ulcer disease) in either partner, which increases the risk of becoming infected with HIV through sexual contact. This is because the same risk behaviors that resulted in the person contracting an STD increase that person's chance of contracting HIV. STDs also can cause genital lesions that serve as ports of entry for HIV, they can increase the number of HIV target cells (CD4+ T cells), and they can cause the person to shed greater concentrations of HIV (CDC, 1998a). For this reason, all sexually active clients, especially women, should be checked regularly for STDs such as gonorrhea and chlamydia. Many STDs that cause symptoms in men are asymptomatic in women. When genital ulcers are treated and heal, the risk of HIV transmission is reduced.

Another factor that increases risk is a high level of HIV circulating in the bloodstream. This occurs soon after the initial infection and returns late in the disease. New drug therapy can keep this level (called viral load) low or undetectable, but this does not mean that other individuals cannot be infected. The virus still exists—it is simply not detectable by the currently available tests. Because the correlation between plasma and genital fluid viral load varies, transmission

may still occur despite an undetectable serum viral load (Liuzzi et al., 1996).

Once HIV passes to an uninfected person who is not taking anti-HIV drugs, the virus reproduces very rapidly. It is known that drug-resistant viruses can be transmitted from one person to another. The treatment implications for a person infected with a drug-resistant virus are not yet known, but treatment will likely be difficult.

There are many misconceptions regarding HIV transmission. For example, HIV is *not* passed from one person to another in normal daily contact that does not involve either exposure to blood or sexual contact. It is not carried by mosquitoes and cannot be caught from toilet seats or from eating food prepared by someone with AIDS. No one has ever contracted AIDS by kissing someone with AIDS, or even by sharing a toothbrush (although sharing a toothbrush still is not advised). Other misconceptions people may have include the following:

- *"It can't happen to me."*—HIV can infect anyone who has sex with, or shares injection equipment with, someone who is infected.
- *"I would know if my sex partner (injection partner) were infected."*—Most people infected with HIV do not look or feel sick and do not even know they are infected.
- *"As long as I get treated for any sexual infections I pick up, I'll be safe."*—No current form of treatment can cure or prevent HIV, and although treating other infections reduces risk, there is still a high chance of getting HIV through unprotected sex or sharing injection equipment.
- *"If I'm only with one sexual partner, and don't share injection equipment, I don't need to worry about HIV."*—This is true only if the partner is uninfected and has no ongoing risk of infection. If the partner is or becomes infected, then anyone who has sex with him

or shares his injection equipment is at high risk for HIV, and the only way to detect infection is to be tested.

■ *"If I douche or wash after sex, I won't get HIV."*—Douching and washing will not prevent HIV.

■ *"If I don't share my own syringe, I won't get HIV."*—HIV can also be spread through shared cookers, filters, and the prepared drug.

Life Cycle of HIV

It is possible to prevent transmission even after exposure to HIV. In San Francisco, postexposure prophylaxis is being offered to people who believe they have high risk for HIV transmission because of exposure with a known or suspected HIV-infected individual. Treatment is started within 72 hours of exposure and includes combination therapy, which may include a protease inhibitor, for a period of 1 month and followup for 12 months.

Once an HIV particle enters a person's body, it binds to the surface of a target cell (CD4+ T cell). The virus enters through the cell's outer envelope by shedding its own viral envelope, allowing the HIV particle to release an HIV ribonucleic acid (RNA) chain into the cell, which is then converted into deoxyribonucleic acid (DNA). The HIV DNA enters the cell's nucleus and is copied onto the cell's chromosomes. This causes the cell to begin reproducing more HIV, and eventually the cell releases more HIV particles. These new particles then attach to other target cells, which become infected. Figure 1-2 illustrates how HIV enters a CD4+ T cell and reproduces.

Measuring HIV in the blood

Physicians can measure the presence of HIV in a person by means of (1) the CD4+ T cell count and (2) the viral load count. The CD4+ T cell count measures the number of CD4+ T cells (i.e., white blood cells) in a milliliter of blood. These are the cells that HIV is most likely to infect, and

the number of these cells reflects the overall health of a person's immune system.

CD4+ T cells act as signals to inform the body's immune system that an infection exists and needs to be fought. Because HIV hides inside the very cells responsible for signaling its presence, it can survive and reproduce without the infected person knowing of its existence for many years. Even though the body can produce sufficient CD4+ T cells to replace the billions that are destroyed by untreated HIV each day, eventually HIV kills so many CD4+ T cells that the damaged immune system cannot control other infections that may make the person sick. This is the late stage of HIV, when AIDS is often diagnosed based on the presence of specific illnesses (i.e., opportunistic infections).

The viral load represents the level of HIV RNA (genetic material) circulating in the bloodstream. This level becomes very high soon after a person is initially infected with HIV, then it drops. Viral load tests measure the number of copies of the virus in a milliliter of plasma; currently available tests can measure down to 50 copies per milliliter, and even more sensitive tests can measure down to 5 copies per milliliter. To explain the relationship between CD4+ T cell count and viral load count and how together they are used to gauge a person's stage in disease progression, a "moving train" analogy can be used. The CD4+ T cell count is used to measure the person's distance to the point of high risk of contracting opportunistic infections, or death. The viral load count is used to measure the rate at which CD4+ T cells are being destroyed. Therefore, the CD4+ T cell count is the train's position on the track, and the viral load is the train's speed toward the outcome (i.e., AIDS and then death).

After a person is infected with HIV, the body takes about 6 to 12 weeks and sometimes as long as 6 months to build up proteins to fight the virus. These proteins are called HIV antibodies (disease-fighting proteins) and are detected by

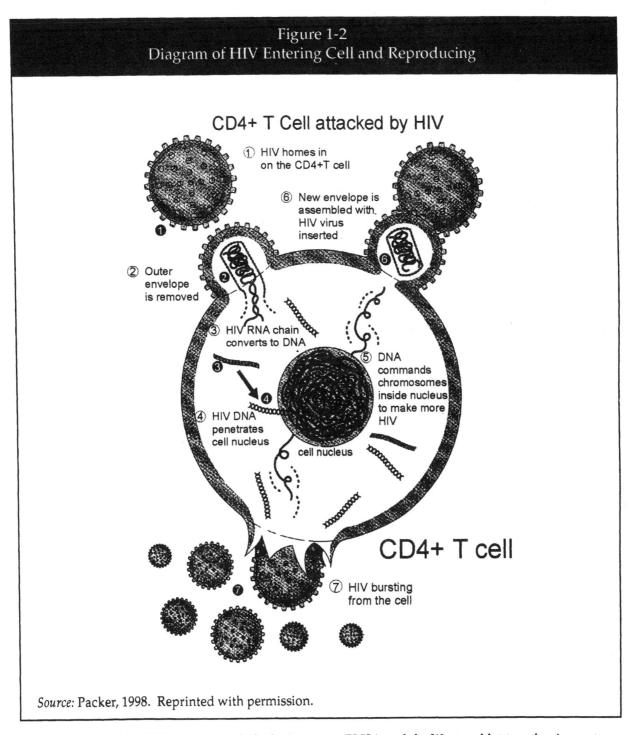

Figure 1-2
Diagram of HIV Entering Cell and Reproducing

CD4+ T Cell attacked by HIV

① HIV homes in on the CD4+T cell

⑥ New envelope is assembled with HIV virus inserted

② Outer envelope is removed

③ HIV RNA chain converts to DNA

⑤ DNA commands chromosomes inside nucleus to make more HIV

④ HIV DNA penetrates cell nucleus

cell nucleus

CD4+ T cell

⑦ HIV bursting from the cell

Source: Packer, 1998. Reprinted with permission.

an HIV test called the ELISA (enzyme-linked immunosorbent assay). The ELISA is very sensitive—it almost always detects HIV if it is there. Rarely, ELISA tests will give false-positive readings (a positive test in someone uninfected). For this reason, a positive ELISA test must always be confirmed with a second, more specific test called the Western blot. According to the CDC, the accuracy of the ELISA and the Western blot together is greater than 99 percent. Rapid HIV tests and home sample collection tests also are options for clients; see Chapter 2 for a more detailed discussion of these types of tests.

The 6 to 12 weeks between the time of infection and the time when an ELISA test for HIV becomes positive are called the "window period." During this period, the individual is extremely infectious to any sexual or needle-sharing partner but does not test positive unless a more expensive viral load test is performed.

The level of virus is determined by using a viral load test; three types of viral load tests are HIV-RNA polymerase chain reaction (PCR), HIV branched DNA (bDNA), and HIV-RNA nucleic acid sequence-based amplification (NASBA). Each of these tests measures the amount of replicating or reproducing virus in the bloodstream; thus a lower value signifies less risk of rapid progression. The best viral load test result is "none detected," although this does not mean the virus is gone, only that it is not actively reproducing at a measurable level.

Disease Progression

Once a person is infected with HIV, she should understand the progression of the disease from initial infection, through the latency period, symptomatic infections, and finally AIDS. The course of untreated HIV is not known but may go on for 10 years or longer in many people. Several years into HIV infection, mild symptoms begin to develop, then later severe infections that define AIDS occur. Treatment appears to greatly extend the life and improve the quality of life of most patients, although estimating survival after an AIDS diagnosis is inexact.

Initial infection

Primary HIV infection can cause an acute retroviral syndrome that often is mistaken for influenza (the flu), mononucleosis, or a bad cold. This syndrome is reported by roughly half of those who contract HIV (Russell and Sepkowitz, 1998) and generally occurs between 2 and 6 weeks after infection. Symptoms may include fever, headache, sore throat, fatigue, body aches, weight loss, and swollen lymph nodes. Other symptoms are a rash, mouth or genital ulcers, diarrhea, nausea and vomiting, and thrush. The CD4+ T cell count can drop very low during the early weeks, although it usually returns to a normal level after the initial illness is over. The

initial illness can last several days or even weeks.

The greatest spread of HIV occurs throughout the body early in the disease. Approximately 6 months after infection, the level of virions produced every day may reach a "set point." A higher set point usually means a more rapid progression of HIV disease. Early treatment may be recommended to reduce the set point, potentially leading to a better chance of controlling the infection.

Alcohol and drug counselors should discuss symptoms that suggest initial HIV infection with their clients and encourage clients to be tested for HIV if they experience such symptoms. This not only will encourage clients who are infected to enter treatment early but also will provide an opportunity for the counselor to help uninfected clients remain that way.

Latency period

After initial infection comes the latency period, or incubation period, during which untreated persons with HIV have few, if any, symptoms. This period lasts a median of about 10 years. The most common symptom during this period is lymphadenopathy, or swollen lymph nodes. The lymph nodes found around the neck and under the arms contain cells that fight infections. Swollen lymph nodes in the groin area may be normal and not indicative of HIV. When any infection is present, lymph nodes often swell, sometimes painfully. With HIV, they swell and tend to stay swollen but usually are not painful.

Early symptomatic infection

After the first year of infection, the CD4+ T cell count drops at a rate of about 30 to 90 cells per year. When the CD4+ T cell count falls below 500, mild HIV symptoms may occur. Many people, however, will have no symptoms at all until the CD4+ T cell count has dropped very low (200 or less). Bacteria, viruses, and fungi that normally live on and in the human body begin to cause diseases that are also known as opportunistic infections.

Early symptoms of infection may include chronic diarrhea, herpes zoster, recurrent vaginal candidiasis, thrush, oral hairy leukoplakia (a virus that causes white patches in the mouth), abnormal Pap tests, thrombocytopenia, or numbness or tingling in the toes or fingers. Most of these infections occur with a CD4+ T cell count between 200 and 500. Symptoms of these infections usually signal a problem with the immune system but are not severe enough to be classified as AIDS. Please refer to Appendix D for a complete checklist of symptoms.

AIDS

In the 1980s, AIDS was defined to include a depressed immune system and at least one illness tied to HIV infection. AIDS-defining conditions are diseases not normally manifest in someone with a healthy immune system. These should prompt a confirmatory HIV test. The additional 1993 AIDS-defining conditions led to the diagnosis of more AIDS cases in women and injection drug users. Since 1993, the list of AIDS-defining conditions has included pulmonary tuberculosis (TB), recurrent bacterial pneumonia, and invasive cervical cancer. HIV-infected persons with a CD4+ T cell count of 200 or less are classified as persons with AIDS (CDC, 1992).

TB and invasive cervical cancer are two AIDS-defining conditions that warrant special mention. Pulmonary TB is the one AIDS-related infection that is contagious to those without HIV. It generally causes a chronic dry cough (sometimes with blood), fatigue, and weight loss. Pulmonary TB requires ongoing treatment for at least 6 months, and close associates of the infected person must be tested for TB. If TB is only partially treated (i.e., the TB patient does not take all of the medications), resistant TB will develop, which can then be passed to others. Although TB, coupled with a positive HIV test,

is an AIDS-defining diagnosis, it also can occur while the CD4+ T cell count is still high. If TB occurs late in the disease after the CD4+ T cell count has dropped, it may not be found in the lungs, and symptoms may include only weight loss and fever, without a cough. It should be noted, however, that the Mantoux PPD test (a test routinely administered to screen for TB by determining reaction to intradermal injection of purified protein derivative) may not be positive if the patient is anergic (i.e., if he has sufficient immune system damage to cause inability to respond to the PPD).

Cervical cancer may progress rapidly in women with HIV but usually is asymptomatic until it is too late for successful treatment. Women who are HIV positive should have Pap tests at least once every 6 months and more often if any abnormality is found.

AIDS symptoms

Most AIDS-defining diseases are severe enough to require medical care, sometimes hospitalization. Some of these diseases, however, can be treated earlier on an outpatient basis if symptoms are reported when they are mild. (Please refer to Appendix C for a complete list of AIDS-defining conditions.)

Cough is a symptom common to several AIDS-related infections, the most frequent of which is *Pneumocystis carinii* pneumonia (PCP—not to be confused with the drug by that name, phencyclidine). PCP is characterized by a dry cough, fever, night sweats, and increasing shortness of breath. Recurrent bacterial pneumonia (i.e., two or more infections within a year) also is an AIDS-defining condition. It often causes a fever and a cough that brings up phlegm. Coughing is also a symptom of TB. As a general guideline, if a cough does not resolve after several weeks, it should be checked by a medical practitioner.

Several skin problems can occur in HIV/AIDS. Kaposi's sarcoma (KS), a rare malignancy outside of HIV disease, may be the best-known skin condition in HIV infection. KS is a cancer of the blood vessels that causes pink, purple, or brown splotches, which appear usually as firm areas on or under the skin. KS also grows in other places, such as the lungs and mouth. KS is highly prevalent among men with AIDS, of whom 20 to 30 percent may develop the condition in contrast to 1 to 3 percent of women with AIDS (Kedes et al., 1997). However, since the introduction of combination anti-HIV therapy, KS is seen less frequently.

Diarrhea is a very common symptom of AIDS. Many AIDS-defining conditions cause diarrhea, including parasitic, viral, and bacterial infections. HIV itself can cause diarrhea if it infects the intestinal tract. Diarrhea also is a common side effect of HIV/AIDS medications. Weight loss can be caused by inadequate nutrition, untreated neoplasms and opportunistic infections (which often are associated with diarrhea), and deranged metabolism (Dieterich, 1997).

Changes in vision, particularly spots or flashes (known as "floaters"), may indicate an infection inside the eye. A virus called cytomegalovirus (CMV) is the most common cause of blindness in people with HIV/AIDS. CMV progresses very rapidly if not treated and is among the most feared of AIDS-related infections. Fortunately, it almost never occurs until the immune system is almost completely destroyed, so it is not usually the first symptom. Counselors can screen for early signs of CMV using the Amsler Grid (see Appendix D). The client also can be taught to screen himself using this screening tool.

A severe headache, seizure, or changes in cognitive function may herald the onset of a number of infections or cancers inside the brain. The two most common brain infections in HIV/AIDS are cryptococcal meningitis, a fungus that usually causes a severe headache, and toxoplasmosis, which can present with focal neurologic deficits or seizure. Seizures also can be caused by the cancer of the central nervous system called lymphoma. Progressive multifocal leukoencephalopathy (PML), a brain disease that causes thinking, speech, and balance problems and dementia also can occur as a result of HIV infection.

End-stage disease

A person with HIV/AIDS can live an active and productive life, even with a CD4+ T cell count of zero, if infections and cancers are controlled or prevented. The newer antiviral medicines can even help the body restore much of its lost immune function. In the past few years, a phenomenon called the Lazarus syndrome has developed among patients with AIDS, wherein, because of optimal drug therapy, someone who had seemed very near death improves and returns to fairly normal function. Untreated, the disease eventually overwhelms the immune system, allowing one debilitating infection after another. Sometimes the possible combinations of medication are no longer effective, the side effects are intolerable, or no further therapy is available.

Hospice care is an appropriate choice for those who have run out of therapeutic options. In hospice care, the individual is treated for pain and other discomforts and allowed to die of the disease. Pain therapy at this stage invariably requires narcotics. It is crucial that the client and other treatment professionals understand that using opiates for pain is entirely different from using them to feed an addiction. The client will develop a need for high doses and will have withdrawal symptoms if the drug is stopped, but will not "get high." If drugs must be stopped (which is uncommon), they can be tapered under medical supervision. See Chapter 2 for a more in-depth discussion of pain management.

Hospice care allows the person with end-stage HIV/AIDS a peaceful death and a chance to address those relationships or experiences that are important. Hospice goals involve maintaining dignity and allowing the client's significant others to dictate how they will cope with this final stage.

Changes in the Epidemiology of HIV/AIDS Since 1995

With the advent of new and effective treatments, the epidemiology of HIV/AIDS is changing. The study of HIV/AIDS epidemiology helps to identify the trends of the disease. Surveillance of AIDS cases since 1996 shows substantial declines in AIDS-related deaths and increases in the number of persons living with AIDS, although the decline is slowing (CDC, 1999b). As people live longer with HIV/AIDS, the ability to use AIDS surveillance data alone to represent trends has diminished. It is difficult but important to track the distribution of prevalence (i.e., existing) and incidence (i.e., new) of both HIV and AIDS cases to detect changes in geographic, demographic, and risk/exposure trends (Ward and Duchin, 1997–1998).

With the mid-year 1998 edition, the CDC started to include information from both HIV infections and AIDS cases in the *HIV/AIDS Surveillance Report* (CDC, 1998c). It should be noted that the number of HIV cases in the report is a conservative estimate of the number of people living with HIV because not all people with HIV/AIDS have been tested (and those who have been tested anonymously are not reported to State health departments' confidential, name-based HIV registries). At the end of June 1999, 30 States and the U.S. Virgin Islands were reporting HIV cases.

This section presents an overview of the trends in the HIV/AIDS pandemic and discusses how the pandemic intertwines with substance abuse. The information is organized to provide a general look at the pandemic in the

United States and its Territories, a discussion of the trends and the populations which are most at risk for contracting the infection, and a regional look at the pandemic (the regions are defined by the CDC). Finally, there is a discussion of special populations and how they are affected by the HIV/AIDS pandemic. For more detail about HIV/AIDS epidemiology, readers are encouraged to visit the CDC's Divisions of HIV/AIDS Prevention Web site, at www.cdc.gov/nchstp/hiv_aids/dhap.htm. The latest CDC HIV/AIDS surveillance reports can be downloaded, and the site provides a wealth of information about the pandemic.

To see the distribution of HIV/AIDS in the United States, see Figures 1-3 through 1-6. Figure 1-3 shows the AIDS rates for male adults and adolescents reported from July 1998 through June 1999. Figure 1-4 shows the number of adult and adolescent male AIDS and HIV cases reported from July 1998 through June 1999. Figure 1-5 illustrates the AIDS rate for female adults and adolescents reported from July 1998 through June 1999, and Figure 1-6 shows the number of female adult and adolescent AIDS and HIV cases reported from July 1998 through June 1999.

Current Trends in the HIV/AIDS Pandemic

Current trends in HIV/AIDS disproportionally affect racial minority populations, especially women, youth, and children within those populations. HIV prevalence is higher among African Americans than in other ethnic groups; from July 1998 through June 1999, African Americans accounted for 46 percent of adult AIDS cases, while representing 12 percent of the total U.S. population. Hispanics accounted for 20 percent of adult AIDS cases from July 1998 through June 1999, while making up only 11 percent of the total U.S. population (CDC 1999b; U.S. Bureau of the Census, 1998). Together, African Americans and Hispanics represent the

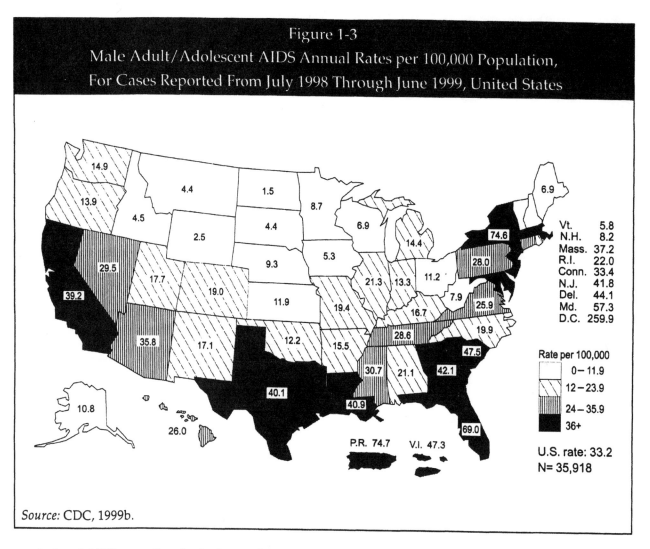

Figure 1-3
Male Adult/Adolescent AIDS Annual Rates per 100,000 Population,
For Cases Reported From July 1998 Through June 1999, United States

Vt. 5.8
N.H. 8.2
Mass. 37.2
R.I. 22.0
Conn. 33.4
N.J. 41.8
Del. 44.1
Md. 57.3
D.C. 259.9

Rate per 100,000
0 – 11.9
12 – 23.9
24 – 35.9
36+

U.S. rate: 33.2
N= 35,918

P.R. 74.7   V.I. 47.3

Source: CDC, 1999b.

majority of AIDS cases thus far in the pandemic (CDC, 1999b, 1999c). In addition, of the HIV cases reported from the 30 States and one Territory from July 1998 through June 1999, 54 percent were among adult and adolescent African Americans, and 10 percent were among adult and adolescent Hispanics. Substance abuse is a primary mechanism by which these vulnerable groups become HIV-infected populations.

It is important to be aware that, although it is customary to categorize cases based on broad ethnic labels, this procedure glosses over fundamental ethnic and cultural differences among people of color and fails to address the underlying economic and social infrastructure that fuels the spread of substance abuse and HIV (National Commission on AIDS, 1992).

Categorizing all persons with African racial heritage as "black" mixes together people of distinct ethnic and cultural heritage (e.g., ethnic descendents of African slaves, Caribbean immigrants) as well as individuals from different socioeconomic groups. Similarly, "Hispanic" refers to a multiethnic and multicultural blend of people from more than 30 geographic regions. Social, political, and economic forces have led to the "ghettoization" of African Americans and Hispanics in the inner cities where there are high rates of drug trafficking, unemployment, poverty, racism, and a lack of access to health care, all of which contribute to high rates of addiction and HIV/AIDS (National Commission on AIDS, 1992). It is within urban, poor, African

Figure 1-4
Male Adult/Adolescent HIV Infection and AIDS Cases
Reported From July 1998 Through June 1999, United States

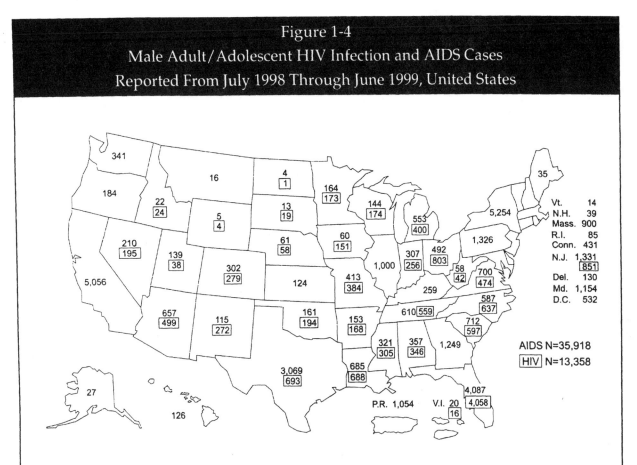

Note: To date, 33 States and Territories are reporting HIV cases; 2 States only report HIV cases in children. A few States use codes in lieu of names; these States' data are not yet included in the CDC's HIV data.
Source: CDC, 1999b.

American and Hispanic communities that HIV/AIDS is most prevalent.

These oppressive socioeconomic factors also have led to high rates of incarceration, sex work, and homelessness for members of African American and Hispanic communities. Drug offenses account for the highest number of Federal crimes for which people are incarcerated (Mumola, 1999). For example, a survey of new commitments to California State prisons found that more than 75 percent of the offenders had histories of drug use (California Department of Corrections, 1998). Not surprisingly, these individuals also have high rates of HIV infection (Stryker, 1993). Sex workers, many of whom are poor, homeless, and substance dependent, are likely to be more concerned with immediate

needs such as housing, food, or substance abuse than HIV or substance abuse prevention and intervention (Kail et al., 1995). This is also true for the homeless or marginally housed who often are dealing with both substance abuse and mental health or mental retardation problems (St. Lawrence and Brasfield, 1995).

However, the highest HIV and AIDS rates among at-risk populations are still found among MSMs (CDC, 1999b), who from July 1998 through June 1999 represented 38 percent of AIDS cases and 30 percent of HIV cases. Minority MSMs especially are at high risk for contracting the infection. See the section "HIV/AIDS Epidemiology Among Groups" later in this chapter for further discussion of HIV/AIDS and MSMs.

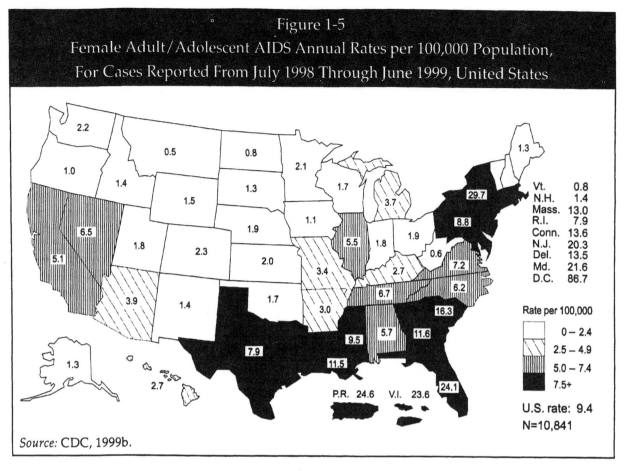

Figure 1-5
Female Adult/Adolescent AIDS Annual Rates per 100,000 Population, For Cases Reported From July 1998 Through June 1999, United States

Vt.	0.8
N.H.	1.4
Mass.	13.0
R.I.	7.9
Conn.	13.6
N.J.	20.3
Del.	13.5
Md.	21.6
D.C.	86.7

Rate per 100,000

	0 – 2.4
	2.5 – 4.9
	5.0 – 7.4
	7.5+

U.S. rate: 9.4
N=10,841

P.R. 24.6   V.I. 23.6

Source: CDC, 1999b.

HIV/AIDS is epidemic among the heterosexual population as well and is fueled by sexual contact with HIV-infected, injection drug-using, or bisexual partners. Heterosexuals located in communities with high prevalence of HIV/AIDS and addiction are at greatest risk for contracting HIV/AIDS from heterosexual contact. This type of heterosexual contact, defined generally as sexual contact with an "at-risk" person (e.g., injection drug users, bisexual man) or an HIV-infected person whose risk was not specified, from July 1998 through June 1999 accounted for about 15 percent of all adult and adolescent AIDS cases and about 17 percent of reported adult and adolescent HIV infection cases (CDC, 1999b). Of these, 61 percent of AIDS cases were women and 39 percent were men; of HIV infection cases, 68 percent were women and 32 percent were men.

From July 1998 through June 1999, there were 4,296 new AIDS cases and 2,321 new HIV cases among women who reported heterosexual contact (CDC, 1999b). Of these, 28 percent of AIDS cases and 21 percent of HIV cases were among women who reported sexual contact with injection drug users, 5 percent of AIDS cases and 6 percent of HIV cases who reported sexual contact with bisexual men, and 66 percent of AIDS cases and 72 percent of HIV cases who reported sexual contact with an HIV-infected person, without reporting the origin of the partner's infection. Of the 2,754 AIDS cases and 1,070 HIV cases for men who reported heterosexual contact, the majority reported sexual contact with an HIV-infected person without reporting the origin of the partner's infection (77 percent of AIDS cases and 80 percent of HIV cases). These data are supported by earlier research that found that HIV infection among heterosexual clients in alcohol abuse treatment, who were primarily male, was

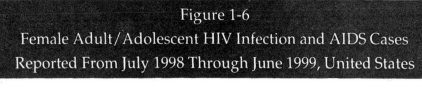

Figure 1-6
Female Adult/Adolescent HIV Infection and AIDS Cases
Reported From July 1998 Through June 1999, United States

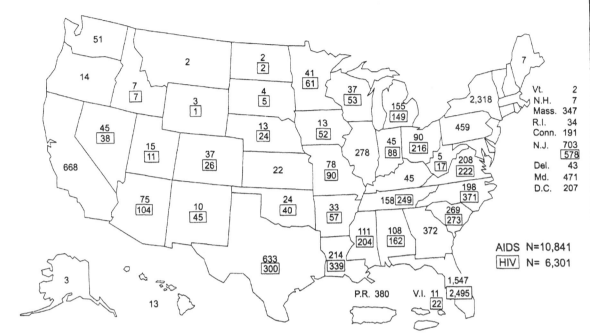

Note: To date, 33 States and Territories are reporting HIV cases; 2 States only report HIV cases in children. A few States use codes in lieu of names; these States' data are not yet included in the CDC's HIV data.

Source: CDC, 1999b.

largely caused by unsafe sexual behaviors (Avins et al., 1994; Woods et al., 1996).

Figures 1-7 and 1-8 illustrate the trend of male and female AIDS cases contracted through heterosexual exposure from 1993 to 1998 by ethnicity. These figures depict only self-identified heterosexual men and women.

Regional HIV/AIDS Epidemiology

Early in the U.S. AIDS pandemic, the Northeast region of the United States had the most AIDS cases, followed by the South, Midwest, and the West (Figure 1-9 contains a breakdown of the States that make up these four regions plus the U.S. Territories, as defined by the CDC). In all regions, AIDS incidence increased through 1994, with the most dramatic increases occurring in the South. Between 1997 and 1998, AIDS

incidence dropped for all regions, but in 1998 the South still had the highest rate (43 percent), followed by the Northeast (28 percent), the West (17 percent), the Midwest (8 percent), and the U.S. Territories (3 percent) (CDC, 1999b). Figure 1-10 demonstrates the change in AIDS incidence of the regions for 1996, 1997, and 1998.

The HIV/AIDS pandemic is evolving differently in different regions of the United States, just as drug use varies from region to region. Therefore, alcohol and drug counselors should become familiar with HIV/AIDS prevalence, incidence, and trends in their local areas, their States, and their regions. Appendix G contains a list of State and Territory departments of health (including addresses, phone numbers, and Web sites where readers

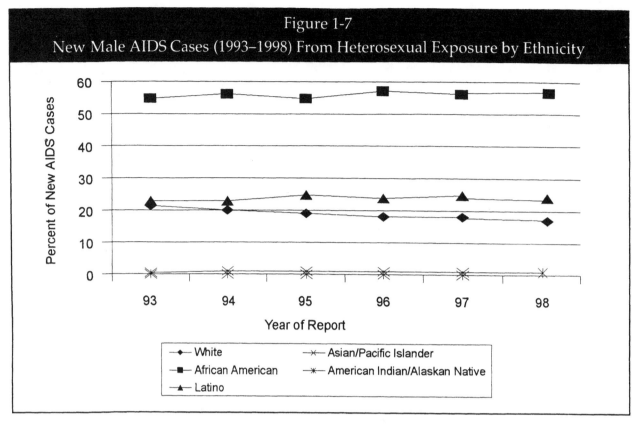

Figure 1-7
New Male AIDS Cases (1993–1998) From Heterosexual Exposure by Ethnicity

Legend:
- ◆ White
- ■ African American
- ▲ Latino
- ✕ Asian/Pacific Islander
- ✻ American Indian/Alaskan Native

can obtain information about their State). When available, State AIDS hotlines also are listed.

The 10 States and Territories reporting the most AIDS cases, in descending order, are New York, California, Florida, Texas, New Jersey, Puerto Rico, Illinois, Pennsylvania, Georgia, and Maryland. The 10 metropolitan areas reporting the highest number of AIDS cases, in descending order, are New York City, Los Angeles, San Francisco, Miami, the District of Columbia, Chicago, Houston, Philadelphia, Newark, and Atlanta (CDC, 1999b). Not surprisingly, these major metropolitan areas also are high-intensity drug-trafficking areas as defined by the Office of National Drug Control Policy (ONDCP, 1998).

HIV Epidemiology Among Groups

Homosexuals
The primary route of HIV transmission for MSMs is through sexual contact, which may occur while the participants are engaged in

substance abuse, including IDU. Within this group, the focus of the pandemic among MSMs has shifted from older, white, urban men to poorer African American and Hispanic men, men with substance abuse problems (including IDU), and young men. Repeated studies have found that MSMs who abuse alcohol, speed, MDMA (3,4-methylene-dioxymethamphetamine), cocaine, crack cocaine, inhalants, and other noninjection street drugs are more likely than those who do not use substances to engage in unprotected sex and become infected with HIV (Paul et al., 1991b, 1993, 1994). One hypothesis about the reason for higher rates of HIV/AIDS among MSMs is that substance abuse may increase sexual risktaking. This is because substance abusers experience decreased inhibition, new learned behaviors (such as using substances and then having unprotected anal intercourse), low self-esteem, altered perception of risk, lack of assertiveness to negotiate safe practices, and perceived powerlessness (Paul et al., 1993).

As of June 1999, more than half of all cumulative male adult and adolescent AIDS cases were among MSMs who reported sexual risk only (57 percent) or sexual risk and IDU (8 percent). Of cumulative HIV cases among adult and adolescent males, 45 percent reported sexual risk only and 6 percent reported sexual risk and IDU (CDC, 1999b). Even though the cumulative total of AIDS cases among MSMs is still highest in white men (62 percent white, 23 percent African American, 14 percent Hispanic), new AIDS cases among MSMs indicate that the disparity between cases among whites and among minorities is narrowing. From July 1998 through June 1999, 53 percent of AIDS cases were among white men, 29 percent were among African American men, and 16 percent were among Hispanic men. Figure 1-11 illustrates the trend of MSM AIDS cases by ethnicity from 1993 to 1998.

As with injection drug users, minority MSMs are disproportionately affected by HIV disease. African American and Hispanic MSMs, compared with their white counterparts, are more likely to inject drugs, to be substance abusers, to be poor, to be paid for sex, and to engage in higher rates of unprotected anal intercourse (National Commission on AIDS, 1992; Peterson et al., 1992). Sociocultural factors, combined with some community values (e.g., machismo, family loyalty, sexual silence) and lack of access to health care and substance abuse treatment, strongly compete with safe sex and drug practices among gay and bisexual men of color (Diaz and Klevens, 1997).

Sex networks and sexual mixing patterns (Renton et al., 1995) are hypothesized to explain the higher risk of HIV infection related to substance abuse among MSMs. MSM substance abusers may form tight groups characterized by

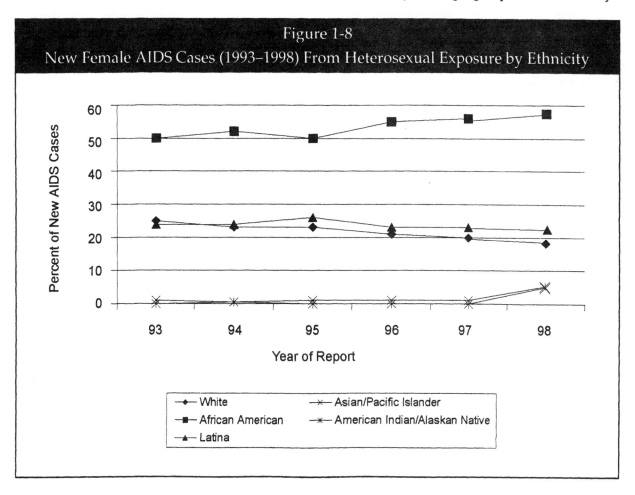

Figure 1-8

New Female AIDS Cases (1993–1998) From Heterosexual Exposure by Ethnicity

Figure 1-9				
CDC Regional Breakdown of U.S. States and Territories				
Northeast	**South**	**Midwest**	**West**	**Territories**
Connecticut	Alabama	Illinois	Alaska	American Samoa
Maine	Arkansas	Indiana	Arizona	Commonwealth
Massachusetts	Delaware	Iowa	California	of the Northern
New Hampshire	District of Columbia	Kansas	Colorado	Mariana Islands
New Jersey	Florida	Michigan	Hawaii	Federated States of
New York	Georgia	Minnesota	Idaho	Micronesia
Pennsylvania	Kentucky	Missouri	Montana	Guam
Rhode Island	Louisiana	Nebraska	Nevada	Puerto Rico
Vermont	Maryland	North Dakota	New Mexico	Republic of the
	Mississippi	Ohio	Oregon	Marshall Islands
	North Carolina	South Dakota	Utah	Republic of Palau
	Oklahoma	Wisconsin	Washington	U.S. Virgin Islands
	South Carolina		Wyoming	
	Tennessee			
	Texas			
	Virginia			
	West Virginia			
Source: CDC, 1999b.				

higher HIV seroprevalence rates, higher sexual mixing, greater IDU, and more trading of sex for money, food, and drugs. These factors are another way to account for higher HIV risk-taking sexual behaviors among MSM substance abusers.

Incarcerated persons

A recent study reported that the confirmed rate of AIDS cases among incarcerated people in State and Federal prisons is more than six times higher than in the general population. About 2.3 percent of all persons incarcerated in the United Sates in 1995 were HIV positive, and about 0.51 percent had confirmed AIDS (MacDougall, 1998; Maruschak, 1997). According to the Bureau of Justice Statistics in the U.S. Department of Justice, in 1997, 57 percent of State prisoners and 45 percent of Federal prisoners said they had used drugs in the month before committing their offense. In addition, 83 percent of State prisoners and 73

percent of Federal prisoners said they had used drugs at some time in the past. Even with these high rates, which increased between 1991 and 1997, substance abuse treatment services declined during the same time period (Mumola, 1999).

In 1991, only 1 percent of Federal prison inmates with substance abuse disorders received appropriate treatment. For those who completed treatment there were no aftercare services in place to help them remain abstinent after they got out of prison (U.S. General Accounting Office, 1998).

Most incarcerated people who have HIV are infected before they enter prison. One study of 46 prisons found an HIV infection rate of 1.7 percent among people entering prison (Withum, 1993). In some correctional facilities, HIV infection rates are as high as 20 percent among women and 15 percent among men. For MSMs, HIV infection rates ranged from 9 to 34 percent;

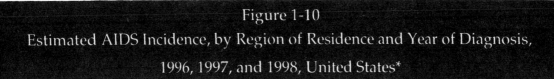

Figure 1-10
Estimated AIDS Incidence, by Region of Residence and Year of Diagnosis,
1996, 1997, and 1998, United States*

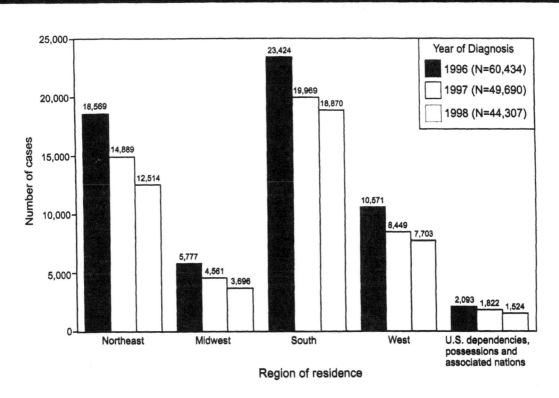

*These numbers do not represent actual cases of persons diagnosed with AIDS. Rather, these numbers are point estimates of persons diagnosed with AIDS adjusted for reporting delays but not for incomplete reporting.
Source: CDC, 1999b.

among injection drug users the infection rate ranged from 6 to 43 percent.

HIV/AIDS and substance abuse interventions implemented in prisons have a great potential to impact the HIV/AIDS pandemic (MacDougall, 1998). Like the HIV-infected population, the incarcerated population has an overrepresentation of minority groups and is characterized by high poverty, overcrowding, IDU, high-risk sexual activities, and poor access to health care. Incarceration presents an opportunity to screen, counsel, and educate inmates about HIV/AIDS, and to provide substance abuse treatment as well. For many incarcerated persons, this may be their

first contact with medical interventions as well as with substance abuse treatment.

When prison inmates return to society, their health status will have an effect on the community to which they return. A study of Hispanic inmates in California found that 51 percent reported having sex within the first 12 hours after release and that they preferred not to use condoms (Morales et al., 1995). In addition, 11 percent reported IDU in the first day after release.

Sex workers

The sex workers who are most vulnerable to contracting and transmitting HIV are street

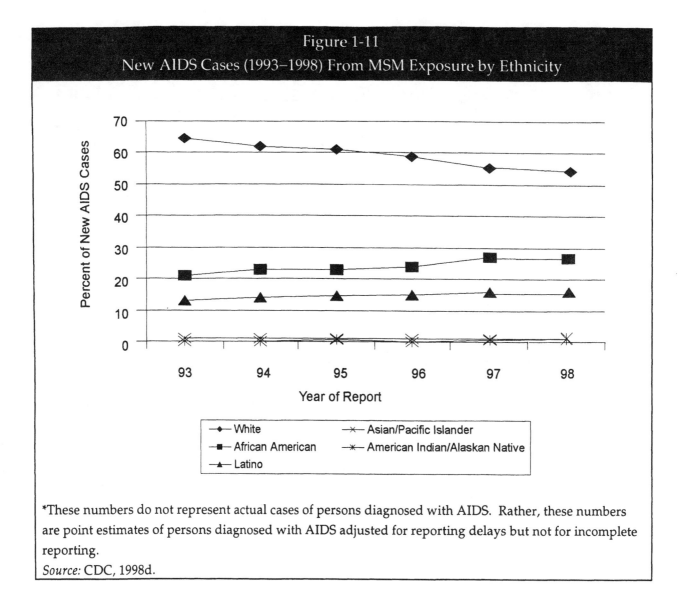

Figure 1-11
New AIDS Cases (1993–1998) From MSM Exposure by Ethnicity

Legend:
- White
- African American
- Latino
- Asian/Pacific Islander
- American Indian/Alaskan Native

(Y-axis: Percent of New AIDS Cases; X-axis: Year of Report — 93, 94, 95, 96, 97, 98)

*These numbers do not represent actual cases of persons diagnosed with AIDS. Rather, these numbers are point estimates of persons diagnosed with AIDS adjusted for reporting delays but not for incomplete reporting.
Source: CDC, 1998d.

workers, who often are poor or homeless, may have a history of childhood abuse, and are likely to be alcohol or drug dependent. A CDC study of female sex workers in six U.S. cities found an HIV seroprevalence of 12 percent, ranging from 0 to 50 percent depending on the city and the level of IDU (CDC, 1987a). A study of male sex workers in Atlanta found an HIV seroprevalence of 29 percent, with the highest rates among those who had receptive anal sex with nonpaying partners (Elifson et al., 1993).

IDU was the main risk factor for HIV infection for female sex workers in six U.S. cities (CDC, 1987a). Female injection drug users who trade sex for money or drugs are more likely to

share needles than female injection drug users who do not engage in sex trading (Kail et al., 1995). The circumstances in which sex workers live also increase their chances of contracting HIV. For example, they may agree to unprotected sex if a client offers more money, if they are desperate for money to buy drugs, or if business has been slow. Violent clients may force unsafe sex, and in many cities police confiscate condoms when they arrest or stop sex workers. HIV prevention outreach to sex workers is difficult because prostitution is illegal. Immediate attention to concerns about food, housing, and drug addiction often take precedence over HIV prevention.

Homeless or marginally housed

Homelessness often occurs in conjunction with substance abuse, chronic mental illness, and unsafe sexual behavior. All of these factors increase homeless people's risk for contracting HIV. A survey of 16 U.S. cities found that 3 percent of homeless people were HIV positive, compared with less than 1 percent of the general adult population (Allen et al., 1994). In other studies, 19 percent of homeless mentally ill men in New York City were HIV positive (Susser et al., 1993), and an 8 percent HIV infection rate was found among homeless adults in San Francisco (Zolopa et al., 1994).

A survey of homeless adults in a storefront medical clinical found that 69 percent were at risk for HIV because of the following factors: (1) unprotected sex with multiple partners, (2) IDU, (3) sex with an injection drug-using partner, or (4) exchanging unprotected sex for money or drugs. Almost half reported at least two of these risk factors, and one fourth reported three or more risk factors (St. Lawrence and Brasfield, 1995). Substance abuse can exacerbate HIV risks because abusers are more likely to forget to use condoms, to share needles, and to exchange sex for drugs. A survey of homeless adults in St. Louis found that 40 percent of men and 23 percent of women reported drug use, and 62 percent of men and 17 percent of women reported alcohol use (North and Smith, 1993).

Adolescents

Because the average period of time from HIV infection to AIDS is about 10 years, most young adults with AIDS were likely infected as adolescents (National Institute of Allergy and Infectious Diseases [NIAID], 1999). Through June 1999 in the United States, 3,564 cases of AIDS in people aged 13 through 19 were reported (CDC, 1999b). In the 13- to 19-year-old age group, 60 percent were male and 40 percent were female. When broken down by ethnic group, 30 percent were white, 49 percent were African American, 20 percent were Hispanic, and 1 percent were Asian/Pacific Islander or American Indian/Alaskan Native.

Most adolescents are exposed to HIV through unprotected sex or IDU. Through June 1999, HIV surveillance data show that there were 4,470 cases reported in the 13- to 19-year-old age group. Of those, 45 percent were male, and 55 percent were female. When broken down by ethnic group, 27 percent were white, 66 percent were African American, 5 percent were Hispanic, and less than 1 percent each were Asian/Pacific Islander or American Indian/Alaskan Native (CDC, 1999b). Half of the infected male adolescents reported exposure through sex with men.

Almost half (42 percent) of female adolescents were exposed to HIV through heterosexual contact. Another significant trend is the number of STDs reported among adolescents: About two thirds of the 12 million cases of STDs reported in the United States each year are among individuals under the age of 25, and one quarter are among teens. This is significant because the presence of an STD can increase the risk of HIV transmission threefold to ninefold, depending on the type of STD (NIAID, 1999).

Adolescents tend to believe they are "invincible" and therefore engage in risky behaviors. Because of this belief they also may delay HIV testing, and, if they do test and are positive, they may delay or refuse treatment. Alcohol and drug counselors who work with adolescents should encourage them to be tested for HIV if they are at risk. Adolescents can be helped by having information about HIV/AIDS explained to them clearly, by drawing out information about behaviors that may have put them at risk for HIV, and by emphasizing the success of newly available treatments.

2 Medical Assessment and Treatment

Treating HIV/AIDS is extremely complex. It can be difficult to keep abreast of the latest recommendations for the care of HIV-infected individuals at a time when knowledge of the nature and course of HIV infection is changing quickly. Therefore, it is important to seek out qualified physicians who have a history of providing services to HIV-infected individuals. This chapter is designed to assist clinicians and medical staff in providing effective medical assessment and treatment of their HIV-infected substance-abusing clients.

It is important that the medical care team have experience with substance-abusing clients because the combination of substance abuse and HIV/AIDS poses special challenges. Practitioners who do not understand the nature of substance abuse may be hesitant to prescribe potent antiretroviral therapy, fearing that substance abusers will not take the medications correctly. There are also special physical considerations for substance abusers. For example, injection drug use (IDU) is associated with very high rates of hepatitis B and C, which can damage the liver. Some medications used to treat HIV/AIDS and its complications can affect treatment for hepatitis, and their use should be planned carefully. Many HIV/AIDS treatment drugs are processed through the liver, and their effects can be either increased or decreased because of hepatitis or chronic alcohol use.

If there is no specialized practice available to the client, alcohol and drug counselors should establish a relationship with a specialty group that can be consulted by the medical care team. The most crucial time for consulting a specialist is when the client is starting, stopping, or changing HIV/AIDS treatment.

Adherence to Medical Care

There is little doubt that adherence to antiretrovirals plays a more important role in long-term outcome than does choice of antiretroviral medications. A client who adheres to the medications will likely have a better outcome, and adherence also is important for preventing the development of drug resistance. Many barriers prevent HIV-infected substance abusers from receiving appropriate, timely medical care (see the section, "Barriers to Care for HIV-Infected Substance Abuse Disorder Clients"). However, once in treatment, their compliance may not be worse than that of other HIV-infected clients (Broers et al., 1994). A client's belief in the effectiveness of anti-retroviral therapy is positively associated with adherence to treatment (Samet et al., 1992). This shows how important it is to educate clients and include them in all aspects of the treatment process. Although a long-term relationship with a provider is based on trust, continuity and availability will also make it more likely that clients take their medications properly.

Health care providers seldom can predict which clients will comply with complex medication schedules. Primary care providers should be aware, however, that a client's relapse into substance abuse is likely to result in noncompliance with medical care. It is important that linkages be maintained between primary care and substance abuse treatment providers so that primary care providers are aware of relapses when they occur; however, it is also important to remember confidentiality rules (see Chapter 9 for more information). Other factors may prevent clients from taking medications as prescribed, such as living in an institution (e.g., a halfway house, homeless shelter, or prison). Psychiatric disorders among drug abusers may also hamper adherence (Ferrando et al., 1996).

Techniques to achieve optimal compliance among HIV-infected clients include the following:

- Simplify drug regimens—twice a day should be the goal.
- Repeat instructions.
- Use written protocols where doses coincide with habits or normal schedule.
- Use a timing device to ensure that medications are taken at the proper time.
- Use lists that clients can post in highly visible places.
- Give positive feedback: provide evidence of effectiveness, such as declining viral load.
- Have support persons (e.g., case managers, family members) reinforce the importance of keeping appointments and adhering to medication regimens.
- Use visual tools, such as pictures of clocks and pills, to help visual learners and those who are illiterate or non–English speaking.
- Encourage attendance at an outpatient HIV/AIDS support group. Hearing from

others who have successfully weathered the uncomfortable side effects and can give support when discouragement or relapse occurs can be highly reinforcing.

The key to encouraging client adherence is education, not only of the clients themselves but also of their families and peers. The client and those who surround her must understand why she is taking these drugs, what they do, and what side effects she may experience. The client should also understand that she may have to take additional medications or use nonmedicinal methods to alleviate the side effects, which can include nausea, vomiting, headaches, rashes, muscle pain, and diarrhea.

The clinician should familiarize the client with the names of all the medications she will be taking, including generic names, brand names, and common abbreviations. It is also important that the medical staff discuss with the client why the timing of the doses is important and how food can affect the ability of the medication to work properly. Staff members should fill out a weekly medication timetable for the client so she can easily see and remember when and how to take her medications.

Because the HIV-infected individual must take antiretroviral medications several times a day for the rest of his life, the drugs must be chosen with care. The choice should be based on the client's daily patterns and on any other medical conditions besides HIV/AIDS. Generally, the fewer doses per day and the fewer restrictions for taking the drugs, the better. (Currently, there is one once-a-day medication available—efavirenz [Sustiva]. Another drug, adefovir dipivoxil [Preveon], has been in development but is not now available.) For example, a person who is using opiates, amphetamines, or cocaine is not likely to be eating regularly, so a medicine that must be taken with food may not be the best option. Before prescribing medications, the medical care team could consult the substance abuse counselor about the client's living patterns. If the therapy is effective, clients who are well will remain so, possibly indefinitely, and those who are ill will generally improve, sometimes becoming well enough to return to or stay at work or begin seeking employment.

Side effects from medications can be difficult or frightening, but the client should not stop taking the medications without first contacting her medical practitioner. Substance-abusing clients are particularly intolerant of unexpected effects such as diarrhea or nausea but usually will continue the medication if they have been informed about such possibilities. Given the tradeoff for a healthier life, most will continue their medications as long as they know that this is less dangerous to them than the HIV itself.

Although injection drug users are one of the groups at high risk for contracting HIV, the majority of them are not in drug treatment. People who provide medical care to HIV-infected substance abusers must work to overcome the barriers that keep many of these clients out of the health care and substance abuse treatment systems and enlist clients who are in these systems to actively participate in their own care.

Supervised Therapy

Substance abuse treatment programs, because of their relatively intense interaction with clients, are in a unique position to help deliver such medication-related services as supervised therapy. Different models for supervised therapy can be effective and should be developed for specific substance abuse treatment settings.

Daily dispensing has been shown to improve adherence to zidovudine (Retrovir—abbreviated as AZT), but its applicability may be limited (Wall et al., 1995). If supervised therapy is already part of a client's substance abuse treatment, it need not be changed because of HIV infection. While important for clients with

tuberculosis (TB), supervised therapy also is a significant issue for clients who have difficulty following antiretroviral and *Pneumocystis carinii* pneumonia (PCP) prophylactic regimens because of homelessness, cognitive impairment, or lack of health insurance or money to obtain medications. This kind of supervision is particularly useful for medications that can be given only once daily or less (e.g., trimethoprim-sulfamethoxazole [abbreviated as TMP-SMX] [Bactrim DS, Septra], fluconazole [Diflucan], dapsone [Dapsone]). A potent once-a-day combination antiretroviral therapy that can be easily administered may soon be available.

Client Empowerment

Adherence to medical care means more than simply taking medications as prescribed. The foremost challenge in providing HIV/AIDS and substance abuse treatment is engaging clients and encouraging them to be active participants in their own care.

Many HIV-infected substance abuse clients may be deeply distrustful of medical providers, and some will refuse or resist treatment for fear that their HIV status will be disclosed. Strict observance of client confidentiality is an essential element of creating an atmosphere of trust in which clients can make the choices that are best for them. Encouraging clients to discuss their fears can help build trust between clients and providers. Client education facilitates client engagement and empowerment, and empowerment results in better adherence to medical care.

The client may also receive help from social support systems that can involve family members, partners, peer support groups, and local AIDS service organizations, which often provide "check-in" telephone calls. It is also likely that the client will respond well to continued positive feedback about her improving condition. For instance, knowing that her viral load has declined while her CD4+

T cell count has increased can help the client continue to tolerate unpleasant side effects (San Francisco AIDS Foundation, 1997b).

The following list of elements of a comprehensive client education program is adapted from *Human Immunodeficiency Virus (HIV-1) Guidelines for Chemical Dependency Treatment and Care Programs in Minnesota* (Pike, 1989). Clients who are HIV infected, whether they are symptomatic or not, should receive education about their disease status, prognosis, and treatment options. All clients with substance abuse disorders, whether HIV infected or not, should receive education about

- The fundamentals of HIV and AIDS
- Strategies for personal risk reduction
- Relevant treatment program policies regarding HIV/AIDS
- Confidentiality rules and expectations
- Benefits of HIV antibody testing
- Overview of local HIV/AIDS resources, including hotlines
- Available medical and social service resources and entitlements, and how to obtain them

Using support groups to connect with other clients facing similar problems can promote empowerment by helping individuals feel less isolated and overwhelmed by their problems. Specific strategies for empowering and engaging clients may include

- Holding support group meetings at the substance abuse treatment facility
- Offering educational sessions for HIV-positive substance abusers in HIV/AIDS and substance abuse treatment settings

Barriers to Care for HIV-Infected Substance Abuse Disorder Clients

Bringing substance abusers with HIV infection into the health care system is a significant challenge. Early treatment provides the maximum potential benefits for both individual and public health (Carpenter et al., 1997; Centers for Disease Control and Prevention [CDC], 1997c). Yet HIV-infected clients often delay seeking medical care. The longest delay occurs in the period of time before testing, which is why getting clients to test is so important. Many clients also delay treatment after they receive positive test results. According to one study, most enter medical care within 3 months of receiving positive test results, but 39 percent delay for more than 1 year (Samet et al., 1998). This study also showed that people with a history of IDU on average delayed entering medical care 19 months longer than those with no history of IDU. In the same study, men who abused alcohol delayed 15 months longer than men who did not. As a result, clients who delayed seeking treatment had lower CD4+ T-lymphocyte counts (also referred to as CD4+ T cells, T-cells, or T-4 helper cells); the median CD4+ T cell count in the study was 280, below the threshold at which HIV/AIDS-related medical therapy should be considered.

Why clients wait so long to seek medical treatment is not well understood. Factors may include lack of financial resources, fear of disclosure, lack of health insurance, lack of social support, difficulty in admitting they may need treatment, an underlying psychiatric disorder, and past problems with the treatment system. Women, in particular, may delay because of responsibilities to care for others or concerns for their children and families. Many parents from low-income families, especially those without a support system, may fear that they will be deemed unworthy because of their substance abuse and subsequently lose custody of their children. Also, individuals' feelings of helplessness about addressing their substance abuse issues may compound a general sense of helplessness about taking care of their health problems. When HIV-infected substance abusers do seek medical attention, they may do so erratically, making excessive use of acute and emergency care services and underusing primary care medical services (Stein et al., 1993).

HIV among incarcerated adults in the U.S. is six times higher than in the general population (Maruschak, 1997). The behaviors that place persons, particularly women, at high risk for incarceration (e.g., substance abuse, commercial sex work) are also behaviors that place them at high risk for contracting HIV. Continuity of medical care for incarcerated persons using anti-HIV medications is critical (Dixon et al., 1993).

Models of Integrated Care

Ideally, all substance abuse treatment programs should be capable of conducting HIV risk assessments and providing basic HIV/AIDS education and counseling to clients. However, this ideal has not always been achieved. Among 2,315 clients interviewed on presentation for addiction treatment in 1992–1993, only 53 percent reported previous HIV testing (Samet et al., 1999). In addition, all programs should provide access to HIV testing and pre- and posttest counseling. If programs cannot provide testing and related counseling onsite, they must have referral relationships with other agencies that will provide these services. For guidance on structuring HIV/AIDS counseling programs, providers should consult the CDC's *Technical Guidance on HIV Counseling* (CDC, 1993).

An integrated approach to caring for HIV-infected substance abuse disorder clients requires developing collaborations and maintaining communication among alcohol and drug counselors, HIV/AIDS medical care providers, and mental health providers. Existing links, such as those established in some managed care organizations, must be developed to expand services and improve access to care (O'Connor et al., 1992a; Selwyn et al., 1989).

The 1993 Substance Abuse Prevention and Treatment Block Grants Interim Final Rule, administered by the Substance Abuse and Mental Health Services Administration, reinforces the importance of links between substance abuse treatment and primary care services, particularly when providing services to injection drug users. For example, the regulations require that injection drug users on a waiting list for substance abuse treatment receive interim services within 48 hours of requesting them. Interim services must include referrals to HIV/AIDS health care services as well as HIV/AIDS counseling and education (see the section "Substance Abuse Prevention and Treatment Block Grant Funding" in Chapter 10).

Primary care staff providing services to HIV-infected substance abuse disorder clients should understand and be responsive to clients' needs (O'Connor and Samet, 1996). They should be aware that a client's relapse into substance abuse may result in noncompliance with medical care. In addition, staff must be sensitive to clients' prior experiences with the medical care community, cultural and language variations and issues related to race and ethnicity, sexual orientation, life experiences, and gender (see the section "Cultural Competency Issues" in Chapter 7).

At each medical visit, primary care providers should ask about the status of the client's substance abuse treatment. Documentation of ongoing substance abuse treatment is important. In certain situations, such as when a client of a program is hospitalized for medical illness, primary care physicians are required to make arrangements to ensure continuation of methadone maintenance. Also, clients need continuous reinforcement of the message that by continuing to abuse substances, they are further damaging their own health as well as placing others at risk of HIV infection (for more information about enhancing client motivation, see TIP 35, *Enhancing Motivation for Change in Substance Abuse Treatment*, [CSAT, 1999d]).

Medical Care Within Substance Abuse Treatment Programs

Chapter 6 provides an overview of substance abuse treatment settings and modalities. Figure 2-1 contains a description of the various models for the provision of medical care commonly found in different substance abuse treatment settings.

Models of Primary Care for a Population With Substance Abuse Disorders

Involving an HIV-infected substance abuser in a primary medical care system that provides ongoing and preventive care can be frustrating (Wartenberg, 1991). It is common for clients to lack primary medical care during periods of intense drug use. Outside of university medical

centers, finding primary care physicians or clinics willing to accept HIV-infected substance abuse disorder clients can be difficult. This is partly because few primary care sites are willing to take on the financial strain of caring for uninsured or underinsured clients. Also, primary care providers generally are not educated on issues related to substance abuse or the evolving specialty of HIV/AIDS care (Samet et al., 1997). The Consensus Panel recommends connecting HIV-infected drug abusers with HIV/AIDS care providers during their substance abuse treatment. Even here, the barriers to primary medical care are apparent.

Existing primary care models should still be evaluated in order to identify how they can be modified and expanded to address the special needs of the HIV-infected, substance-abusing population (O'Connor et al., 1992b; Samet, 1995). To date, there is only one study of outcomes for clients seen in substance abuse treatment settings who are referred to available

---

Figure 2-1
Models of Medical Care in Substance Abuse Treatment Programs

There is considerable variation in the levels of medical care provided by substance abuse treatment programs.

- *Inpatient treatment programs* generally have fairly extensive onsite medical capabilities for providing medical care to clients or are closely affiliated with a nearby medical center. These programs can provide only acute, short-term medical care. Some *residential treatment programs* are affiliated with a medical center, but many have only a loose affiliation.
- *Intensive outpatient treatment programs* may be located in or closely affiliated with a hospital or medical center.
- *Social model programs*, whether residential or day and evening programs, have no medical capabilities and may be only loosely affiliated with a medical facility. These programs generally concentrate on providing psychosocial services.
- *Methadone maintenance programs* are required to have a medical director, although this individual's active clinical presence may be minimal. Nursing staff is onsite primarily to dispense methadone or LAAM (levo-alpha-acetyl-methadol). Some methadone programs have started to develop more comprehensive onsite primary medical care services, although wide variations persist. These programs serve clients who have used heroin or other opiates.
- *Therapeutic communities* are residential and generally have minimal onsite medical capabilities.

community primary care resources (Stein et al., 2000). One study that compared onsite with offsite primary care for a small group of subjects found that onsite care provided in a substance abuse treatment setting had significant continuity-of-care advantages (Umbricht-Schneiter et al., 1994).

Onsite systems

Well-defined models exist for providing primary care to HIV-infected substance abuse disorder clients (Figure 2-2). Methadone treatment programs that provide onsite primary care medical services (whether sharing the same space or the building next door) often have been hospital- or university-affiliated programs and have benefited from a close association with affiliated medical specialists (O'Connor et al., 1992b; Selwyn et al., 1989; Sorensen et al., 1989). Onsite systems enhance client followup and adherence to therapies.

Referral systems

The practice of distributing clients from substance abuse treatment programs to various clinical sites for primary medical care is called a *distributive care system*. Optimally, primary care should be multidisciplinary, with social workers, physicians, physicians-in-training, nurses, mental health professionals, and alcohol and drug counselors included in the treatment staff. A case manager may be helpful in facilitating communication among treatment personnel (see Chapter 6 for more information). For newly diagnosed clients, linkage to accessible medical care is important to prevent delay in seeking care. Counselors and nurses must continue to encourage early entry into treatment for those people who are reluctant or face barriers such as lack of transportation or child care.

Communication

When clients are sent to referral sites for primary medical care, a communication system should be in place to ensure that appointments are kept and that information about medical care is sent back to the referral point. A memorandum of understanding between the referral site and the primary care provider is recommended to ensure that this feedback occurs systematically. Forms for transfer of confidential information should be signed by clients at their initial visits to both primary care and substance abuse treatment sites (see Chapter 9 for additional information). The 1993 Substance Abuse Prevention and Treatment Block Grants Interim Final Rule requires States to coordinate substance abuse

---

Figure 2-2
Components of Onsite Medical Systems

The most successful onsite medical systems provide a range of medical services, including

- Health maintenance and prevention
- Screening for infectious diseases (hepatitis, syphilis)
- HIV counseling and testing
- Prophylaxis against TB and HIV-related opportunistic infections
- Antiretroviral therapy
- Immunizations (pneumococcal, *Haemophilus influenzae*, hepatitis B)
- Family planning and pregnancy services
- Treatment of episodic illness, hospital followup, and coordination of care

Source: Batki and London, 1991; O'Connor et al., 1992b; Selwyn et al., 1993; Umbricht-Schneiter et al., 1994.

disorder prevention and treatment activities with other services, including HIV/AIDS services. MOUs may be used as evidence that such coordination is being sought.

Contractual arrangements

Some HIV/AIDS services may have contractual arrangements with other health care facilities. For example, clients with identified health problems, such as positive tuberculin skin test results, may be sent to a local hospital with which the referring facility has a contractual arrangement. The contractual arrangement guarantees that the client will be seen and specifies services to be rendered. Unlike referrals, a contractual arrangement contains a built-in mechanism that ensures continuity of care. Detoxification programs often have such an arrangement with medical providers.

Recommended elements of a contractual arrangement for primary medical care services are described in Figure 2-3.

Medical Standards Of Care

This section describes a range of practices endorsed by Consensus Panel members of this TIP. Where specific treatment recommendations exist or where data strongly indicate that a particular intervention is better than alternative treatments, this information is clearly stated. Where there are arguments for and against a particular intervention, both the advantages and disadvantages are provided.

The Consensus Panel wishes to provide clinicians treating HIV-infected substance-abusing clients with current information on which to base clinical decisions that are in the best interests of their clients. This section also provides basic information to treatment personnel who are not physicians. Many excellent online sources of information about current HIV/AIDS care are listed in Appendix F, with special reference to primary care and outpatient management.

Classification of HIV Infection And AIDS

See Appendix C for a description of the clinical categories of HIV and AIDS. See Chapter 1 for a discussion of the origins and development of HIV and AIDS.

Benefits of Early Intervention

The best time to treat HIV is as early as possible. The sooner an HIV-infected individual receives treatment, the more likely his survival will be

---

Figure 2-3
Recommended Elements of a Contractual Arrangement
For Primary Medical Care Services

The following are services that substance abuse treatment facilities should consider including in a contractual arrangement for primary medical care services:

- Phlebotomy (drawing blood samples)
- Clinical laboratory services
- Access to physician and midlevel providers (e.g., nurse practitioner, physician's assistant)
- Diagnostic and treatment services, such as radiology, specialty medical clinics, and hospitalization

At a minimum, freestanding substance abuse treatment units that have no physician on staff and provide no screening services for HIV should have an individual trained in HIV issues available for triage and referral when necessary.

prolonged and his symptoms less dire. In the 1980s and early 1990s, researchers focused on determining the best time to begin HIV treatment. Initially, this was thought to be the stage at which a CD4+ T cell count of 500 is reached. However, due to the inadequacy of viral suppression, the virus quickly developed resistance and resumed reproduction, and the benefits were lost. Now, however, combinations of three or more different medicines are used to treat HIV, each medicine working in a different way to fight the virus. Figure 2-4 illustrates how drug therapy works at various stages in the life cycle of HIV. Most researchers agree that an HIV-infected individual with a detectable viral load who is ready to begin treatment should do so at once. The availability of new antiretroviral agents and rapid acquiring of new information have led to updates in treatment guidelines on a regular basis. Some clinicians prefer to wait until the CD4+ T cell count drops below 500 or the viral load rises above 10,000 (CDC, 1998h). Before beginning HIV treatment, however, the client must be ready to commit to taking these medicines every day for the rest of her life (i.e., must be in a stage of "treatment readiness"). Any deviation from the medication schedule can foster the development of drug resistance and hasten the appearance of AIDS.

The client should also be mentally and emotionally ready to undergo treatment because compliance will depend on his willingness to adhere to the medication schedule. Self-efficacy theory (Bandura, 1977) describes the necessity that an individual believe not only that an action will achieve its desired goal but also that he will be able to perform the action effectively. If the individual receives reinforcement from many sources that the medications are effective and that it will be possible to take them correctly, he is more likely to make the attempt. Substance abuse treatment professionals can play a key role in this process. With their understanding of the day-to-day realities of their clients' lives (e.g., barriers such as homelessness), alcohol and drug counselors can aid the clinician in choosing a drug regimen that the client will be able to follow.

Drug Resistance

Although combination therapy is the most effective treatment to date, once an individual begins this form of treatment, she cannot stop taking any of the medications because the virus can then develop resistance to that medication and possibly to other related antiretroviral medications. Resistant viruses can be transmitted to others and may make treatment difficult or impossible. Although combination therapy can be complex, the counselor should strongly discourage the client from taking only some of the pills, taking "drug holidays" (which was a common practice and recommendation with AZT monotherapy), or skipping doses because these practices lead to resistance. If there is a need to discontinue any antiretroviral medication for an extended time, clients should be advised of the theoretical advantages of stopping *all* anti-HIV medications rather than continuing one or two agents.

Resistance occurs when a virus no longer responds to a drug. All viruses have the ability to learn from and possibly outwit human immune system defenses. As HIV multiplies, it makes random changes in its genetic code, which allow it to escape human immune system defenses and the suppressive effects of anti-HIV therapy. An anti-HIV drug regimen that is not followed properly can speed up this process. When a therapy does not completely suppress HIV replication, the virus produces mutations that can replicate despite the presence of anti-HIV medications. If unchecked, these mutations will significantly change the original virus, and this new, stronger version of the virus is considered to be drug resistant.

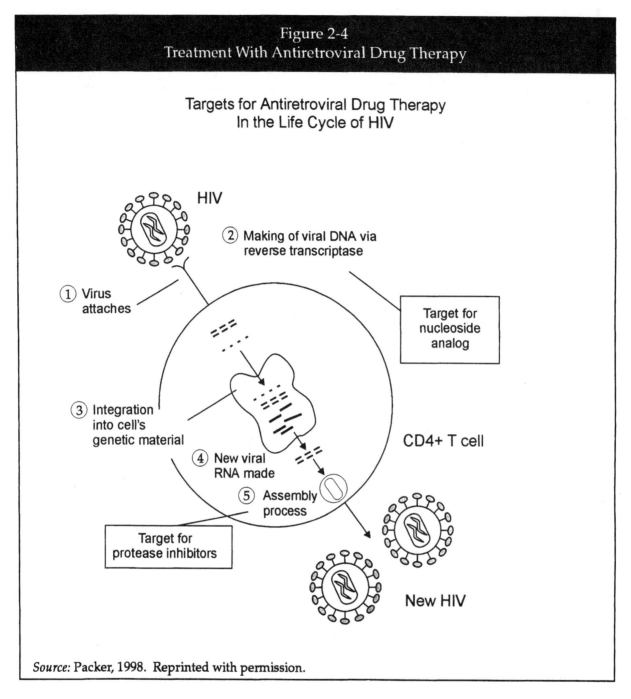

Figure 2-4
Treatment With Antiretroviral Drug Therapy

Targets for Antiretroviral Drug Therapy
In the Life Cycle of HIV

Source: Packer, 1998. Reprinted with permission.

Cross-resistance occurs when a virus develops resistance to one medication, which automatically makes it resistant to other related medications. When HIV develops resistance to indinavir (Crixivan), for instance, it can also become resistant to ritonavir (Norvir). If resistance develops to one protease inhibitor (PI), then it is likely that HIV has become cross-resistant to other PIs (San Francisco AIDS Foundation, 1997b). Resistance and cross-resistance have become the most serious setbacks in the struggle against HIV/AIDS since the development of combination therapy.

Postexposure Prophylaxis

Postexposure prophylaxis (PEP) is an HIV treatment administered within 72 hours after exposure to HIV. An individual who has been exposed to the virus can prevent it from becoming established in her body if she treats it very quickly. PEP involves taking a multidrug combination that will stop the virus before it damages the immune system.

When someone is exposed to HIV, his immune system cells carry the virus to the lymph nodes, where it begins to rapidly replicate. Within 3 to 5 days, new virus particles then spill out into the bloodstream and flood the body. This is the stage of acute HIV infection that PEP is aimed to prevent. If this can be averted, the individual may be able to clear the virus, and his immune system can safely destroy what remains (CDC, 1998f).

PEP must begin before the individual tests HIV positive and before HIV is detected on a blood viral load test. However, early treatment even after this 3- to 5-day "window of opportunity" can still slow the advance of the disease. The standard PEP treatment is a combination of three antiretroviral medications.

PEP is not a "morning-after" drug. It requires a month of daily treatments, which can produce unpleasant side effects. It is expensive, and it is not FDA-approved. Because of these factors, many insurance plans do not cover it. Also, there are concerns within the HIV treatment field that using powerful anti-HIV drugs too often may create resistance in the virus. Consequently, PEP should be administered only to health care workers who have received significant occupational exposure and in cases of accidental sexual exposure (for example, if a condom breaks or someone is raped) (San Francisco AIDS Foundation, 1997a).

Testing for HIV

Counseling and testing prior to and after HIV antibody testing has multiple goals. It is used to explain the limitations of the HIV test, to help persons assess their risks, to encourage and reinforce behavior change, and to refer infected individuals to clinical care. All counseling

should be performed by a counselor trained in HIV counseling. Test results should be discussed face to face with the client (rather than by telephone or mail), and appropriate precautions must be taken regarding confidentiality of test results and potential adverse effects of testing, such as psychological stress.

Testing for HIV is a difficult decision and always an individual one. Because more effective HIV therapy is now available, an individual has more treatment choices. Treating HIV when it is discovered late is more difficult. Typically, it takes a few weeks to obtain results from standard HIV tests; unfortunately, many people who are tested do not return to learn their results. However, new rapid HIV tests are being developed (e.g., OraSure™) that can produce reliable results in hours instead of days; this may substantially increase the number of individuals who learn about their HIV status (CDC, 1998h). The sensitivity and specificity of rapid HIV tests are comparable to enzyme immunoassay tests.

Another testing option is home sample collection (HSC) tests, which allow people to test themselves for HIV. Currently, two HSC tests have been approved by the FDA. The user performs a finger stick and mails the specimen, identified by an anonymous code number, directly to the laboratory. The user later calls a toll-free number to obtain test results, counseling, and referrals (Branson, 1998). All positive home tests should be confirmed by a supplemental test.

If a person at high risk is unprepared for a positive result or unwilling to consider treatment, an HIV test may not be helpful. On the other hand, if a person has an overwhelming fear or preoccupation with HIV, it may be wise to test, even if the risk is fairly low. For those clients who may be unprepared for a positive test result, pretest counseling may be necessary. Usually more than one pretest counseling session is held to better prepare the client before she takes the test. Another alternative is group counseling for preparing clients for HIV testing before formal pretest counseling begins.

HIV testing may be either anonymous or confidential, depending on the local laws, or both types of testing may be available. Confidential testing means that the person tested will give his name, which is reported to the State health department. Anonymous testing means that the person does not have to give his name, and no name is reported to anyone. There is much controversy surrounding HIV reporting systems.

By the beginning of 1999, 30 States had established name-based reporting systems for HIV. Of these, 11 also eliminated their anonymous testing sites. New York's law, passed in 1998, includes a partner notification provision. Three other States use unique identifier systems, where, instead of by name, clients are identified by a code combining their gender, race/ethnicity, birth date, and social security number. Three more States introduced HIV reporting bills in the 1998 legislative session that never became laws (CDC, 1999a; Fuentes, 1999). Supporters of name-based reporting, including the CDC, believe that these programs will help generate more accurate statistics concerning the spread of HIV. Opponents argue that these systems will deter people at high risk from being tested. For example, populations such as immigrants or women may not be tested because of the social risk involved in disclosure (Shelton, 1998). Alcohol and drug counselors and HIV primary care personnel should be aware of the reporting requirements in their States.

Before testing, the client's level of risk for HIV should be considered. This level can be determined by how often the client has engaged in risky behaviors. Anyone with a history of drug use should be tested because the seroprevalence in this group is much higher than in the general population. Someone who has a higher number of lifetime sexual partners is at higher risk for HIV, especially if she has engaged in high-risk behaviors. Anyone with a sexually transmitted disease (STD) should be tested. Whatever a person's risk level, it is important to remember that it only takes one exposure to HIV to become HIV-infected.

Certain symptoms might also indicate the need for an HIV test. If someone who has engaged in risky behavior has flulike symptoms, this might indicate a recent infection with HIV and the need for testing. Shingles (herpes zoster) also is a common early sign of HIV infection, causing a painful rash that occurs in a line on only one side of the body. Oral thrush in a nonpregnant adult also indicates immune dysfunction, as does chronic diarrhea, night sweats, weight loss, or fevers. Recurrent vaginal yeast infections are a common sign of HIV infection in women. TB is increasingly problematic among those with HIV infection and can occur even when the immune system is in good condition. Symptoms of TB include a chronic cough and fever.

After initial infection, there often is a long period of time (several years) during which an infected person may appear and feel healthy. Unfortunately, this means that the signs of later stage HIV disease will be the first signals that something is wrong. Many people, especially injection drug users, are hospitalized for HIV-related pneumonia or other serious diseases before they even discover they have HIV.

Significance of CD4+ T cell counts and HIV RNA (viral load)

CD4+ T cell counts

CD4+ T cells are the subset of white blood cells in the immune system that are specifically targeted by HIV. Although HIV also infects other types of cells, the virus's effects on CD4+ T cells cause most of the immunosuppression characteristic of HIV disease.

CD4+ T cell counts generally are the markers for the stage of a client's HIV disease. A normal CD4+ T cell count ranges from 500 to 1,400 (Laurence, 1993). Although they reflect the overall status of the immune system and are presumed to reflect the stage of illness, CD4+ T cell counts can fluctuate over time. Results can also vary among different laboratories and be affected by factors such as coexisting illnesses and time of day. (Measuring CD4+ T cell counts during acute coexisting illness is not generally recommended.) To obtain the most accurate information about trends in a client's CD4+ T cell levels over time, counts should be taken twice initially at intervals a few days apart and periodically thereafter. To increase reliability and consistency of results, tests should be done at the same laboratory each time, if possible. The CD4+ T cell *percentage*, or the percentage of lymphocytes that are CD4+ helper cells, is an additional measurement often performed as part of basic CD4+ lymphocyte subset studies. The CD4+ T cell percentage, which includes the CD4+ helper cell count, may show less variability than the CD4+ T cell count. Long-term therapy may be based on the results of these tests.

It is important to remember that CD4+ T cell counts are only an indirect measure of viral activity; they measure the effects of the virus on the target cell, not the activity or virulence (capability of causing disease by breaking down protective mechanisms of the host) of the virus itself. Viral load tests, described in the next section, quantify viral levels in blood and determine strain type and other indicators of virulence.

Despite their limitations, CD4+ T cell measurements are useful for indicating points at which treatment decisions should be made. The average yearly decline of CD4+ T cell counts in HIV-infected clients is 30 to 90 cells per year; however, the rate of decline can vary (Mellors et al., 1997). Some clients' CD4+ T cell counts decline rapidly, while others remain stable for long periods. There is no evidence that CD4+ T cell counts decline more rapidly in HIV-infected substance abusers than in other HIV-infected populations (Graham et al., 1992; Margolick et al., 1992; Saag, 1994).

Viral load testing

The plasma HIV RNA level has been shown to be the strongest predictor of the progression to AIDS (Mellors et al., 1997). The test measures the number of viral particles per milliliter of plasma. As with CD4+ T cell counts, test results can vary depending on many factors. Viral load testing should not be done during a coexisting infection or within 4 weeks of a vaccination. Currently available commercial test kits can measure down to 50 copies per milliliter, and more sensitive viral load assays are available with a sensitivity of 5 copies (U.S. Department of Health and Human Services [DHHS] and the Henry J. Kaiser Family Foundation, 1997).

Quantification of HIV RNA is the best method of monitoring the client with HIV infection, particularly when antiretroviral therapy has begun. However, viral load tests are expensive, and some insurance plans do not cover repeated use of these tests. Higher levels of HIV RNA suggest greater viral replication and correlate with the number of acutely infected cells as well as with an accelerated rate of disease progression. Therefore, reducing the viral load as closely as possible to undetectable levels is the optimal goal. By using viral load data along with the client's CD4+ T cell count, clinicians can estimate the time to AIDS or death for clients who choose not to take or are unable to take antiretroviral medications.

Initial Assessment

Medical care provided to HIV-infected individuals varies depending on the stage of the infection, but all clients should receive evaluation and followup (O'Connor et al., 1994b; O'Connor and Samet, 1996). Assessment of the behaviors associated with HIV transmission, such as unsafe sex and substance abuse practices, is an important part of the initial client assessment.

At the initial assessment and periodically thereafter, substance-abusing clients should receive risk assessments and comprehensive medical examinations. These examinations can be performed onsite or at another facility through referral or a contractual arrangement.

Medical History

A thorough medical history is an important first step that helps the clinician proceed to clinical evaluation and formulate a treatment plan. Taking the history may occupy an entire client visit, particularly if it is combined with education and counseling. When taking a medical history, health professionals should consider the following:

- If the HIV test occurred elsewhere, it might be helpful to begin by asking when the client took the test and why. This question could yield information about the client's medical history and risk behaviors.
- Questions about drug use and sexual practices should be explicit, clear, open-ended, and nonjudgmental.
- Documentation of the positive HIV test result, if performed elsewhere, should also be obtained and noted in the record. If there is any suggestion that previous HIV test information is not accurate (e.g., repeatedly normal CD4+ T cell counts and undetectable virus), the HIV test should be repeated.
- Sometimes the risk history will indicate the duration of the client's infection. If so, the provider may want to discuss the usual latency period of HIV with the client and the implications of the client's history in determining the stage of the disease and the prognosis. Clients should be counseled about risk reduction and encouraged to notify past and present sexual or drug use

contacts of their HIV status (see Chapter 4 for more information about risk reduction).

- Contact notification is a difficult issue for many clients, but most people cooperate once they understand that their contacts may be at serious risk. Often, State health departments assist people in locating and notifying contacts (see Chapter 9 for more information about notification).
- Ask questions about specific symptoms of HIV infection (e.g., fevers, night sweats, diarrhea, weight loss, lymphadenopathy, thrush, vaginitis, or skin changes) or symptoms suggesting undiagnosed AIDS-defining conditions (e.g., mental state changes, visual changes, severe headaches, chronic diarrhea, shortness of breath, or difficulty swallowing).
- Questions about past medical history should be certain to cover previous diagnoses and treatment of TB, syphilis, genital herpes and herpes zoster, hepatitis B and C, purified protein derivative testing, recurring bacterial pneumonia, and (in women) abnormal Pap smears. STDs are common in substance abusers, particularly among women involved in commercial sex work or the exchange of sex for drugs.
- The client's immunization history should be recorded.
- Mental health issues should be discussed, including past psychiatric treatment and hospitalizations, chronic use of prescribed or nonprescribed psychotropic medications, and the client's current mood. Anxiety and depression are common in this population, often predating the HIV diagnosis (see Chapter 3 for more information on mental health treatment).
- Specific information should be collected about the client's social situation, including functional status, housing, employment, health insurance, and social support from family members or significant others. These

questions may identify urgent social needs and prompt immediate referral to a social service agency or provider.

- A complete social history should be taken, including family genogram, financial information, assessment of coping styles and skills, current losses and grief issues, spiritual assessment, educational factors, cultural issues and beliefs about HIV status and substance abuse, and emotional assessment.

- At the conclusion of the visit, a tuberculin skin test with anergy panel should be done, a set of laboratory tests performed or ordered, and one or more needed immunizations given. At the next visit, a full physical examination can be done, and lab results reviewed.

Physical Examination

Although HIV and its complications may involve nearly every organ, the HIV-directed general physical exam should focus on (1) the skin, (2) the eyes, (3) the mouth, (4) the anogenital region, (5) the nervous system, (6) the lymphatic system, and (7) client weight and temperature. Knowledge of a client's immune status may also direct the physician toward screening other areas. For example, the eyes should be examined for retinitis in clients with very low CD4+ T cell counts. If the client has particular complaints or other chronic conditions such as diabetes or asthma, the exam should focus on those conditions.

Skin

- The skin may be affected early in the course of HIV infection and in many cases may have been the reason why HIV testing was originally done.
- Bacterial agents may cause folliculitis, impetigo, and bacillary angiomatosis. Injection drug users may have infected tracks, skin abscesses, or cellulitis.

- Topical fungal infections are common (e.g., candidiasis, angular cheilitis at corners of lips).
- *Molluscum contagiosum*, pearly papules most often found on the genitalia and face, may lead to serious cosmetic concerns. Warts are also common.
- Herpes, both simplex and zoster, may be the initial indication of HIV disease and often is more severe in clients who are HIV positive.
- Many clients suffer from xerosis (dry skin) or chronic itchiness.
- Inflammatory conditions such as seborrheic dermatitis, psoriasis, and eosinophilic folliculitis are common and often difficult to treat.
- Kaposi's sarcoma, now a relatively rare complication, presents as oval purplish nodules and plaques, most often on the trunk, legs, or hard palate. This disease is more common in men than in women.
- Biopsy is the appropriate step to evaluate any skin lesion that does not respond promptly to standard therapy.

Eyes

- Direct ophthalmoscopy of the optic fundi, preferably with dilation of the pupils, should be done for clients who have CD4+ T cell counts below 100 (on a regular basis if they are asymptomatic and immediately if any eye complaint arises).
- Cytomegalovirus retinitis is characterized by red or orange patches, or "floaters," on the retina and can progress quickly to blindness by affecting the macula or leading to retinal detachment. Any visual complaints that cannot be simply explained should be directed to an ophthalmologist (see Appendix D for a copy of the Amsler grid).

Mouth

- The oral cavity should be checked at every clinical visit. Any oral lesion can affect nutrition, and many cause extreme discomfort. Periodontal disease can be aggressive in persons with HIV disease, and it is important to stress regular dental care (every 6 months) and good oral hygiene.

- Oral candidiasis, or thrush, most often appears as white plaques on the buccal mucosa and tonsillar areas. Without treatment, thrush often spreads throughout the mouth; in persons with advanced disease, candidiasis can affect the esophagus, leading to severe pain on swallowing and the need for prolonged systemic treatment. When it involves only the mouth, thrush may be asymptomatic and should be treated with antifungal agents. Angular stomatitis commonly is associated with mucosal candidiasis.

- Hairy leukoplakia, a lesion related to Epstein-Barr virus, often presents as a white plaque on the side of the tongue and can be confused with thrush. Sandpapery to the gloved hand, leukoplakia may grow in size and cause difficulty in chewing, but sometimes it spontaneously regresses.

- Ulcerations that appear on keratinized epithelium—lips, tongue, hard palate—are most likely herpetic; ulcers on the buccal mucosa are most often aphthous.

Anogenital region

- A baseline anal inspection is essential for all clients. HIV-infected persons with a history of receptive anal intercourse are at increased risk for *papillomavirus*-associated anal squamous cell cancer.

- The clinician also should check for anal discharge, warts, herpetic ulcers, hemorrhoids, fissures, and traumatic tears. Fissures, traumatic tears, and what the client might consider hemorrhoids may be recurrent genital herpes.

- The clinical role of the anal Pap smear remains undefined.

- Clients with HIV may be at risk for other STDs such as syphilis, chlamydia, gonorrhea, herpes simplex, and chancroid.

- In uncircumcised clients, it is important to retract the foreskin to check for *candida balanitis* and chancroid.

- The testicles should be palpated for tenderness, epididymal swelling (a sign of gonococcal or chlamydial infection), and masses.

- The intertriginous areas may have tinea.

- In women, the external genitalia should be inspected for warts, ulcers, and vesicles.

- Other sexually transmitted infections that are less common in this population but must be considered in women include gonorrhea, chlamydia, and syphilis.

- HIV-infected women are at high risk for cervical dysplasia and cervical cancer (see the women's health issues section later in this chapter about cervical abnormalities).

Nervous system

- A brief, structured cognitive exam, such as the Mini Mental State Examination (see Appendix H), should be performed at regular intervals on all clients, particularly those with advanced disease (see also Chapter 3).

- The clinician must consider affective disorders and alcohol or drug use when interpreting the common complaint of memory difficulty.

- The other essential part of the neurologic exam involves an evaluation for neuropathy, a problem that may be HIV related but often is medication related.

- Documenting ankle-jerk reflexes and vibratory sensation in the distal extremities is critical before starting antiretroviral therapy.

Lymphatic system

Most HIV-infected persons have palpable lymph nodes at some point during the course of disease. Such nodes—which may involve multiple sites—do not predict disease progression but often cause discomfort and distress. Clients should be reassured that these nodes are common and often spontaneously increase and decrease in size. If a client experiences a rapid or continuous enlargement, worsening pain, or drainage in a particular node, it should be examined to rule out an opportunistic infection or malignancy. In the case of unexplained constitutional symptoms, node biopsies can be useful to search for evidence of systemic infection.

Weight and temperature

- Weight loss often suggests undiagnosed opportunistic infections, rapidly progressive HIV disease, depression, or substance abuse.
- Because weight loss is an early and meaningful sign of deteriorating clinical status, the client's weight should be measured at each visit.
- Lipid distribution and weight gain due to PIs should be checked.
- Fevers may indicate an underlying opportunistic infection and should be looked for at each visit.
- A current trend in nutritional management of HIV infection is bioelectrical impedance analysis (BIA). This quick and simple procedure can show the ratio of lean muscle mass to body fat and weight. It is no longer sufficient to look at total weight loss to indicate potential problems with nutrition.

Laboratory Tests

Before antiretroviral therapy is initiated in any client, certain laboratory studies should be done. The suggestions listed here should be adapted to the particular circumstances of a client and physician.

- **HIV RNA (viral load).** Viral load testing is the essential parameter that influences decisions to initiate or change antiretroviral

therapies. Using quantitative methods, the clinician should measure plasma HIV RNA levels at the time of diagnosis and every 3 to 4 months thereafter in the untreated client. Ideally, viral load testing should be performed twice before therapy is started to ensure accuracy and consistency of measurement. Only one measurement is needed in clients with advanced disease. To gauge the effect of therapy, viral load should be checked 4 to 8 weeks after initiation of therapy. The indications for plasma HIV RNA testing are shown in Figure 2-5.

- **CD4+ T cell counts.** As noted above, CD4+ T cell counts at present are the standard test to assess the level of immune dysfunction in HIV-infected clients. It is preferable to perform two CD4+ T cell tests a few days apart to help determine a baseline and assess clients' eligibility for antiretroviral therapy. CD4+ T cell counts should be measured every 3 to 6 months after diagnosis.

- **Blood counts.** A complete blood count (CBC) can alert the clinician to blood abnormalities common in HIV-infected clients, including leukopenia and thrombocytopenia. In clients receiving particular antiretroviral agents, the frequency of CBCs is determined by the need to monitor for hematologic toxicity. For example, in symptomatic clients not on AZT, CBCs can be repeated at 3- to 6-month intervals; in asymptomatic clients not on AZT, repetition every 6 months to a year is advised.

- **Purified protein derivative.** Tuberculin skin testing should be performed in HIV-infected persons annually. In early stages of HIV infection, reactivity to the skin test is usually maintained. As HIV disease advances, response may be blunted or absent (anergy). A reaction greater than or equal to 5 mm indication is considered positive for defining

Figure 2-5		
Indications for Plasma HIV RNA Testing*		
Clinical Indication	**Information**	**Use**
Syndrome consistent with acute HIV infection	Establishes diagnosis when HIV antibody test is negative or indeterminate	Diagnosis**
Initial evaluation of newly diagnosed HIV infection	Baseline viral load "set point"	Decision to start or defer therapy
Every 3–4 months in clients not on therapy	Changes in viral load	Decision to start therapy
4–8 weeks after initiation of antiretroviral therapy	Initial assessment of drug efficacy	Decision to continue or change therapy
3–4 months after start of therapy	Maximal effect of therapy	Decision to continue or change therapy
Every 3–4 months in clients on therapy	Durability of antiretroviral effect	Decision to continue or change therapy
Clinical event or significant decline in CD4+ T cells	Association with changing or stable viral load	Decision to continue, initiate, or change therapy

* Acute illness (e.g., bacterial pneumonia, TB, herpes simplex virus, PCP) and immunizations can cause increases in plasma HIV RNA for 2–4 weeks; viral load testing should not be performed during this time.

** Plasma HIV RNA results should be verified with a repeat determination before starting or making changes in therapy. HIV RNA should be measured using the same laboratory and the same assay.

Source: CDC, 1998j; Freedberg et al., 1994.

TB infection. In populations with a high prevalence of TB, a skin test may be falsely negative. HIV-infected persons have a high risk of developing active TB if they have positive skin tests, and they require treatment.

■ **Screening chemistries**. Annual routine screening chemistries are recommended. Testing at 2- to 4-month intervals is indicated in clients receiving medications with potential liver, kidney, and muscle toxicity. Liver function tests must be checked more frequently because of the high risk of exposure to hepatotoxic agents. Hepatitis viruses, alcohol, and several of the antiretroviral agents commonly elevate transaminases (ritonavir in particular;

didanosine [Videx] is contraindicated with a history of pancreatitis; indinivar raises the total bilirubin).

■ **Syphilis**. Annual serologic screening for syphilis is recommended in sexually active persons.

■ **Toxoplasmosis**. Baseline testing is useful to identify clients with past exposure to toxoplasma who may benefit from prophylaxis against this infection. Without prophylaxis, these clients have about a 30 percent chance of developing cerebral toxoplasmosis in the course of their HIV infection (especially when the CD4+ T cell count drops below 100). Annual testing is advised in clients without prior exposure.

- **Hepatitis B virus (HBV).** The prevalence of past exposure to HBV approaches 90 percent in many HIV-infected substance abuse populations in the United States (O'Connor et al., 1994b). Because of the high cost of the HBV vaccine, it is more cost-effective to first screen clients for exposure to this virus to determine if vaccination is necessary. Vaccination is indicated for HIV-infected clients without previous exposure (i.e., all markers negative).

- **Hepatitis A and C.** Injection drug users are at risk for hepatitis A (HAV) infection (although the reason for this has not been determined) and hepatitis C (HCV) infection, which, like HBV, is parenterally transmitted. HCA usually is benign and self-limited; HCV may be treated with injected interferon-alpha and ribavirin, but this treatment is expensive, only modestly effective, and often causes unpleasant side effects. Even so, it may be helpful to determine the presence of prior viral hepatitis in clients likely to be exposed to the increasing numbers of hepatotoxic medications used to treat HIV disease. This may be particularly important for HCV, which appears to persist as a chronic, active infection and is more common than HBV. It also is recommended that injection drug users receive hepatitis A vaccine (CDC, 1999e).

- **Chest x-ray.** A chest x-ray generally is optional in the initial client evaluation, although some clinics and physicians require a TB chest x-ray before they will see a client for the first time. Routine chest x-rays can provide a baseline when clients present with respiratory symptoms, but no studies support this recommendation. Chest x-rays may also be useful in clients with a past history of pulmonary disease or heavy smoking.

Evaluating Symptomatic Illness

Clinicians providing care to HIV-infected substance abusers must be familiar with the clinical manifestations of HIV disease and also be aware that these manifestations can be difficult to distinguish from common medical complications of substance abuse. Differential diagnoses in HIV-infected substance abusers can be challenging because both HIV infection and substance abuse have clinical effects on a wide range of organ systems. It is important to consider the possibility of adverse drug reactions or interactions for those clients who are taking HIV medications (see the section, "Pharmacologic Interactions," later in this chapter). To provide optimal care to this population, clinicians must be fully aware of the combined medical effects of substance abuse, HIV infection, and HIV medications (O'Connor et al., 1994a). Figure 2-6 lists the common symptoms that may be related to either HIV infection or substance abuse.

Anorexia, weight loss, and fatigue may be complications of chronic cocaine use, caused by HIV infection, symptoms of specific AIDS-related opportunistic infections (e.g., *mycobacterium avium complex* [MAC], cytomegalovirus, TB, or side effects of medications). Tachycardia, flulike illness, fatigue, abdominal pain, and diarrhea may be symptoms of drug withdrawal, particularly opioid withdrawal, or they may be symptoms of acute or chronic HIV-related conditions.

Chest pain, coughing, and shortness of breath may be symptoms of crack cocaine use, bacterial pneumonia, or HIV-related pulmonary infections such as PCP. Bacterial endocarditis with fever, night sweats, and chest pain or other pulmonary effects may result from unsterile intravenous injection or may indicate HIV-related opportunistic infection. Heavy cigarette

Figure 2-6		
Medical Complications of Substance Abuse That May Affect Differential Diagnosis of Injection Drug Users With HIV		
Possible Diagnoses		
Symptoms	**HIV Related**	**Substance-Abuse Related**
Constitutional: ■ Anorexia ■ Weight loss ■ Fever ■ Night sweats ■ Diarrhea	■ HIV infection ■ MAC ■ Cytomegalovirus ■ TB	■ Cocaine use ■ Methamphetamine use ■ Injection-related bacterial infections ■ TB ■ Heroin withdrawal
Pulmonary: ■ Chest pain ■ Cough ■ Shortness of breath	■ Bacterial pneumonia ■ PCP	■ Cocaine use ■ Marijuana use ■ Tobacco use ■ Aspiration pneumonia ■ TB ■ Pulmonary embolism
Neurologic: ■ Altered mental state ■ Psychosis ■ Seizures ■ Focal deficits ■ Peripheral neuropathy	■ HIV infection ■ Toxoplasmosis ■ Cryptococcosis ■ Progressive multifocal leukoencephalopathy (PML) ■ Human T-lymphotropic retrovirus type 1 (HTLV-1)	■ Intoxication and withdrawal from heroin ■ Methamphetamine-induced psychosis ■ Cocaine ■ Alcohol ■ Benzodiazepines ■ Drug-related chronic encephalopathy ■ Pyogenic central nervous system infection ■ Trauma ■ Alcoholic polyneuropathy
Dermatologic: ■ Pruritus ■ Rash	■ HIV dermatitis ■ HIV-related thrombocytopenia	■ Drug-related pruritus ■ Chronic hepatitis ■ Cellulitis ■ Alcohol/heroin-induced thrombocytopenia ■ Lymphedema
Miscellaneous: ■ Lymphadenopathy ■ Uremia	■ HIV-related lymphadenopathy ■ HIV-related nephropathy	■ Localized infection ■ Heroin nephropathy
Source: O'Connor et al., 1994b.		

smoking in injection drug users may also make it difficult to interpret symptoms such as shortness of breath or the results of pulmonary function tests. HIV and its related opportunistic infections commonly affect the nervous system, resulting in conditions such as HIV-related dementia, CNS cryptococcosis, toxoplasmosis, and HIV-related peripheral neuropathy. Drug intoxication or withdrawal also can affect consciousness, cognition, and behavior. Heroin and cocaine use may cause stroke syndromes and other cerebrovascular diseases. Alcoholic, nutritional, and traumatic peripheral neuropathy syndromes may also be more common in substance abusers than in the population as a whole.

Psychiatric complications

In 1998 the prevalence of depression among HIV-infected persons was estimated at 30 to 40 percent. It may be higher among persons with substance abuse disorders and those symptomatic with AIDS. Increasing symptoms, progressive disability, and decline in function may bring sadness, anxiety, fear, insomnia, and a feeling of being overwhelmed. Substance-dependent persons may have few coping resources (other than substance abuse). Grief over the loss of loved ones (who may also have had AIDS) can be severe. Clinicians should make every effort to make definitive diagnoses. Situational anxiety or depressive symptoms can be treated with supportive psychotherapy. Support groups, both HIV-related and others, and encouragement toward social and family interaction are important parts of treatment. Pharmacologic interactions may be needed in severe, persistent sleep disturbances, major depression, generalized anxiety, and posttraumatic stress disorders.

Pharmacologic Aspects

HIV disease is now seen to fit the pattern of a chronic disease (with complications and remissions) rather than an illness that appears suddenly and progresses rapidly to death. Clients periodically need acute care inpatient resources, especially in the latter stages of the disease. However, as clients experience longer asymptomatic periods between illnesses, the emphasis increasingly is on ambulatory management and primary care for HIV infection.

Medications to control HIV infection have become more available. The most effective treatment is a combination of three or more different medications. Most often, two of the medications are nucleoside reverse transcriptase inhibitors (NRTIs), and the third can be either a nonnucleoside reverse transcriptase inhibitor (NNRTI) or a PI. Combination therapy with three or more medicines generally reduces the viral load to near or below the level of detection. There are currently six FDA-approved NRTIs, one nucleotide, five PIs, and three NNRTIs, and thus many potential combinations would seem to be possible. However, once a medication from a certain class is used (e.g., PIs, NRTIs), the likelihood increases that the virus will develop resistance to some or all other drugs in that class, so the options quickly become very limited. This is known as cross-resistance. For this reason, it is widely believed that the best chance for success in HIV treatment is with the first treatment regimen, which is why adherence and followup are so critical.

All the medications administered in combination therapy have side effects and specific requirements for use. For example, AZT may be given with lamivudine (Epivir, also known as 3TC) as the two NRTIs. These both can be taken either with or without meals. A possible side effect of AZT is anemia. The clinician may add the PI indinavir, which cannot be taken with food or with other medications and also requires the client to drink a great deal of water because it causes kidney stones. A newly described side effect of PIs is weight gain in the trunk, while the arms and legs become thinner (lipodystrophy), and for women the central distribution of weight often causes breast enlargement.

Care strategies have incorporated both antiretroviral therapy and a wide range of prophylactic regimens to effectively prevent opportunistic infections. A recent study found, however, that preventive interventions such as TB prophylaxis and pneumococcal vaccine were used by only about 30 percent of eligible clients, and use of preventive interventions was lowest among HIV-infected injection drug users (Glassroth et al., 1994).

Little is known about interactions of HIV medications with street drugs, and a specialist should be consulted about interactions, even for over-the-counter drugs. PIs have the greatest potential for interacting with other drugs. For example, PIs can prevent amphetamines from leaving the system, which then build up to toxic or deadly levels. Heroin, on the other hand,

may be metabolized more quickly (Horn, 1998). See Figure 2-7 for a listing of interactions between HIV medications and street drugs.

Antiretroviral Therapy

The goal of antiretroviral therapy is to improve the length and quality of the client's life. None of the medications currently available to treat HIV-infected clients is a cure, but, used in combination, they can decrease viral replication, improve immunologic status, delay infectious complications, and prolong life. The ideal time to begin antiretroviral therapy remains debatable; immune damage occurs over time, which suggests that all HIV-infected people may eventually benefit from treatment. However,

Figure 2-7
Interactions of HIV Medications With Street Drugs

Drug	Interaction and Effects
Ecstasy	3- to 10-fold buildup of 3,4-methylene-dioxymethamphetamine (MDMA) in the blood, bruxism (teeth grinding), palpitations, joint stiffness, dehydration. Possibility of liver and kidney damage. May be deadly.
Speed/Methamphetamine	2- to 3-fold buildup of methamphetamine in the blood, increased anxiety, manic behavior, shortness of breath, racing heart beat, and dehydration.
Heroin	Heroin is metabolized more quickly; less "hit," less "buzz," withdrawal symptoms.
Special K (ketamine hydrochloride)	Buildup of ketamine is likely; increased sedation, disorientation, and hallucinations. Effects last longer.
Cocaine	Little is known about cocaine's interaction with PIs as no studies have been conducted, but if an individual has HIV, smoking, shooting, or even snorting cocaine may compromise the immune system. In one test-tube study, cocaine made HIV reproduce 20 times faster than normal.
GHB (gamma hydroxybutyric acid)	Combining GHB with the antiprotease drugs is another unknown. Like many recreational drugs, GHB may suppress the immune system.

Source: Adapted with permission from Horn, 1998.

given that the virus has not been eradicated, antiretroviral medications once started must be taken for the rest of the client's life.

Although there is theoretical benefit to treating asymptomatic clients with CD4+ T cell counts greater than 500, no long-term benefit has yet been demonstrated. Those with high CD4+ T cell counts and very low HIV RNA levels may consider delaying therapy. The major dilemma confronting clients and providers is that the antiretroviral regimens with the greatest potency in viral suppression and CD4+ T cell count preservation are the most medically complex and are associated with a wide array of side effects and drug interactions (see the section, "Pharmacologic Interactions"). The decision to begin antiretroviral therapy in the asymptomatic client is difficult and often involves multiple visits to review treatment options. The factors to consider include (1) client willingness and readiness to begin therapy and remain adherent; (2) the degree of immunodeficiency; (3) the risk of disease progression as determined by plasma HIV RNA; (4) the risk of side effects; (5) the ongoing treatment of other medical conditions, such as diabetes; (6) barriers to care, such as lack of insurance and unstable housing; and (7) stability in drug use patterns and substance abuse treatment (see Figure 2-8). It is important to remember that combination therapies do not work for everyone, even for those who do follow the directions. Many long-term survivors of HIV have experienced very little improvement on the new medications. Once the client has decided to undergo treatment, the goal of therapy should be to suppress plasma viral load to undetectable levels. Based on current data, the preferred treatment regimen is two nucleoside analogs and one PI (Figure 2-9). Alternative regimens have been used, including two PIs together with one or two NRTIs or substituting an NNRTI for the PI in a three-drug regimen. Monotherapy, the standard of care before 1995, is now outdated. If a client is only on one medication,

---

Figure 2-8
Risks and Benefits of Early Initiation of Antiretroviral Therapy
In the Asymptomatic HIV-Infected Client

Potential Benefits

- Control of viral replication and mutation, reduction of viral burden
- Prevention of progressive immunodeficiency; potential maintenance or reconstitution of a normal immune system
- Delayed progression to AIDS and prolongation of life
- Decreased risk of selection of resistant virus
- Decreased risk of certain drug toxicities (such as anemia)

Potential Risks

- Reduction in quality of life from adverse drug effects and inconvenience of current maximally suppressive regimens
- Earlier development of drug resistance
- Limitation in future choices of antiretroviral agents due to development of resistance
- Unknown long-term toxicity of antiretroviral drugs
- Unknown duration of effectiveness of current antiretroviral therapies

> ### Figure 2-9
> ### Recommended CD4+ T Cell Testing Frequencies and Thresholds for
> ### Initiation of Antiretroviral Therapy
>
> **Testing Frequency**
>
> - CD4+ T cell count = 500 and over: Every 6 months
> - CD4+ T cell count < 500 but > 50: Every 3 months
> - CD4+ T cell count < 50: Many experts see no need for testing (except in relation to initiation of new antiretroviral therapy, to observe whether therapy results in an increased CD4+ T cell count)
>
> | Antiretroviral Therapy Clinical Category | CD4+ T Cell Count and HIV RNA | Recommendation |
> | --- | --- | --- |
> | Symptomatic (i.e., AIDS, thrush, unexplained fever) | Any value | Treat |
> | Asymptomatic | CD4+ T cells < 500/mm³
or
HIV RNA > 10,000 (bDNA)
or   > 20,000 (RT-PCR) | Treatment should be offered. Strength of recommendation is based on prognosis for disease-free survival and willingness of the client to accept therapy.* |
> | Asymptomatic | CD4+ T cells > 500/mm³
and
HIV RNA < 10,000 (bDNA)
or   < 20,000 (RT-PCR) | Many experts would delay therapy and observe; however, some experts would treat. |
>
> *Some experts would observe clients whose CD4+ T cell counts are between 350 and 500/mm³ and HIV RNA levels < 10,000 (bDNA) or < 20,000 (RT-PCR).
> *Source:* CDC, 1998i.

the provider should examine this further and educate the client on current standards of care.

Highly Active Antiretroviral Therapy

Highly active antiretroviral therapy (HAART) is a combination of antiretroviral regimens that incorporates at least three antiretroviral drugs. Treatment with HAART has resulted in longer survival and improved quality of life for many people with HIV. This therapy is now considered the standard of care by most HIV specialists.

Resting CD4+ T cells are among the "safe havens" where HIV may persist for years interwoven into the cells' genes despite aggressive three-drug antiretroviral therapy. New therapies to attack these "safe havens" are under study. In resting CD4+ T cells taken from the bloodstream of a small number of study clients receiving interleukin-2 plus HAART, researchers were unable to find HIV that was capable of replicating, even when they looked for the virus in millions of cells with sensitive laboratory procedures (Folkers, 1998).

HAART may be beneficial at all stages of HIV disease, from initial exposure through acute and chronic infection and when AIDS symptoms are present. In general, people at earlier stages of HIV disease receive the most long-lasting benefits from HAART, particularly those individuals who have never undergone HIV treatment. Those with advanced AIDS and those who have used anti-HIV drugs for years generally benefit less from HAART. For reasons that are not yet completely understood, some HIV-infected persons cannot tolerate the side effects of therapy with PIs or do not benefit from them (San Francisco AIDS Foundation, 1997c).

A typical HAART regimen includes a PI when used with two NRTI analogs. Many three- and four-drug combinations can reduce HIV to very low levels for sustained periods. For example, the NNRTI class of medication may be added to or substituted for a PI in combination with two NRTI analogs. Some physicians recommend using didanosine plus hydroxyurea, an anticancer drug, in combination with a PI and an additional NRTI analog. When beginning anti-HIV therapy with ritonavir (six 100-mg capsules twice a day for a total of 1,200 mg daily) and nevirapine (Viramune) (one 200-mg tablet daily for 2 weeks, then twice daily), these drugs are first administered at lower doses, then slowly increased to lessen the possibility of side effects. Medications used in the treatment of HIV (including those expected to become available shortly) are summarized in Figure 2-10. Figure 2-11 presents a schedule and side effects for NRTIs, NNRTIs, and PIs.

Nucleoside analogs

AZT, the first approved antiretroviral agent, taken in combination with didanosine or lamivudine is more effective than AZT alone in slowing progression to AIDS and prolonging survival. AZT plus lamivudine with or without a PI has been recommended for prevention of HIV infection after a needlestick or sexual exposure. AZT alone given to pregnant HIV-infected women at 14 to 34 weeks of gestation reduces transmission of the virus to their babies from 26 to 8 percent, but many clinicians now favor combination treatment for pregnant women. Adverse effects include anemia, neutropenia, nausea and vomiting, headache,

and muscle aches. For many substance abusers, the side effects of AZT mimic substance withdrawal, especially from opioids.

Lamivudine used with AZT decreases viral load and may decrease the emergence of AZT-resistant isolates. It also is commonly used in combination with stavudine (abbreviated as D4T) (Zerit) and didanosine. Side effects include headache, nausea, diarrhea, abdominal pain, and insomnia. Lamivudine and AZT have been combined into a single pill (Combivir) for convenience.

Stavudine is most often used as a substitute for AZT in initial combination therapy, or after failure of AZT-containing regimens. When combined with didanosine or lamivudine, stavudine has potent effects. It causes dose-related peripheral sensory neuropathy, which often disappears when the drug is stopped and may not recur when it is restarted at a lower dose. Subjective complaints are infrequent and include headache, gastrointestinal intolerance with diarrhea, or esophageal ulcers. Liver function tests may increase, and pancreatitis has occurred but is rare.

Didanosine is mainly used in combination with AZT and stavudine, plus a PI or NNRTI. Treatment-limiting toxicities of didanosine include peripheral neuropathy, pancreatitis, and diarrhea. Severe lactic acidosis and retinal depigmentation also can occur. Clients with a history of pancreatitis should avoid didanosine. Onset of abdominal pain should prompt an evaluation for possible pancreatitis. Miscellaneous side effects include rash, marrow suppression, hyperuricemia, hypokalemia, hypocalcemia, and hypomagnesemia.

Zalcitabine (Hivid) can be used in combination with AZT but is the least potent of the nucleoside analogs. Side effects include peripheral neuropathy, rash, stomatitis, esophageal ulceration, and pancreatitis.

Abacavir (Ziagen) is used primarily in combination with AZT and lamivudine. It may be part of a regimen containing a PI. The side

Figure 2-10 Summary of HIV Medications					
Generic Name	**Trade Name**	**Drug Class**	**Abbreviation**	**Usual Dosage**	**Common Side Effects (Comments)**
Abacavir	Ziagen	NRTI	1592U89	300 mg b.i.d.*	Hypersensitivity reaction, nausea, vomiting, malaise, headache, diarrhea, or anorexia; rarely clients may develop lactic acidosis with severe hepatomegaly and steatosis
Didanosine	Videx	NRTI	ddI	400 mg b.i.d. (125 mg b.i.d. if <60 kg)	Pancreatitis, peripheral neuropathy, diarrhea (take on empty stomach)
Lamivudine	Epivir	NRTI	3TC	150 mg b.i.d.	Anemia, gastrointestinal upset
Stavudine	Zerit	NRTI	D4T	40 mg b.i.d. (30 mg b.i.d. if <60 kg)	Peripheral neuropathy
Zalcitabine	Hivid	NRTI	ddC	0.75 mg t.i.d.**	Peripheral neuropathy, stomatitis and aphthous esophageal ulcers, pancreatitis, hepatitis
Zidovudine	Retrovir	NRTI	AZT, ZDV	300 mg b.i.d.	Bone marrow suppression, gastrointestinal upset, headache, myopathy
Zidovudine/ Lamivudine	Combivir	NRTI		1 tablet b.i.d. (150 mg lamivudine + 300 mg zidovudine)	Myopathy, lactic acidosis, severe hepatomegaly with steatosis, headache, gastrointestinal upset, malaise, fatigue, nasal symptoms, cough, musculoskeletal pain, fever/chills, anorexia, abdominal pain/cramps, neuropathy, insomnia, depression, rash, dizziness, myalgia, arthralgia
Delavirdine	Rescriptor	NNRTI	DLV	400 mg t.i.d.	Rash
Efavirenz	Sustiva	NNRTI	DMP-266	600 mg qd	Dizziness, vivid dreams, dissociation feeling
Nevirapine	Viramune	NNRTI	NVP	200 mg qd x14d, then b.i.d.	Rash

Figure 2-10 (continued) Summary of HIV Medications					
Generic Name	Trade Name	Drug Class	Abbreviation	Usual Dosage	Common Side Effects (Comments)
Amprenavir	Angenerase	PI	VX-478	1,200 mg b.i.d.	Rash, headache
Indinavir	Crixivan	PI	MK-639 IDV	800 mg q8 hr	Kidney stones, hyperbilirubinemia (take on empty stomach)
Nelfinavir	Viracept	PI	AG-1343 NFV	1,250 mg t.i.d.	Diarrhea (take with food)
Ritonavir	Norvir	PI	ABT-538 RTV	600 mg b.i.d.	Asthenia, nausea, diarrhea, vomiting, anorexia, abdominal pain, taste perversion (liquid), and circumoral and peripheral paresthesias; occasionally clients develop hepatitis; multiple important drug reactions
Saquinavir	Fortovase (soft gel capsule), Invirase (hard gel capsule)	PI	Ro3T-8959 SQV-SGC	1,200 mg t.i.d, or 1,800 mg b.i.d.	Take with meal or up to 2 hours after meal
*b.i.d., two times a day **t.i.d., three times a day					

effect of greatest concern is a hypersensitivity reaction that appears within the first 6 weeks of therapy, most commonly in the second week. Fever, nausea and vomiting, malaise, diarrhea, and sometimes rash occur. These symptoms intensify with each dose to the point of intolerability. If abacavir is discontinued because of hypersensitivity, rechallenge can result in serious, rapid, and possibly deadly recurrence of symptoms.

Nonnucleoside reverse transcriptase inhibitors

Like NRTI analogs, these drugs inhibit reverse transcriptase but by a different mechanism.

Neviripine (Viramune) acts synergistically with nucleosides but must be combined with other medications to avoid rapid development of resistance. Trials of neviripine with AZT and didanosine have been effective in lowering HIV RNA to undetectable levels for up to 1 year.

Figure 2-11
Summary of HIV Medication Schedules for NRTIs, NNRTIs, and PIs

NRTIs—must use two, along with another drug at the same time

Medication	Dosage	Common side effects
AZT, ZDV (Retrovir) Combivir is one pill containing AZT and lamivudine; it is not a different drug.	Take 2 or 3 times daily, with or without food.	May cause anemia. Some are afraid to take AZT because for many years it was used alone, but clients died anyway. In combination it can be far more effective. Do not combine with stavudine.
Stavudine (Zerit)	Take 2 times daily, with or without food.	If numbness or tingling develops in the toes, see a medical professional. Do not combine with AZT.
Lamivudine (Epivir)	Take 2 times daily, with or without food.	Active against hepatitis B. Discontinuing in the face of persistent hepatitis B can result in a flareup of hepatitis B. Do not combine with zalcitabine. Can be combined with AZT and called Combivir; can also be combined with didanosine.
Didanosine (Videx)	Take 1 or 2 times daily, *without* food.	If numbness or tingling develops in the toes, see a medical professional. If persistent abdominal pain with or without vomiting develops, see a medical professional immediately.
Zalcitabine (Hivid)	Take 3 times daily, with or without food.	If numbness or tingling develops in the toes, see a medical professional. Combines with AZT.
Abacavir (Ziagen)	Take 2 times daily.	Warning: Fatal hypersensitivity reactions have been associated with therapy with abacavir. If symptoms of hypersensitivity occur (fever, rash, fatigue, gastrointestinal upset), client should discontinue use as soon as possible. It should not be restarted following such a reaction because more severe symptoms will recur within hours and may include life-threatening hypotension and death (from Ziagen package insert).

NNRTIs—must use with at least two NRTIs

Medication	Dosage	Common side effects
Efavirenz (Sustiva)	Take once daily, with or without food.	Vivid dreams, dissociation. See medical professional if rash appears.
Nevirapine (Viramune)	Start once a day, then take 2 times daily, with or without food.	See medical professional if rash appears.
Delavirdine (Rescriptor)	Take 3 times daily, with or without food.	See medical professional if rash appears.

Figure 2-11 (continued)		
Summary of HIV Medication Schedules for NRTIs, NNRTIs, and PIs		
PIs—must use with at least two NRTIs		
Medication	**Dosage**	**Common side effects**
Ritonavir (Norvir)	Take 2 times daily, best with food.	Often causes nausea and diarrhea, may cause numbness around the mouth. Multiple important drug reactions.
Nelfinavir (Viracept)	Take 3 times daily, best with food.	Often causes nausea and diarrhea.
Indinavir (Crixivan)	Take 3 times daily, *without* food, drink plenty of water.	Often causes kidney stones, some nausea and diarrhea.
Saquinavir (Fortavase)	3 times daily, *must* take with food.	Some nausea and diarrhea.

Delavirdine (Rescriptor) acts synergistically with nucleosides and PIs. It should be used in combination with at least two other medications. The main side effect is a rash.

Efavirenz (Sustiva) also acts synergistically with nucleosides and PIs. It can be given in one daily dose and is used by many physicians as a first-line treatment for HIV. Side effects include rash and central nervous system disturbances, of which the most common is "disconnected" sensations such as confusion, abnormal thinking, impaired concentration, depersonalization, abnormal dreams, and dizziness. Other side effects include somnolence, insomnia, amnesia, hallucinations, and euphoria.

Protease inhibitors

PIs prevent the cleavage of protein precursors, which is essential for HIV maturation, infection of new cells, and replication. In clients with advanced HIV infection, a PI has led to marked improvement and prolonged survival. However, all PIs can cause increased bleeding in hemophiliacs, hyperglycemia, and new onset or worsening of diabetes.

Ritonavir is a potent HIV inhibitor, and when given to clients with advanced disease

who are being treated with nucleosides, decreases progression to death compared with placebo (8 percent versus 5 percent) (Cameron et al., 1998). Common side effects include nausea (sometimes severe), diarrhea, asthenia, circumoral and peripheral anesthesia, altered taste, renal failure, and elevation in cholesterol and triglycerides.

Indinavir is a potent PI when used with AZT (or stavudine) and lamivudine, lowering the rate of disease progression and mortality more than two nucleoside analogs alone. This triple combination effect has been durable; an early fall in plasma HIV RNA to undetectable levels can last more than 2 years. Kidney stones have been reported in 4 percent of clients, and asymptomatic elevation of indirect bilirubin occurs in about 10 percent of clients.

Nelfinavir (Viracept) is active in combination with many other nucleosides and PIs. Diarrhea has been the main side effect.

Saquinavir (Fortovase) combined with Ritonavir and a NRTI analog has been clinically effective. Diarrhea, nausea, abdominal pain, and increased aminotransferase activity can occur. The hard gel capsule is Invirase, and the soft gel capsule is Fortovase. Fortovase was introduced in November 1997 as the preferred formulation due to improved bioavailability.

Hundreds of clinical trials have confirmed the durable reduction in HIV RNA levels using three-drug combinations. Although the number of medication combinations is growing and new plans for initial and second-line therapies continue to evolve, client compliance remains a major concern. In addition to developing simple regimens, it is appropriate for the clinician to choose antiretrovirals at least in part on the basis of their side effects. For example, in clients with preexisting pancreatitis, didanosine should be used with extreme caution. For those with neuropathy, didanosine, zalcitabine, and stavudine should be used with caution.

Altered body fat distribution occurs commonly in persons with HIV on long-term antiretroviral therapy. Once thought to be seen only in PI users, changes in body dimensions—including increase in abdominal girth and breast size and wasting of leg muscles—have been noted in many patients independent of PI use and may be especially common in those who are on NNRTIs. The underlying mechanism for these troubling symptoms remains unclear, and an effective therapy is elusive (Gervasoni et al., 1999).

Changing antiretroviral therapy

Criteria for changing therapy include (1) suboptimal initial reduction in HIV RNA level, (2) reappearance of viremia after suppression to undetectable levels, (3) persistent and progressive decline in CD4+ T cells, (4) development of intolerable side effects, or (5) inability to remain adherent. In all cases, the clinician must determine whether the treatment failure is caused by imperfect adherence (due to toxicity, lack of resources, or client's lack of understanding), altered absorption or metabolism of one or more drugs in a combination, multidrug pharmacokinetics, or viral resistance to one or more agents. When the decision to change therapy is based on HIV

RNA, a second viral load test is needed before the decision is made.

In general, it is preferable to change all the drugs used in the failing combination, except in those instances when viral loads are undetectable and a side effect can be traced to a specific medication. In some cases where the viral load is not suppressed completely, it may be best to continue the present regimen because it has been partially effective and the client's options are limited. If the initial combination therapy was effective but the client later developed detectable viral loads, second-line (salvage) combinations are less likely to be effective.

Clients temporarily discontinue antiretroviral therapy for many reasons (Singh et al., 1996). However, there are no studies estimating the number of doses, days, or weeks missed that would increase the likelihood of drug resistance. If clients must discontinue any antiretroviral medication for an extended time, stopping all their medications simultaneously may minimize the chance of developing resistant viral strains.

Combination therapy commonly requires the client to take large numbers of pills, up to 20 per day. Arranging schedules to take medication with or away from meals, timing doses, having access to refrigeration, and keeping adequately hydrated can be a full-time job. This may be difficult for clients who are homeless, currently using drugs, relapsing, and so on, and these issues must be assessed prior to changing regimens.

Resistance to antiretroviral agents

Drug resistance remains an obstacle to achieving the full benefits of antiretroviral agents. HIV's rapid replication rate fuels continual production of HIV variants (mutations) that thrive under the selective pressure of antiretroviral therapy. Combination therapy that suppresses HIV replication can delay the emergence of drug-resistant virus. However, a viral load below the limit of detection does not always mean that viral replication has completely halted, particularly in areas such as lymph nodes. Assays to measure whether HIV can grow despite the presence of a specific medication (resistance assays) are now available, but their application remains to be established.

Pharmacologic Interactions

HIV infection does not change the need for medications to treat substance abuse. The most common medications used to treat substance abuse are methadone, disulfiram (Antabuse), buprenorphine (Buprenex), and naltrexone (ReVia). In addition, benzodiazepines, barbiturates, clonidine hydrochloride, and other medications commonly are used in detoxification. These medications can be used by HIV-infected substance abusers in the same way they are used by uninfected clients. Neither maintenance nor detoxification treatment need be altered by the presence of HIV infection.

Interactions with methadone

The best-documented interaction between substance abuse medication and HIV infection medication is that of methadone with rifampin (Rifadin), a drug used to treat TB or, less commonly, MAC (Kreek et al., 1976). Rifampin causes a faster breakdown of methadone in the liver and a faster decrease in plasma methadone level. This results in rapid onset of classic opioid withdrawal symptoms, usually within several days of taking rifampin. Increasing clients' daily methadone doses will prevent this outcome. Typically, the dosage is increased by 10 mg every 1 to 2 days, beginning on the day rifampin is started and increasing as needed to prevent symptoms of opioid withdrawal, titrated to prevent this oversedation. It often is necessary to continue this pattern until the dosage is at least 50 percent greater than the original daily dose. It is important for the client or the physician to inform the methadone program of changes in the client's medication.

Rifabutin (Mycobutin) is a medication structurally related to rifampin and frequently used for prophylaxis and treatment of MAC in HIV-infected clients. Rifabutin may have a pharmacologic interaction with opioids similar to that of rifampin.

Phenytoin (Dilantin) and phenobarbital (Phenob) have a similar but less dramatic effect on plasma methadone levels, causing opioid withdrawal symptoms over a period of days to weeks. It may be necessary to increase methadone dosage, but usually this increase does not have to be as great or as rapid as for rifampin. Other interactions are in Figure 2-12.

When therapy with rifampin or phenytoin is discontinued, methadone doses should, in most cases, gradually be lowered to avoid oversedation. Clients usually arrive at a final stable dose that is higher than the original dosage level before the other medications were introduced (Selwyn and O'Connor, 1992).

Interactions with antiretroviral agents

No clinically significant interactions have been found between AZT and either methadone or disulfiram. One study suggested, however, that elimination of AZT may be slower in methadone-maintained clients compared with a control group not receiving methadone. However, this study found no evidence that clinical toxicity from AZT was worse in the methadone-maintained group (Schwartz et al., 1990).

Only a few studies have investigated the interactions of other antiretrovirals with methadone. Early laboratory studies showed that ritonavir and indinavir may increase methadone levels; nevirapine may decrease methadone levels, and saquinavir has no effect.

Figure 2-12
Methadone Interactions With HIV Medications

Significantly Reduces Methadone Levels
- Rifampin
- Dilantin
- Phenobarbital

Reduces Methadone Levels
- Carbamazepine
- Ritonavir
- Rifampin
- Neviripine
- Efavirenz

May Raise Methadone Levels
- Alcohol
- Delavirdine
- Fluconazole

May Affect Methadone Levels
- Nelfinavir

No Significant Effect on Methadone Levels
- Clarithromycin/Azithromycin
- Didanosine
- Lamivudine
- Saquinavir
- Stavudine
- Trimethoprim/Sulfamethoxazole
- Zalcitabine
- AZT

Source: Gourevitch and Friedland, 1999a.

However, only one study has been reported using client plasma levels; here, ritonavir decreased methadone levels by 35 percent, the opposite of what was expected from laboratory studies. Two case reports of nelfinavir decreasing methadone levels have been documented. Further work on drug interactions is needed because in vitro data may not accurately predict in vivo results. If drowsiness or other symptoms associated with methadone excess are reported, clinicians might consider lowering methadone dose using trough methadone blood levels to guide treatment. Similarly, trough levels can be used to establish whether withdrawal symptoms are due to increased methadone metabolism (Gourevitch and Friedland, 1999a).

Pain Management

Managing acute and chronic pain in HIV-infected, substance-abusing clients can be a challenging clinical problem (Selwyn and O'Connor, 1992). Although providers may have well-founded concerns about potential drug-seeking behavior, these concerns may interfere with clinical judgment about the appropriateness of using narcotic analgesics. Like other clients, substance abusers often are undertreated for acute pain. Medication for pain control, including narcotics, should never be withheld merely because a client has a history of substance abuse.

As with all clients in pain, the provider's primary goal is to maximize comfort while minimizing side effects. Local measures (rest, heat, ice, analgesic rubs) should be used as a first line of pain treatment where appropriate. If these measures fail to adequately relieve the pain, a systematic pharmacologic approach is recommended. Initially, over-the-counter medications such as aspirin, acetaminophen (Tylenol), and nonsteroidal anti-inflammatory agents should be used, with dosages increased as needed. Caution must be used in employing acetaminophen in clients with liver diseases such as hepatitis C, as it can worsen liver disease.

If these medications prove inadequate for pain relief, narcotic analgesia may be necessary. Because of their tolerance for narcotics, clients with opiate use disorders generally require higher doses of narcotic analgesia and more frequent dosing intervals for effective pain control. This is especially true for clients maintained on methadone. See also the section below, "Use of Unapproved Medications or Alternative Therapies."

Agents used for persistent neuropathic pain include anticonvulsants (phenytoin, carbamazepine [Tegretal], gabapentin [Neurontin]), tricyclic antidepressants (amitriptyline [Elavil], desipramine [Norpramin]), or topical agents (capsaicin [Capzasin]). These agents may be used alone or in combination with other analgesics. Acupuncture may be particularly helpful in some cases of neuropathic pain.

The treatment plan and the reason for using narcotics for pain control must be clear to both provider and patient. It is important not only that the patient know that her pain is taken seriously but also that narcotic use will not be extended beyond a time-limited period required for analgesia. Late-stage clients with AIDS who have chronic, severe pain syndromes may require long-term analgesia. Attempting to manage pain in methadone-maintained clients by increasing their daily dose of methadone is a common error. Instead, if narcotic analgesics are indicated, providers should continue the client's usual methadone dose and add a shorter acting narcotic for acute pain control. Pentazocine (Talwin) and other mixed opiate agonist–antagonists should not be used for analgesia in methadone-maintained clients because they may precipitate withdrawal.

Chronic pain management in substance abuse disorder clients is most effective if there is close primary care followup and coordination of a treatment plan with substance abuse treatment professionals. Pain management specialists should be consulted as needed to examine alternative management strategies (Selwyn and O'Connor, 1992).

Interventions

Currently, no validated protocol for HIV/AIDS pain therapy exists. Because clients with HIV/AIDS often have pain problems similar to clients with cancer, the World Health Organization's (WHO's) "cancer pain analgesic ladder" is a useful starting point for managing pain in HIV-infected persons.

1. The first step of the WHO treatment ladder is to use acetaminophen (Tylenol) or a nonsteroidal anti-inflammatory drug (NSAID) (e.g., ibuprofen, naprosyn). Long-term use of NSAIDs is not recommended because of gastrointestinal and renal side effects and toxicities. Caution should be employed when using acetaminophen in clients with liver disease.

2. Step two of the ladder adds a "weak opioid" such as codeine, oxycodone, hydrocodone, or dextropropoxyphene to acetominophen or an NSAID. This regimen is useful for mild to moderate pain.

3. The third step is to add an adjuvant (drugs that may either enhance the effect of the opiate or have independent pain-relieving activity). Examples of adjuvants include corticosteroids, antidepressants, anticonvulsants, and antihistamines.

4. Step four should be used for clients with severe pain intensity. At this stage, clinicians recommend the use of a strong opioid like morphine, fentanyl/duragesic patches, hydromorphone, or methadone. Medication dosages should be individually titrated and scheduled around the clock with extra doses provided for "breakthrough" pain.

Additional points are as follows:

■ In any setting, the quality of pain control is influenced by the training, expertise, and experience of clinicians.

■ Always treat the underlying cause of the pain. Treating the cause of pain (infection, tumor, etc.) is the single best method of pain relief.

■ Decisionmaking about pain control should include the input and preferences of the client and family.

- When initiating pain treatment, the least invasive route for medication administration should be selected first. This is usually the oral route, unless contraindicated for some reason.
- Continually evaluate the response to the regimen or plan. Change the drug, schedule, dose, and route; prevent and treat side effects of the pain medication as often as needed.
- Establish clear directions about whom the client or caregiver should notify in case of problems.
- Pain management should be reevaluated at points of transition in the provision of services (i.e., from hospital to home) to ensure that optimal pain management is achieved and maintained.
- Effective pain management requires collaboration across disciplines and among clinicians.
- Effective pain relief should be accomplished by developing a regimen or plan that *prevents* pain.
- Do not interrupt HIV treatment as a deliberate consequence of methadone maintenance disruptions (i.e., do not hold antiretroviral treatment "hostage").

Special Considerations for Substance-Abusing Clients

When opioids are required for pain control, the dual diagnosis of HIV/AIDS and a substance abuse disorder produces a challenge for even the most experienced clinician. Specific principles, listed below, must be followed to ensure fair assessment of the pain complaint (e.g., clients may fabricate pain to obtain drugs) and to provide the best chance of achieving satisfactory pain relief (Portenoy and Payne, 1992).

- When developing a pain treatment plan, distinctions must be made among (1) clients who are actively using illicit opioids and receiving treatment for pain, (2) former drug abusers who no longer use drugs, and (3) clients in methadone maintenance (Fultz and Senay, 1975).
- Clients actively abusing heroin or prescription opioids and those on methadone maintenance should be assumed to have some degree of drug tolerance, which necessitates higher starting doses and more frequent dosing intervals of pain medication than in the nonaddicted client.
- Choose a medication route and formulation that are less likely to be diverted or abused (e.g., controlled-release oral or transdermal [patch] drug).
- Set firm limits on the ability of the client to negotiate for escalating doses of opioid.
- Use adjuvant medications to enhance opioid analgesia.
- Acting out and noncompliance are frequent responses to poor pain management.
- Clients who are actively abusing drugs often manifest psychological disorders that influence pain perception (depression, anxiety), requiring concomitant treatment.
- In clients who have abused drugs in the past or for those on methadone maintenance programs, the combined stress of HIV/AIDS and pain may manifest itself in the reappearance of substance abuse behaviors.
- Nonopioid analgesics should never be substituted for opioid analgesics to treat severe pain in the suspected or known substance abuser.

Reducing Risk of Medication Abuse

Setting clear limits and devising a consistent treatment plan help reduce the risk of medication abuse by substance-abusing clients. The following strategies are recommended:

- Designate one care provider to dispense prescriptions for controlled drugs.
- Dispense limited amounts of controlled drugs (e.g., 1 week's supply or less).

- Advise clients that lost or stolen prescriptions will not be replaced (see also "Abuse of Psychiatric Medications" in Chapter 3).

Informal verbal "contracting" with patients about the need to discuss symptoms openly and not seek prescriptions from multiple providers should occur once trust in the primary care relationship is established. Discussing the risks of serious drug interactions may allow patients to understand provider concerns.

Abuse of intravenous infusion lines

Clients symptomatic with AIDS are frequently prescribed narcotic analgesics and may even have an indwelling intravenous line for infusion therapy. Injection drug users are at very high risk of using this indwelling intravenous line to administer heroin, cocaine, and other drugs of abuse. It is therefore essential that clients with such lines who are at risk for misuse be cared for in residential health care settings, including hospice-based home care, where adequate monitoring and support can be provided.

Clinical Trials Enrollment

Good physician–client relationships can foster client participation in clinical trials. Ongoing efforts are needed to educate clients and their families about the importance of clinical trials and to alleviate any suspicion of the medical profession. Clinicians should be aware that HIV-infected substance abusers in abstinence-based treatment programs may be reluctant to participate in clinical trials of unapproved medications because such participation reminds them of taking illicit drugs. Also, recovering substance abusers in abstinence-based treatment programs may not want to take drugs of any kind.

Specific efforts should be made to incorporate more clients with substance abuse disorders, women, and minorities into HIV clinical trials. All of these groups currently are underrepresented.

To avoid conflicts of interest, it is recommended that the clinician responsible for the clinical trial not be the client's primary care provider, if possible. When a client enters a trial, followup mechanisms for results must be in place so that this information is available to substance abuse treatment staff.

Use of Unapproved Medications And Alternative Therapies

In the face of life-threatening, chronic illness, when a cure is not available, many clients will seek unapproved medications or alternative therapies. Care providers must be aware that HIV-infected clients may be using alternative or complementary therapies, for example, acupuncture, meditation, and vitamin and herbal dietary supplements. According to one study of clients with HIV in Boston (Fairfield et al., 1998), these clients used alternative therapies at a high rate; they frequently visited alternative therapy providers, incurred substantial expenditures, and reported improvement with these treatments.

Unless a therapy is known to be harmful, however, clients need not be discouraged from trying it. Clinicians have a responsibility to find out, in a nonjudgmental manner, what alternative or unapproved therapies clients are using and then to obtain as much information as possible about these therapies. This information should be shared with clients, emphasizing that the risks and benefits of these therapies cannot always be predicted. Certain alternative therapies (e.g., acupuncture, meditation, herbal teas) may actually help to decrease clients' reliance on or need for controlled substances, narcotic analgesics, sleeping medication, and so forth.

Unsupervised antibiotic use can complicate the diagnosis and treatment of bacterial infections in HIV-infected substance abuse disorder clients. Clinicians should specifically ask clients about unsupervised antibiotic use because clients may not consider the information relevant to their medication or drug use histories (Selwyn and O'Connor, 1992).

Prophylaxis Against Opportunistic Infections

Current strategies for HIV/AIDS care include the use of prophylactic regimens to help prevent specific opportunistic infections. As clients survive for longer periods with lower CD4+ T cell counts, it is important to develop additional prophylactic regimens for infections that occur at more advanced stages of HIV (Figure 2-13). A recent review summarizes current practice regarding prophylaxis of opportunistic infections in HIV-infected clients (CDC, 1997c).

Because of the range of medications that an HIV/AIDS patient may take, another critical strategy for HIV/AIDS care is to designate someone (other than the physician) as a medication "case manager." This person would communicate with all the specialists a patient is seeing and monitor all the drugs prescribed so that no harm is done to the patient.

Pneumocystis Carinii Pneumonia

Pneumocystis carinii pneumonia (PCP) was the first opportunistic infection for which prophylactic regimens were developed. Since the late 1980s, widespread use of PCP prophylaxis has resulted in a dramatic decrease in incidence of this opportunistic infection. However, despite the availability of effective prophylaxis, PCP is still the most common opportunistic infection; many clients who develop PCP are unaware of their HIV status and hence are not receiving prophylaxis.

The risk of PCP increases significantly when a client's CD4+ T cell count drops to around 200.

It is recommended that all clients with CD4+ T cell counts of 200 or below receive ongoing PCP prophylaxis. Because of their high risk of progressing to AIDS, HIV-infected clients with histories of oral candidiasis or other AIDS-defining infections should be offered PCP prophylaxis regardless of their CD4+ T cell levels. This includes clients who have had PCP before because there is a high rate of recurrence of PCP (more than 30 percent within 1 year).

Trimethoprim-sulfamethoxazole (TMP-SMX) (Bactrim DS, Septra) is the most effective anti-PCP medication (Bozzette et al., 1995). A single daily dose of one double-strength tablet is most commonly prescribed, although thrice-weekly dosing may be adequate. A daily single-strength tablet may also be effective and may improve adherence.

Clients who comply with this prophylactic regimen have only a 5-percent chance of developing PCP. Additionally, clients taking TMP-SMX for PCP prophylaxis may also decrease their chances of contracting cerebral toxoplasmosis and pyogenic bacterial infections. This may be especially important for HIV-infected substance abusers who are at high risk for sinusitis, bacterial pneumonia, and endocarditis.

For clients who cannot tolerate TMP-SMX, dapsone is a reasonable alternative. Dapsone, however, can cause hemolytic anemia in clients who are deficient in the enzyme glucose 6-phosphate dehydrogenase (G6PD), especially people of African descent. Therefore, clients must be screened for this deficiency before beginning therapy. The minimal effective dose of dapsone is unknown; regimens of 50 mg per day, 100 mg per day, and 100 mg three times per week are common.

Aerosolized pentamidine, in a single dose of 300 mg per month, is another option for PCP prophylaxis. The advantages of aerosolized pentamidine are that it has little, if any, systemic

Figure 2-13
Prophylactic Regimens

Pneumocystis carinii pneumonia (PCP)

Indications. All clients with CD4+ T cell counts of 200 or below; all clients with oral candidiasis, recurrent bacterial infections, TB, and chronic constitutional symptoms; and all clients with a history of PCP, regardless of CD4+ T cell count, should receive PCP prophylaxis.

Dosage. TMP-SMX is the most effective prophylactic agent. One double-strength tablet daily (160 mg TMP + 800 mg SMX) is commonly prescribed. One double-strength tablet 3 times weekly is also acceptable; however, daily dosing may promote adherence. One single-strength tablet daily (80 mg TMP + 400 mg SMX) may also be effective. Dapsone (50 mg per day, 100 mg per day, 100 mg 3 times weekly) is an alternative for clients who cannot tolerate TMP-SMX. Aerosolized pentamidine (NebuPent), 1 x 300 mg monthly by nebulizer, is an option in settings with adequate ventilation.

Side effects. TMP-SMX: rash, leukopenia, nausea/vomiting, liver function abnormalities, fever. Side effects are usually dose related. HIV+ clients should be monitored for sulfonamide allergy because they have a high incidence of allergic and/or other reactions to this class of drug. Dapsone: rash, nausea/vomiting, anemia. Aerosolized pentamidine: cough, bronchospasm, metallic taste. Desensitization and rechallenge protocols for TMP-SMX.

Complications. TMP-SMX: Stevens-Johnson syndrome, mucous membrane ulceration, hepatitis, serum sickness (infrequent). Dapsone: hemolytic anemia in G6PD-deficient clients. Peripheral neuropathy or other nervous system effects (infrequent). Pentamidine: Breakthrough PCP, extrapulmonary pneumocystosis.

Management of pregnant clients. Same indications as for clients who are not pregnant. TMP-SMX should be given until 36 weeks' gestation, then give aerosolized pentamidine to prevent neonatal exposure to sulfonamides.

Toxoplasmosis

Indications. Positive antitoxoplasma antibody test, especially for clients with CD4+ T cell counts < 100 and/or a history of HIV symptomatic disease.

Dosage. TMP-SMX (see "PCP Prophylaxis," above) has been suggested by several studies to offer protection against toxoplasmosis. Dapsone (100 mg 3 times weekly) plus pyrimethamine (Daraprim) (50 mg 1 time weekly) is an alternative for clients who cannot tolerate TMP-SMX.

Side Effects. TMP-SMX: See "PCP Prophylaxis," above. Pyrimethamine: Rash and anemia or leukopenia are possible but unlikely at 50 mg/week dose.

Mycobacterium avium complex (MAC)

Indications. Clients most at risk are those with late-stage HIV disease (CD4+ T cell count < 50).

Dosage. Azithromycin 1,200 mg weekly or clarithromycin 500 mg twice daily. Rifabutin is approved for prophylaxis; 300 mg daily has been shown to be effective. Rifabutin for MAC prophylaxis is contraindicated in clients with active TB; exclude active TB before initiating therapy. Rifabutin has multiple potential drug interactions.

Side Effects. Nausea/vomiting, gastrointestinal distress, rash, brown-orange discoloration of urine (rifabutin only). Rifabutin may interact adversely with other HIV medications (fluconazole, clarithromycin) and may accelerate methadone and other opioid metabolism.

| **Figure 2-13 (continued)** |
| **Prophylactic Regimens** |

Cryptococcosis
Indications. Infrequent complication of HIV infection.
Dosage. Fluconazole may have a prophylactic effect, but routine prophylaxis could promote the development of resistant fungi (e.g., candida species).

Herpes simplex virus (HSV)
Indications. Recurrent HSV infection (most common in the genital area). Likelihood of recurrence increases with declining CD4+ T cell count. No strict threshold for initiation of prophylaxis.
Dosage. VAL Acyclovir (Zovirax) 500 mg two or three times a day

toxicity, and it may be the only medication a client can tolerate. However, it is clearly inferior to TMP-SMX for persons with CD4+ T cell counts below 50. Secondary breakthrough rates of PCP in clients on pentamidine may exceed 15 percent a year. In addition, extrapulmonary pneumocystosis, where clients show evidence of PCP infection outside the lung, has been seen. These manifestations occur more commonly in clients receiving only inhaled pentamidine rather than systemic prophylaxis with TMP-SMX or dapsone.

Pentamidine should be administered only in settings with adequate ventilation that are consistent with CDC standards. Not only can pentamidine administration produce bronchospasm and cough, but the coughing has been associated with transmission of TB in inadequately ventilated settings. Some substance abuse treatment programs offering onsite aerosolized pentamidine use specially designed sputum induction and pentamidine administration booths equipped with strong exhaust systems and high-efficiency particulate air filters to decrease the risk of contamination.

Side effects

TMP-SMX is well tolerated, with a low incidence of side effects. However, clients with HIV infection have a higher risk of allergy to sulfonamides than other client populations and must be monitored for adverse effects. Possible side effects, which tend to be dose related, include fever, rash, leukopenia, anemia, nausea, and vomiting. Serious reactions such as Stevens-Johnson syndrome, mucous membrane ulceration, hepatitis, and serum sickness are unlikely but potentially serious.

Clients on dapsone may experience rash, gastrointestinal upset, and anemia. Less common side effects include mental state changes and peripheral neuropathy. Sulfa allergy is generally not a contraindication to dapsone. Many clients who have developed rashes on TMP-SMX are able to tolerate dapsone without adverse effects; however, they should be monitored as part of routine followup.

Prophylaxis during pregnancy

The current standard of care is to offer a pregnant woman PCP prophylaxis if she would be so treated if not pregnant (e.g., CD4+ T cell count less than 200, or preexisting HIV-related disease). Although the possible risks or benefits to the fetus are uncertain, it has become standard to use TMP-SMX until 36 weeks of gestation and then change to aerosolized pentamidine to prevent neonatal exposure to sulfonamides (which can cause jaundice in the newborn).

Toxoplasmosis

Cerebral toxoplasmosis, another common opportunistic infection in clients with AIDS, occurs most frequently in people who previously had a positive antitoxoplasma antibody test. Serologic testing for toxoplasma antibody is recommended as part of the basic primary care approach to HIV infection, in order to detect clients at high risk for this opportunistic infection.

For clients with CD4+ T cell counts below 100, a positive antitoxoplasma antibody test is reason to consider toxoplasmosis prophylaxis. TMP-SMX also offers protection against the development of toxoplasmosis, but for clients who cannot tolerate TMP-SMX it has been suggested that dapsone plus pyrimethamine may provide effective prophylaxis against toxoplasmosis as well as PCP. Practitioners may also want to remind clients who own cats that changing cat litter without gloves and a mask may put them at higher risk for toxoplasmosis. Clients with a history of toxoplasmic encephalitis and other diseases from toxoplasmosis are maintained on chronic suppressive therapy with sulfadiazine (Sulfadine) and pyrimethamine plus folinic acid.

Mycobacterium Avium Complex

Clients with AIDS also are at risk for infection with atypical mycobacteria, especially MAC. This is a late-stage complication of HIV disease that generally occurs in its disseminated form (e.g., in the blood) only in clients with CD4+ T cell counts less than 50. As clients survive longer with low CD4+ T cell counts, prevention and treatment of this common complication will be increasingly important. Started at CD4+ T cell counts of 75 to 100, there are three options for prophylaxis against MAC. The macrolide antibiotics, clarithromycin (Biaxin) (500–1,000 mg daily) and azithromycin (Zithromax) (1,200 mg once a week), are effective. The rifampin-like drug rifabutin also is approved for prophylaxis (300 mg daily). Rifabutin, like rifampin, causes accelerated metabolism of methadone; as a result, caution should be

exercised in prescribing rifabutin to methadone-maintained clients. Rifabutin may also interact with other HIV medications. For a list of methadone interactions with HIV medications, see Figure 2-12.

Because of the potential for adverse drug interactions and the overload of daily pills for clients with low CD4+ T cell counts, some clinicians opt to wait until the CD4+ T cell count drops to 50 before initiating prophylaxis for MAC, and others do not use prophylaxis at all. Because MAC generally responds well to treatment (although treatment usually requires two medications), prophylaxis options should be discussed.

Cryptococcosis

Cryptococcal meningitis is a relatively infrequent complication of HIV infection, but it is one of the more common AIDS-defining opportunistic infections of the CNS. Treatment of cryptococcal meningitis has been greatly aided by the introduction of new systemic triazole antifungal medications such as fluconazole and itraconazole (Sporanox). These agents have made it possible to shorten the initial course of intravenous therapy with amphotericin B for cryptococcosis and certain other systemic fungal infections (e.g., histoplasmosis) and have allowed chronic suppressive therapy with oral agents that do not require chronic intravenous administration.

Because cryptococcosis is not a common infection (occurring in fewer than 10 percent of clients with AIDS), routine prophylaxis is not cost-effective. However, intermittent prescription of triazoles for the more common oral candidiasis may unintentionally be leading to the decrease in cryptococcal disease.

Routine prophylaxis of cryptococcosis carries a risk of promoting development of resistant organisms, including resistant *candida* and other fungal species. In addition, in parts of the country where histoplasmosis and coccidioidomycosis are more common fungal complications of AIDS, the use of fluconazole has not been associated with decreased risk of occurrence of these infections.

Herpes Simplex Virus

HIV-infected clients with herpes simplex virus (HSV) may be prone to recurrent genital HSV infection, and those symptomatic with AIDS may develop widespread cutaneous disease. There is no strict threshold for initiation of prophylaxis. Clients may receive chronic prophylaxis with acyclovir (Zovirax) (generally from 1,000 to 1,500 mg daily in two or three doses) or famciclovir (Famvir) (500 mg twice daily) as might be given to clients without HIV infection. The likelihood of recurrent HSV infection increases with a declining CD4+ T cell count. Acyclovir, taken together with antiretroviral therapy, may benefit late-stage AIDS clients (Stein et al., 1994; Youle et al., 1994), although this remains controversial.

Cytomegalovirus

There has been much interest in potential prophylactic agents against cytomegalovirus (CMV), which, like MAC, has been increasingly common in clients surviving for longer periods of time at low CD4+ T cell counts. CMV most commonly causes retinitis, which can lead to blindness if untreated, and may also cause neurologic, gastrointestinal, adrenal, pulmonary, and other systemic diseases.

An oral form of ganciclovir (Cytovene), used as a prophylactic, may reduce CMV incidence although data on its effectiveness are conflicting. This medication has low serum levels that may promote CMV resistance; it has many side effects, requires careful monitoring, and requires the client to take many pills. In addition, initial retinitis is rarely sight-threatening; therefore, primary prophylaxis is not widely recommended. Currently, the treatment options for active CMV are intravenous ganciclovir, foscarnet (Foscavir), cidofovir (Vistide), or intraocular formivirisen.

Bacterial Infections

Researchers noted the presence of bacterial pneumonia and sepsis in injection drug users before the HIV/AIDS pandemic, but they occur more frequently in HIV-infected substance abusers. Bacterial pneumonia in this population is most often caused by *Streptococcus* pneumonia and *Haemophilus influenzae*. Both bacterial pneumonia and related bacteremia tend to occur in the earlier stages of HIV and can be predictors of subsequent HIV-related illness in previously asymptomatic clients. Drug smoking and cigarette smoking may account for at least some of the increased risk. Persons with HIV develop invasive pneumococcal disease at a rate of 150 to 300 times higher than uninfected persons.

Bacterial endocarditis is a well-recognized complication of IDU. Several studies have suggested that HIV infection may aggravate the frequency and severity of endocarditis, and others have shown a similar endocarditis course in HIV-positive and HIV-negative drug abusers (Nahass et al., 1990). Active injection drug users also are at risk for a variety of serious bacterial infections involving the skin, soft tissues, bones, joints, central and peripheral nervous systems, and other anatomical sites. Proper needle hygiene and skin disinfection before drug injection may help prevent some of these complications.

Sexually Transmitted Diseases

STDs are common in substance abusers, especially crack cocaine abusers. Women and men involved in commercial sex work or the exchange of sex for drugs have particularly high rates of STDs.

Baseline assessment should include taking the client's history of STDs and any involvement in sex-for-sale or sex-for-drugs transactions. Inspection for genital and perianal lesions should be part of the baseline physical examination. Serologic testing for syphilis, including both treponemal and nontreponemal tests (e.g., Venereal Disease Research Laboratory and fluorescent treponemal antibody-absorption, should be included in the initial laboratory testing screen.

Female substance abusers should be offered a complete pelvic examination and testing for gonorrhea, chlamydia, and HSV as well as the more common bacterial vaginosis, trichomonas, and candidiasis. (See section on women's health issues below.) Women should also have Pap smears at least annually because of the risk of cervical cancer.

Syphilis

HIV-infected clients with primary and secondary syphilis should receive three weekly doses of benzathine penicillin or treatment with supplemental antibiotics (e.g., amoxicillin or ampicillin with or without probenecid) in some cases.

While lumbar puncture and cerebrospinal fluid (CSF) examination would be required to formally rule out neurosyphilis in persons with latent syphilis, a more practical plan for treatment of an HIV-infected substance abuse population is as follows:

- Treat all latent-syphilis HIV-infected clients.
- Reserve lumbar puncture and CSF examination for clients with neurological complications or whose followup serologic tests do not indicate a clear response to antibiotic therapy.
- Have a low threshold to refer clients for further diagnostic workup or treatment as indicated.

Hepatitis

Evidence of infection with HBV and hepatitis C virus (HCV) has been found in more than two thirds of long-term injection drug users (Esteban et al., 1989; Stimmel et al., 1975). Chronic

substance abusers are also at increased risk for infection with hepatitis A virus (HAV) and hepatitis delta virus (HDV), which coexists with HBV. Concurrent alcohol use may also cause liver-function abnormalities, thus complicating clinical diagnoses. Because many commonly used HIV medications—including TMP-SMX, pentamidine, dapsone, rifampin, and ritonavir—may cause liver toxicity, liver function tests are required.

There is no consistent evidence that coexisting chronic HBV infection adversely affects the course of HIV disease or, conversely, that HIV disease adversely affects coexisting HBV infection. However, individuals who are coinfected with HIV and HBV may have higher blood levels of HBV than individuals who are not HIV infected. Consequently, these coinfected individuals may be at higher risk of transmitting HBV infection. HIV does seem to accelerate the course of HCV infection, leading to more rapid progression to cirrhosis (Soto et al., 1997).

Drugs used in treating HIV and its complications affect HBV (lamivudine, famciclovir, interferon-alpha) and HCV (interferon). Ribavirin, which is used in the treatment of HCV, should not be used with AZT. Flares of HCV have been reported with initiation of potent antiretroviral therapy. Rebound of HBV can occur in clients with HBV when they stop taking lamivudine.

Nervous System Disease

Clinicians caring for HIV-infected clients must frequently assess clients for altered mental state and other neurologic and neuropsychiatric syndromes. Differential diagnosis in such clients may include HIV-related dementia or encephalopathy, specific opportunistic infections affecting the CNS, metabolic or toxic encephalopathy, and the effects of substance abuse (see also Chapter 3).

In HIV-infected clients, underlying neurologic conditions associated with substance abuse can obscure or complicate diagnosis of the varied causes of peripheral nervous system disease.

HTLV-I and HTLV-II

These retroviruses are "cousins" of HIV. Human T-lymphotropic retrovirus type 1 (HTLV-I) has been associated with adult T-cell leukemia/lymphoma and with certain chronic degenerative neurologic diseases. Human T-lymphotropic retrovirus type 2 (HTLV-II) is less clearly associated with specific disease outcomes.

In the United States, infection with HTLV-I and HTLV-II is concentrated among injection drug users. Seroprevalence studies in the mid-1980s found that more than one-third of substance abusers in selected groups sampled in the New York City metropolitan area and in the southeastern United States were infected with HTLV-I or HTLV-II.

In at least one study, HTLV-II coinfection was associated with rapid progression of HIV disease in substance abusers infected with both viruses (Page et al., 1990). Clinicians caring for HIV-infected substance abusers should suspect coexisting HTLV-I or HTLV-II infection and consider serologic testing in clients with degenerative neurologic disease, T-cell leukemias, or rapidly progressing HIV disease.

Malignancies

Three types of cancer—Kaposi's sarcoma, malignant lymphoma, and invasive cervical cancer—are considered AIDS-defining conditions under the classification system for HIV infection and AIDS established by the CDC in 1993 (see Appendix C). HIV-infected substance abusers are at relatively low risk for Kaposi's sarcoma; however, malignant lymphomas have been documented in this population. Persistent generalized lymphadenopathy is common in HIV-infected clients, and palpable lymphadenopathy is common in injection drug users, particularly those who continue to inject drugs. Nevertheless, the presence of large (greater than 2 cm), firm, tender, or rapidly growing lymph nodes in an HIV-infected injection drug user should always prompt further diagnostic evaluation. The women's issues section in this chapter provides discussion of cervical cancer. In addition to these AIDS-defining cancers, other malignancies have been found to occur with greater frequency in HIV-infected substance abusers. These non–AIDS-defining cancers (reported in several case studies and one population-based study) include solid tumors of the lung, head and neck, and gastrointestinal tract, of which lung tumors are the most common (O'Connor et al., 1994b).

Immunizations

The CDC recommends that HIV infection be considered an indication for pneumococcal vaccination because of the markedly increased risk of pneumococcal pneumonia among HIV-infected clients. The effectiveness of this vaccine in clients with severely weakened immune systems is questionable, but it has been found to provide moderate immunity when given in the earlier stages of HIV infection.

Vaccination against *H. influenzae* type B should also be considered because HIV-infected individuals, particularly injection drug users, are at increased risk for *H. influenzae* pneumonia.

Vaccination for viral influenza is potentially useful for two reasons:

1. HIV-infected clients are known to be at increased risk of pulmonary infection with bacteria that commonly complicate influenza.
2. Because symptoms of influenza may mimic those of opportunistic infections, minimizing the incidence of influenza may

prevent unnecessary diagnostic evaluations for other HIV-related conditions.

The CDC also recommends that all HIV-infected individuals and the health care workers who provide their care should receive the hepatitis B vaccine. Clients with HIV infection, if they have not already been exposed to HBV, are at high risk of acquiring it and are more likely than non–HIV-infected individuals to become chronic HBV carriers. Furthermore, HIV-infected HBV carriers may be more infectious because they are likely to have higher blood levels of HBV (see information under "Laboratory Tests"). A complete HBV serologic profile should be part of the baseline assessment of all substance abusers with or at risk for HIV infection, and clients who are negative for HBV antibody markers should be considered eligible for HBV vaccine.

All the vaccines mentioned above are more effective when administered early in the course of HIV infection. The benefits outweigh the risks, and there is little evidence that these vaccines are harmful to HIV-infected clients.

Other immunizations

Few data exist on the safety or effectiveness of vaccinating HIV-infected adults for diphtheria, tetanus, mumps, rubella, polio, and measles. Inactivated polio, diphtheria, and tetanus

vaccines are likely to be safe. Because these infections may cause illness in clients with suppressed immune systems, vaccination appears warranted according to standard guidelines for their use in non–HIV-infected adults.

Vaccination with the live, attenuated mumps, rubella, and measles vaccines may pose a greater risk to HIV-infected persons, and the benefit is less certain. However, these vaccines are used routinely in HIV-infected children whose immune systems are not suppressed, and in recent years the measles vaccine has been safely given to HIV-infected adults during local measles epidemics (see Figure 2-14).

Women's Health Issues

Primary care providers should be aware that, in general, the incidence of gynecological disorders is likely to be higher among female substance abusers than among non–substance-abusing women (DeHovitz et al., 1994; Millstein and Moscicki, 1995). Some disorders (such as STDs) result indirectly from substance abuse, while others may result from living conditions that influence the overall health status of women, such as the lack of regular medical care.

Vaginitis

Drug-using women, with and without HIV infection, have high rates of vaginitis. The most

---

Figure 2-14
Immunizations in HIV-Infected Clients

- The CDC recommends immunization of HIV-infected individuals against pneumococcal pneumonia, influenza, and hepatitis B.
- *Haemophilus influenzae* type B vaccine and hepatitis A vaccine may also be considered.
- HIV-infected clients are likely to benefit from and unlikely to be harmed by immunization against polio (using killed polio vaccine), diphtheria, and tetanus.
- Measles vaccination should be considered for HIV-infected substance abuse disorder clients at risk of contracting measles.
- Immunization is more effective in clients who are not severely immunocompromised.

Source: CDC, 1993.

common causes include bacterial vaginosis followed by candidiasis and trichomonas, with no difference in incidence between HIV-positive and high-risk (e.g., drug-using) women. Among HIV-infected women, the risk of severe or refractory vaginal candidiasis increases with a declining CD4+ T cell count, but in most cases the treatment is the same as for HIV-negative women.

Cervical abnormalities

Since 1993, invasive cervical cancer has been considered an AIDS-defining condition. HIV-infected women are at high risk for cervical dysplasia and cervical cancer associated with human papillomavirus. Women who are current or former substance abusers constitute approximately 50 percent of AIDS cases in women in the United States. Clinicians treating substance-abusing women should therefore be particularly alert to the possibility of cervical cancer.

A cervical Pap test should be performed at least yearly, and abnormalities should be evaluated with colposcopy. Facilities treating HIV-infected women must either provide Pap smears and gynecologic followup onsite or have contractual arrangements for provision of these services.

Pregnancy

A large number of women become pregnant after they are diagnosed with HIV disease. There is no evidence that HIV disease progression is accelerated during pregnancy, after an abortion, or in the postpartum period (Alliegro et al., 1997). A woman's options should be discussed in a way that empowers her to make her own decision about whether to continue the pregnancy with optimal prenatal care or seek a termination. The infant initially will have a positive HIV antibody test result because of the presence of maternal antibodies in its blood. New DNA-PCR tests of infants'

blood can diagnose HIV infection in infants soon after birth.

Maternal–fetal transmission of HIV can occur at any stage of gestation, although it is believed to occur primarily during labor and delivery. Use of AZT during pregnancy and in the neonate postpartum decreases the rate of vertical transmission of HIV by 65 percent. AZT does not appear to have any adverse fetal effects. Cesarean sections in HIV-infected women show a reduction in risk of transmission to the newborn as well (International Perinatal HIV Group, 1999).

Treatment providers should note that the 1993 Substance Abuse Prevention and Treatment Block Grants: Interim Final Rule requires prevention and treatment programs to link pregnant clients with prenatal services. See Chapter 4 for more information about pregnancy and HIV.

Nutrition

Substance abuse treatment personnel must be aware of the special nutritional needs of HIV-infected substance abusers. Poor oral intake and malabsorption of nutrients, caused by diarrhea and alteration of levels of endogenous anabolic hormones (especially in men), contribute to wasting. Staff should also be familiar with guidelines concerning nutritional supplements and with interventions to address the causes of inadequate food consumption. (See Figure 2-15 for a summary of factors that must be considered in relation to the client's food consumption.) Clients who are losing weight and for whom oral nutritional supplements are inadequate or ineffective should be referred to an HIV specialist. There are different nutritional concerns for clients on PIs, such as weight gain, "protease paunch," and elevated triglyceride levels. Significant weight loss is a predictor of poor survival. It is important to combine approaches to weight loss, including treating

Figure 2-15
Factors Hindering Food Consumption in HIV-Infected Clients

Problem	Intervention
Anorexia (poor appetite)	Small, frequent meals; calorie- and protein-dense foods; relaxation techniques before meals; appetite stimulants (e.g., Megestrol acetate). Must investigate HIV medications as a potential cause of anorexia (e.g., ritonavir).
Nausea	Cold, bland, dry foods. Investigate HIV medications as a possible cause.
Vomiting	Liquid diet (temporarily). Eat when asymptomatic; antiemetics as needed.
Diarrhea	Use of bulking agents; fluid replacement.
Early satiety	Small, frequent meals.
Dysphagia (difficulty swallowing)	Evaluate for oral diseases, opportunistic infection, and CNS disease. Soft, blenderized or pureed foods or baby foods as tolerated; calorie- and protein-dense supplements.
Odynophagia (pain when swallowing)	Same as for dysphagia, plus avoidance of foods that cause pain (soda bubbles or citrus, spicy, or rough-textured foods).
Difficult or painful chewing	Same as for dysphagia and odynophagia, plus sucralfate slurry or viscous lidocaine swish before meals.

Source: New York State Department of Health AIDS Institute; adapted from Rakower and Galvin, 1989.

underlying illness, attention to nutrition, and correcting metabolic abnormalities that cause loss of muscle mass. This can be particularly challenging for inpatient treatment centers because the schedules for snacking and eating will have to be more flexible, and the usual rules may not work for someone who is HIV positive and in substance abuse treatment.

Cigarette Smoking

Smoking is highly prevalent among substance abusers. HIV-infected smokers are more likely to develop bacterial pneumonia, oral candidiasis, and hairy leukoplakia, and heavy smokers are more likely to develop these conditions than are light smokers. Smoking cessation strategies should be pursued in substance-abusing populations (Conley et al., 1996).

3 Mental Health Treatment

Individuals with substance abuse disorders, whether or not they are HIV infected, are subject to higher rates of mental disorders than the rest of the population. In some studies of substance abusers, the lifetime prevalence of such disorders is as high as 51 percent (Kessler et al., 1996). However, the percentage of HIV-infected substance abusers with psychiatric disorders has not been ascertained. One study found that 79 percent of HIV-infected injection drug users in treatment required psychiatric consultation and 59 percent had psychiatric disorders other than substance abuse. Forty-five percent of these individuals had organic mental disorders, such as cognitive impairment, anxiety disorders, and mood disorders (Batki et al., 1996). Another study of inner-city adult HIV/AIDS clinics concluded that rates of psychiatric distress in patients of these clinics were much higher than in the general population or in other outpatient medical clinics (Lyketsos et al., 1996). There is some evidence that certain psychiatric disorders such as depression and antisocial personality disorder may be more common among HIV-infected persons with substance abuse disorders than among HIV-infected gay men (Ferrando and Batki, 1998).

Evidence is mounting that psychiatric disorders are common in persons with HIV/AIDS. Preliminary data from the Federal HIV/AIDS Mental Health Services Demonstration Program show high levels of co-occurring substance abuse and psychiatric disorders (the program is administered by the Center for Mental Health Services [CMHS] and funded jointly by CMHS, the Health Resources and Services Administration, and the National Institute of Mental Health). More than 5,000 persons with HIV/AIDS received services in 11 projects across the country between 1994 and 1998. The demographic characteristics of those served mirror the emerging profile of the pandemic: large numbers of disadvantaged minorities, persons with substance abuse disorders, women, and heterosexuals. As the health care delivery system plans for the 21st century, it confronts the complex challenge of designing and implementing cost-effective programs for persons with HIV/AIDS that provide medical, mental health, and substance abuse treatment.

Counselors working with HIV-infected substance abusers should be aware of the variety of both HIV- and substance-induced psychiatric symptoms. It is also important to recognize that psychiatric symptoms may be caused by substance abuse, HIV/AIDS, or the medications used to treat HIV/AIDS, as well as by pre-existing psychiatric disorders.

Linkages With Mental Health Services

Programs that integrate substance abuse and mental health treatment provide both mental health and substance abuse services in the same setting, with the same team of clinicians, and with common treatment plans. However, integrated programs are not always possible or available. Therefore, substance abuse treatment programs that do not have the resources to adequately assess and treat mental illness should be closely linked to mental health services to which clients can be referred. Also, many mental health services are not equipped to treat substance abuse disorders but can refer clients to substance abuse treatment programs. Open lines of communication will enable personnel in both locations to be informed about clients' treatment plans and progress (see Chapter 9 for a discussion of confidentiality issues). Treatment staff should maintain contact with the client and continue treatment during and after the psychiatric referral. Providing concrete assistance, such as transportation to the psychiatric referral site, may increase the likelihood of clients' success in following through on referrals to psychiatric services.

Because it may be difficult for any one clinician to address the complex mental health and counseling needs of HIV-infected substance abusers, the care of these clients is likely to involve multiple providers. A coordinated, holistic approach should be taken to address the multiple problems of this population. (Chapter 6 includes a discussion of how case management can provide this approach.)

Common Mental Disorders in HIV-Infected Clients

Neuropsychiatric effects of HIV infection are relatively common and can significantly influence treatment planning for substance abuse disorders (American Society of Addiction Medicine, 1998). In general, mental disorders of concern in HIV-infected substance abusers may be divided into three broad categories:

- Substance-induced mental disorders
- HIV-related mental disorders
- Medication-related mental disorders

Mental disorders may fall into one or more of these categories. Following is a discussion of common mental disorders among individuals with HIV infection, particularly those with concurrent substance abuse disorders (Ferrando and Batki, 1998). (Terms used are those found in the *Diagnostic and Statistical Manual of Mental Disorders*, 4th ed. [DSM-IV].)

Adjustment Disorders

Often characterized by anxious or depressed mood, adjustment disorders tend to be time-limited (i.e., 3 to 4 weeks) responses to acute stresses, such as receiving news of HIV infection or experiencing worsened disease severity, a partner's diagnosis or death, job loss, or other life event. Stages of adjustment to the stress of life-threatening HIV infection have been described as similar to the stages of adjustment to other illnesses. These stages generally begin with a crisis and then progress to acceptance and adaptation.

Sleep Disorders

Sleep disorders can result from substance abuse, psychiatric disorders, or physical illness. Sleep disorder in the form of insomnia is a common problem associated with some types of substance abuse such as intoxication from central nervous system stimulants (e.g., cocaine or methamphetamine) or withdrawal from central nervous system depressants such as alcohol, benzodiazepines, or from opioids such as heroin. Occasionally, maintenance on methadone can be associated with insomnia.

Psychiatric illness is a common cause of sleep disturbance. Depression is most often associated with insomnia, although less commonly it can lead to excessive sleep.

Anxiety disorders also are associated with insomnia, and posttraumatic stress disorder commonly leads to sleep disturbance in the form of nightmares and other symptoms.

Medical illness such as pulmonary disease or the side effects of medications such as bronchodilators can lead to insomnia. Finally, HIV disease itself appears to be associated with an increased incidence of sleep disorders (Wiegand et al., 1991).

Depressive Disorders

Depression is common among patients with substance abuse disorders, even without the impact of HIV/AIDS. Depression is a common response to learning that one is HIV infected or is becoming more ill, and also may be related to substance abuse or to withdrawal. For example, clients may become depressed for prolonged periods of time after withdrawal from use of alcohol, opiates, stimulants, and other substances (Kanof et al., 1993).

Mania

Mania occurs frequently in clients who are HIV positive. In one study of an HIV/AIDS medical clinic, the incidence of mania was as high as 8 percent (Lyketsos et al., 1993). Mania also can be a complication of substance abuse, particularly the use of cocaine and other stimulants. It can be difficult to determine whether mania is induced by substance abuse or HIV infection (Lyketsos et al., 1993; Mirin et al., 1988).

Dementia

Dementia can be defined as the loss of cognitive and intellectual functions without impairment of consciousness and characterized by disorientation, impaired memory, and disordered judgment. Dementia may occur because of chronic alcoholism, head trauma, and numerous other causes, in addition to HIV disease.

Differentiating these dementias can be difficult. All forms of dementia can be present with cognitive, behavioral, and motor abnormalities. However, effective HIV treatment, particularly highly active antiretroviral therapy (HAART), substantially decreases the occurrence of dementia. AIDS dementia complex (ADC) is a severe form of dementia and is one of the most challenging and anxiety-provoking manifestations of HIV disease for the client and his significant others, as well as for the treatment provider.

The diagnosis of dementia in the HIV-infected substance abuser is based on the presence of significant and disabling impairment of functioning. Usually, impairment occurs in three areas:

- Cognitive functioning (e.g., memory disturbance)
- Behavioral functioning (e.g., altered behavior such as agitation or psychosis)
- Motor functioning (e.g., gait disturbance, incontinence)

A neuropsychological examination is a necessary part of the assessment of dementia. However, a brief cognitive capacity examination such as the Mini Mental State Examination (MMSE) should not be relied upon to diagnose dementia (see Appendix H for a copy of the MMSE), although poor performance on such a screening instrument may indicate that dementia is present and that further testing is advisable.

HIV-related neurocognitive loss usually progresses gradually. Figure 3-1 indicates the degrees of impairment that may be seen at different stages in the course of dementia.

Early signs and symptoms of neurocognitive impairment include

- Short-term memory loss (e.g., forgetting appointments, misplacing items, forgetting to take important medications)

Figure 3-1
Abbreviated San Francisco General Hospital Neuropsychiatric
AIDS Rating Scale (NARS)

Cognitive/Behavioral Domains

NARS Staging	Orientation	Memory	Motor	Behavioral	Problem Solving	Activities of Daily Living (ADLs)
0 (normal)	Fully oriented	Normal	Normal	Normal	Can solve everyday problems	Fully capable of self-care
0.5 (minor)	Fully oriented	Complains of memory problems	Fully ambulatory; slightly slowed movements	Normal	Has slight mental slowing	Slight impairment in business dealings
1 (mild)	Fully oriented but may have brief periods of "spaciness"	Mild memory problems	Balance, coordination, and handwriting difficulties	More irritable, labile, or apathetic and withdrawn	Difficulty in planning and completing work	Can do simple ADLs; may need prompting
2 (moderate)	Some disorientation	Memory moderately impaired; new learning impaired	Ambulatory but may require a cane	Some impulsivity or agitated behavior	Severe impairment; poor social judgment; gets lost easily	Needs assistance with ADLs
3 (severe)	Frequent disorientation	Severe memory loss; only fragments of memory remain	Ambulatory with assistance	May have an organic psychosis	Judgment very poor	Cannot live independently
4 (end stage)	Confused and disoriented	Virtually no memory	Bedridden	Mute and unresponsive	No problem-solving ability	Nearly vegetative

Source: The NARS was developed by A. Boccellari, Ph.D.; J.W. Dilley, M.D.; and I. Barlow, M.D., Department of Psychiatry, San Francisco General Hospital, in collaboration with S. Hernendez and B. Haskell, San Francisco Department of Public Health. This figure was adapted from Price and Perry, 1994; Hughes et al., 1982; and the American Academy of Neurology, 1991.

- Loss of visual, spatial, and fine motor coordination (e.g., impaired handwriting, difficulty assembling objects or equipment)
- Cognitive slowing (e.g., taking longer to speak or to understand, appearing "slow" in interviews)
- Mood changes (e.g., mild apathy, depression, hyperactivity)

In later stages of dementia, major impairments become obvious, such as

- Mutism or unresponsiveness to speech
- Agitation, hallucinations, paranoia, or other delusions
- Severe neurological problems (incontinence, inability to walk)

The risk of dementia and other cognitive deficits is highest in HIV-infected clients who are severely immunocompromised. The CD4+ T cell count is a useful index of an individual's risk for AIDS dementia. Generally, dementia is most likely to occur in clients with CD4+ T cell counts below 200 (Boccellari et al., 1993a, b). Neuropsychological testing can establish what stage of impairment a patient has reached, and this information is helpful in treatment planning, treatment expectations, and placement decisions. HIV-related dementia has been reported to respond to treatment with zidovudine (AZT) (Retrovir) and also to treatment with HAART (see Chapter 2).

Delirium

Delirium is an altered state of consciousness manifesting in confusion, disorientation, disordered cognition and memory, agitation, faulty perception, and autonomic nervous system activity. Delirium is an emergent medical problem with a high mortality rate and requires immediate investigation of its cause and immediate initiation of treatment. Sudden development of mental confusion associated with acute encephalopathy or delirium can stem from many sources, including infection,

substance intoxication or withdrawal, toxicity from medication, or metabolic disturbances. Delirium is more common than dementia in HIV-infected substance abusers.

Psychosis

Psychotic symptoms may be seen in advanced HIV/AIDS dementia or in delirium and can be difficult to differentiate from substance-induced hallucinations and delusions (e.g., paranoid psychosis resulting from the use of "crack" cocaine).

Personality Disorders

HIV-infected substance abusers have higher rates of maladaptive personality traits. These generally correlate with early onset of the substance abuse. Antisocial traits also are common. Traits and actual personality disorders may require a more directive and supervisory role for the treatment team. For information on the interaction of personality disorders with substance abuse treatment, see TIP 9, *Assessment and Treatment of Clients With Coexisting Mental Illness and Alcohol and Other Drug Abuse* (CSAT, 1994b).

It is possible that HIV-infected individuals are more susceptible to the side effects of psychotropic medications than are non–HIV-infected persons. Medical staff should therefore exercise restraint in prescribing sedatives, antipsychotics, antidepressants, or antianxiety agents for their HIV-infected clients.

Cognitive Impairment and Adherence to Treatment

Both substance abuse and HIV infection may cause cognitive impairment that can reduce adherence to medical care. The care provider should take into account any possible cognitive impairment when beginning client education. For example, it is important to allow clients time to recover from the acute effects of substance intoxication or withdrawal. Clients' ability to understand the content of counseling sessions should be assessed before the counseling occurs (Forstein, 1992).

To determine the substance abuse and mental health treatment needs of persons with HIV/AIDS, the care provider must understand the impact HIV infection has on the brain itself. Even during the early stages of infection, brain function associated with tasks related to memory, attention, concentration, planning, and prioritizing may be affected by the HIV virus. The client who complains of forgetfulness, gets lost on the way to appointments, or has difficulty adhering to schedules or medication dosing should be carefully assessed. These symptoms of possible cognitive impairment could be the result of HIV/AIDS or they could result from other mental health and substance abuse disorders such as depression, substance-induced dementia, or mental retardation. Poorly controlled diabetes or liver disease can also lead to cognitive impairments. It may not be possible to determine the cause of the impairment, but recognizing its presence and its effects on functioning are essential to knowing how best to help the client.

Neuropsychological testing can search for the presence of specific cognitive impairments. Screening and testing instruments assess intellectual functioning, reading and math skills, speed of mental processing or problemsolving, and status of long- and short-term memory and recall. The neuropsychologist interprets the test results to help formulate a diagnosis when symptoms are complex and to assess previous and current capabilities relating to memory, attention, problemsolving, concentration, and the ability to plan and prioritize.

Communication between medical and counseling staff will help to ensure that cognitively impaired clients are not perceived as deceitful or manipulative. Care providers must keep in mind that cognitively impaired clients' nonadherence to treatment may be a result of the impairment and not caused by denial, resistance, or unwillingness to accept care.

Medication-Related Mental Disorders

Psychiatric symptoms in HIV-infected substance abusers may result from the use of prescription medication. For example, high doses of AZT can produce anxiety, insomnia, or hyperactivity. Similarly, efavirenz (Sustiva) is associated with a variety of central nervous system symptoms, such as very vivid dreams or nightmares (see the section below on drug interactions). The use of steroids in HIV/AIDS treatment also has risen, and these medications may induce psychosis.

In cognitively impaired substance abusers with late-stage HIV disease, memory and other cognitive functions may be worsened by certain combinations of medications, particularly central nervous system depressants such as benzodiazepines (e.g., diazepam [Valium]) and anticholinergic medications such as the tricyclic antidepressants (e.g., amitriptyline [Elavil]). The interaction of some antiretroviral agents, such as the protease inhibitor ritonavir (Norvir), can interfere with the metabolism of benzodiazepines, antipsychotics, and other medications, further aggravating the adverse effects of the antiretroviral agents in the central nervous system.

Assessment and Diagnosis

Assessment and diagnosis of mental illness in HIV-infected substance-abusing clients is a daunting challenge because of these clients' complex problems. It is important to evaluate clients' behavior in context. For example, acute depression is relatively common among clients who have just learned they are HIV positive. This type of time-limited adjustment disorder can lead to worsened substance abuse. In turn, depression can be made more severe or prolonged by substance abuse.

It can be difficult to determine whether substance abuse preceded a client's psychiatric disorder or vice versa. Substance abuse may occasionally be an attempt at self-medication in response to an underlying psychiatric disorder (Khantzian, 1985). Although mental disorders may predate substance abuse, generally the reverse is true. Because an accurate and complete history cannot always be obtained from the client, corroborative sources of information (such as the client's significant others or a previous health care provider) are essential to a complete assessment. Making inquiries of collaborative sources of information will mean disclosing the client's substance abuse or HIV/AIDS status, and the client's written consent is required. See Chapter 9 for more information on consent issues.

Figure 3-2 outlines the major categories of information necessary for a basic mental health assessment.

History Taking

Assessment of the HIV-infected substance abuse treatment client should begin with rapport and trust building and then proceed to a psychosocial history that is as judgment free as possible. The assessment should move from open-ended questions to more specific questions. This questioning should acknowledge and respect gender, ethnic, and cultural differences, as well as sexual orientation. The provider also should keep in mind that history taking may require more than one sitting, depending on the emotional and mental capacity of the client. Many clients with comorbid disorders cannot or will not tolerate long questioning sessions.

A complete medical history focusing on both HIV/AIDS and substance abuse should be taken when a client enters treatment. A recent physical examination and laboratory test results

should be readily accessible because they may help in assessment of the client's counseling needs. For example, a CD4+ T cell count below 200 informs the mental health or counseling professional that the client is at higher risk for HIV-related dementia (Boccellari et al., 1994). Clients should be reassessed periodically. Fluctuating health status and functional capacity mean that clients' treatment needs will change over time.

Mental State Examination

A comprehensive mental state examination can detect mental disorders. The cognitive portion of the mental state examination can be performed by using standardized questionnaires such as the MMSE (see Appendix H). The most important part of the mental state exam is the section regarding cognitive impairment and danger to self or others (Cockrell and Folstein, 1988; Folstein et al., 1975).

It is helpful to have a psychiatrist or psychologist perform the examination, but most general practitioners are familiar with the basic components of a brief mental state examination. Nursing staff and counselors can also be taught to administer screening exams. A well-designed screening exam will assist clinicians in asking appropriate questions. In addition to the MMSE, other examinations such as the Beck Depression Inventory may be useful in assessing the severity of depressive symptoms (Beck, 1993). Repeated mental state examinations will help determine changes in a client's cognitive or behavioral status.

Treatment Goals

It is essential to set realistic treatment goals that correspond to the client's functional capacities. For example, immediate abstinence from substances may be an excessive expectation of severely psychologically disturbed substance abusers, and treatment programs may have to consider a range of goals for such clients.

Figure 3-2 **Initial Mental Health Assessment for the HIV-Infected** **Substance Abuse Treatment Client**	
1. Developmental/Social History ■ Childhood trauma or illness ■ Education ■ Employment ■ Sexual orientation ■ Relationship history ■ Current support system/social network **2. Family** ■ Family relationships ■ Family psychiatric history ■ Family substance abuse history **3. Medical History** ■ HIV history: Date of diagnosis ■ Stage of disease according to CDC classification system (see Chapter 2) ■ Most recent CD4+ T cell count ■ Most recent viral load ■ HIV-related illnesses ■ Other medical illnesses ■ Current medications **4. Substance Abuse History** ■ Age of onset of substance abuse ■ Substance abuse description: 　◆ Types of substances 　◆ Amounts 　◆ Frequency 　◆ Route of administration ■ Past or current substance abuse treatment ■ Involvement with self-help (e.g., Alcoholics Anonymous, Narcotics Anonymous)	**5. Psychiatric History** ■ Age of first psychiatric problems ■ Outpatient treatment ■ Inpatient treatment ■ Past and current diagnosis/diagnoses ■ Past and current medications and responses **6. Current Psychiatric Symptoms** ■ Behavior (e.g., agitation) ■ Appearance of psychomotor retardation ■ Cognitive: 　◆ Level of arousal/alertness 　◆ Attention/concentration 　◆ Orientation 　◆ Memory 　◆ Calculation ■ Mood (e.g., depression) ■ Mania ■ Emotional instability ■ Anxiety (acute or chronic) ■ Symptom pattern (episodic; e.g., panic attacks vs. generalized) ■ Psychotic symptoms (e.g., thought disorder) ■ Hallucinations ■ Delusions **7. Danger to Self or Others** ■ Ability to care for self ■ Suicidality ■ Assaultive/homicidal ideation

Cultural Sensitivity

Therapeutic interventions must be sensitive to the culture and ethnicity of the client population. Whenever possible, therapists and support group leaders should share the culture of their clients and should speak the same language. Cultural compatibility among therapists, case managers, service providers, and clients is important in creating an atmosphere of trust in which sensitive issues, such as family support and group mores, can be addressed.

Cultural factors may have to be taken into consideration in the assessment of psychiatric symptoms. For example, some individuals may have strong spiritual beliefs that can be labeled delusional if their cultural context is not understood.

Generally, the clinician's best guide is the client's significant others or the community context. If the client's beliefs are consistent with her community or culture, it is less likely that she is delusional (Perez-Arce et al., 1993). See Chapter 7 for further discussion of cultural issues.

Pharmacologic Treatment For Psychiatric Disorders

Standard pharmacologic approaches may be used to treat psychiatric disorders in HIV-infected substance abuse clients, with some specific considerations. Without exception, a medical and psychiatric diagnostic evaluation should always be carried out before medication is provided.

Some substance abuse treatment staff may have concerns regarding pharmacologic interventions because they believe that psychiatric medications may place clients at risk for relapse to substance abuse. Although these concerns must be acknowledged, it is necessary to distinguish between medications and drugs of abuse. An approach that withholds psychiatric medications when they are appropriate deprives clients of the opportunity to benefit from a legitimate and necessary treatment option.

Medications for Psychiatric Disorders in HIV-Infected Substance Abusers

When prescribing medications to HIV-infected substance abusers, physicians should use a graduated approach that increases the level and type of medication slowly, a step at a time. Low doses of safer and less abusable medications should be tried first, and higher doses or less safe agents used only if the initial approach is ineffective. Figure 3-3 offers a guide to appropriate pharmacologic therapy for clients with HIV/AIDS and substance abuse disorders. For more in-depth information about pharmacology and mental illness, see TIP 9, *Assessment and Treatment of Patients With Coexisting Mental Illness and Alcohol and Other Drug Abuse* (CSAT, 1994a).

Figure 3-3
Use of Medications for Psychiatric Disorders in HIV-Infected Substance Abusers

A hierarchical or stepwise strategy should be followed in prescribing medications to HIV-infected substance abusers. Low doses of safer and less abusable medications should be tried first, and higher doses or less safe agents used only if the initial approach is ineffective.

Sleep Disorders
When treating sleep disorders in patients who have HIV/AIDS and substance abuse disorders, choose an approach that minimizes abuse potential.

First Tier
- Simple "sleep hygiene" aids such as a glass of warm milk, a warm bath, meditation, or soothing music are the first recommended ways to deal with insomnia.

Figure 3-3 (continued)
Use of Medications for Psychiatric Disorders in HIV-Infected Substance Abusers

Second Tier

■ Trazodone (Desyrel) is an antidepressant and sleeping medication with no known abuse potential and low adverse effects. Dosage can start at 25 to 50 mg at bedtime and increase as needed to 100 to 200 mg. Side effects include hypotension (low blood pressure) and very rarely priapism (persistent painful erection). (Priapism occurs in fewer than 1 in 4,000 men taking trazodone.)

■ Doses of Hydroxyzine (Vistaril, Atarax) or diphenhydramine (Benadryl) can start at 25 to 50 mg at bedtime and increase to 100 to 150 mg. These medications are generally moderate in abuse potential, but they can cause anticholinergic side effects, such as dry mouth and lowering of the seizure threshold if given in very high doses (over 250 mg per day).

■ Mirtazapine (Remeron) is a sedating antidepressant. In the lower end of this dose range (15 mg taken at bedtime), mirtazapine can be effective in helping initiate sleep. Side effects include weight gain. Mirtazapine is probably safer than antihistamines or tricyclics (see below).

■ Doses of tricyclic antidepressants (TCAs) such as amitriptyline or doxepin (Sinequan) for sleep can start at 25 to 50 mg at bedtime. TCAs have numerous adverse effects (see "Mood Disorders" section below) and are often lethal in overdose amounts (> 1 g [1,000 mg]). These antidepressants also are often abused by patients in methadone programs (especially amitriptyline).

■ Sedating antipsychotic medications such as chlorpromazine (Thorazine) should be used only in the presence of psychotic or manic symptoms, never for insomnia alone.

Third Tier

■ If the medications listed above fail, a brief course of benzodiazepines should be considered, preferably on a short-term basis (ideally, for less than 2 weeks). They should be moderately short acting, such as temazepam (Restoril) and lorazepam (Ativan), to minimize accumulation of medication and resultant sedation. An alternative agent that shares most of the properties of benzodiazepines, but may be somewhat less abusable, is zolpidem (Ambien).

■ Ultra-short-acting agents such as triazolam (Halcion) should be avoided because they may cause withdrawal psychosis and confusion, including memory loss. Be cautious when prescribing long-acting medications such as diazepam (Valium) because of their cumulative effects. Flurazepam (Dalmane) also can have cumulative effects and may cause morning confusion ("hangover"). Caution is also urged with alprazolam (Xanax), which may be more abusable than other benzodiazepines and is associated with considerable rebound anxiety.

Anxiety

Chronic anxiety

First Tier

■ Alternatives to pharmacologic intervention include relaxation techniques, meditation, supportive psychotherapy, and counseling, as well as stress management and reduction, and possibly acupuncture. Some of these approaches should be tried before medications are introduced.

Second Tier

■ Buspirone (Buspar) is a nonabusable medication for chronic anxiety, such as in generalized anxiety disorder. Buspirone is not effective in the treatment of acute anxiety, as it takes at least 2 weeks to act.

Figure 3-3 (continued)
Use of Medications for Psychiatric Disorders in HIV-Infected Substance Abusers

- Selective serotonin reuptake inhibitors (SSRIs), such as sertraline (Zoloft), fluoxetine (Prozac), and paroxetine (Paxil), have been shown to be effective in the treatment of panic disorder. Due to their delayed onset of action, SSRIs are not effective for treating acute anxiety.

- TCAs such as imipramine (Tofranil) also are alternatives to potentially dependence-producing agents such as the benzodiazepines and have been demonstrated to be effective for treating both generalized anxiety disorder and panic disorder. They are not effective for acute anxiety.

- Patients must be warned that it is usually necessary to take buspirone, SSRIs, or TCAs for at least 2 weeks before antianxiety effects are felt.

Third Tier

See third-tier section of Sleep Disorders above with the same cautions for the use of benzodiazepines: Choose relatively short-acting medications for limited-time use and at limited dosages.

Acute anxiety

- Other possible alternatives to the benzodiazepines for treatment of acute anxiety disorders are beta-blockers such as propranolol (Inderal) and the antihypertensive agent clonidine. However, clonidine may pose a danger of overdose and should be dispensed in limited amounts (e.g., 1 week's supply). Hydroxyzine (Vistaril, Atarax) can also be used in doses of 25 to 50 mg in the daytime as needed as an antianxiety agent, although it is highly sedating. If these fail, then short-term use (less than 2 or 3 weeks) of benzodiazepines may be indicated.

- Antipsychotics should not be used to treat anxiety if there is no evidence of psychosis, mania, or severe dementia. (Whenever possible, psychotherapy, such as cognitive–behavioral therapy, should be tried before moving on to pharmacological treatments for panic disorder.)

Panic attacks

First Tier

- A nonbenzodiazepine medication such as an SSRI (e.g., sertraline) or if an SSRI fails, then a TCA, such as desipramine, should be administered. Dosing should start very low and then advance gradually to levels approaching those used to treat depression. For example, sertraline should be begun at no more than 25 mg per day, but may be increased to 50 or 100 mg per day; fluoxetine should be started at 10 mg per day and may be increased to 20 mg per day; paroxetine should be started at 10 mg per day and increased to 30 if needed. TCAs may have to be started as low as 10 mg per day and gradually increased over several weeks to as much as 150 mg per day if needed. Response takes 2 to 4 weeks. TCAs have numerous moderately troublesome side effects (see "Mood Disorders" section below) and can be lethal in overdose amounts (> 1 g [1,000 mg]).

Second Tier

- If SSRIs or TCAs are ineffective, too risky, or not tolerated because of adverse effects, benzodiazepines should be used. Alprazolam is probably the most frequently used benzodiazepine, but may not be the best choice in patients with substance abuse disorders because of its relatively short duration of action and the need for multiple daily doses. Diazepam or chlordiazepoxide (Librium) may be preferable because they may produce slower onset of side effects. Any benzodiazepine is likely to be effective when used in divided doses totaling approximately 10 to 60 mg per day of diazepam or its equivalents.

- See "Sleep Disorders" section for the risks of benzodiazepine use.

Mood Disorders

Major depressive disorders
First Tier

- The initial approach should include supportive psychotherapy (individual or group) and possibly peer-based supportive counseling. If these approaches fail, however, pharmacologic interventions should be made readily available to the substance abuse disorder patient with HIV/AIDS.
- A careful evaluation must always be done before medications are prescribed. Mood disorder patients are at risk of suicide. Patients also should be warned that it usually is necessary to take medications for at least 2 weeks before antidepressant effects are felt.

Second Tier

- The SSRI antidepressants—fluoxetine, 20 mg per day; sertraline, 100 to 200 mg per day; paroxetine, 20 to 50 mg per day; citilopram (Celexa) 20 to 40 mg per day; and fluvoxamine (Luvox) 100 to 300 mg per day—are all safe and effective. They tend to be nonsedating and generally are safe even in overdoses. They are usually the most tolerable antidepressants. Side effects in 10 to 20 percent of patients may include jitteriness, insomnia, muscle tightness or twitching, mild appetite loss, and mild gastrointestinal illness, as well as some loss of sexual interest and delayed orgasm or ejaculation.
- Trazodone also is safe but its sedating properties limit its usefulness. Patients can rarely take it in large enough doses or in the divided doses necessary for antidepressant effectiveness. However, it can be useful as a sleeping medication.
- Bupropion (Wellbutrin SR) is a non-TCA that is generally safer in overdose than the TCAs. It is more complicated to use than the SSRIs because it must be given in two divided doses totaling 200 to 300 mg per day. Bupropion tends to increase the risk of seizures more than other antidepressants. Other side effects include jitteriness and insomnia. There is a lower incidence of sexual adverse effects with bupropion than with other antidepressants. Note: bupropion levels are increased by coadministration of the protease inhibitor ritonavir.
- Nefazodone (Serzone) is also a non-TCA, and is generally better tolerated than TCAs. It may be helpful for patients who experience sleep difficulties or adverse sexual effects because of SSRIs. Nefazodone generally is given in at least two doses per day, with a daily dose ranging from 300 to 600 mg/day. Side effects may include light-headedness, visual disturbance, and mild sedation.
- Mirtazapine is yet another non-TCA. It is sedating and is associated with weight gain, but has few adverse effects on sexual functioning and can be given in a single nighttime dose ranging from 15 to 45 mg per day.
- Citalopram was recently approved by the FDA for use as an antidepressant. The drug is a new addition to the SSRIs, which are now considered the preferred agents for treatment of this condition. The most common adverse effects of citalopram are nausea, dry mouth, increased sweating, somnolence, and insomnia. A few men have reported difficulty with ejaculation and temporary impotence. No serious cardiovascular side effects have been reported with use of the drug during clinical trials. Some patients may experience a slight weight loss during therapy. The incidence of

Figure 3-3 (continued)
Use of Medications for Psychiatric Disorders in HIV-Infected Substance Abusers

some adverse events increases as the dose of drug increases. Citalopram can be administered in either 20 or 40 mg doses daily.

Third Tier

■ TCAs are not addictive, but they have a number of troublesome side effects, including dry mouth and short-term memory loss. Other side effects—blurry vision, constipation, tremor, and low blood pressure—may contribute to falls, weight gain, and oversedation. Side effects may be offset by low dosages. HIV-infected patients may be more sensitive to side effects. Substance-abusing patients may be more likely to request TCAs that have sedating effects, such as doxepin and amitriptyline.

■ All of the TCAs are lethal in overdose and should not be given to unmonitored suicidal patients.

Fourth Tier

■ Psychostimulants may be useful for late-stage AIDS patients with severe psychomotor retardation (Fernandez, 1990). Some dramatic, rapid improvement has been observed.

■ Methylphenidate (Ritalin) is the safest and easiest to manage of the psychostimulants. Methylphenidate and amphetamines such as dextroamphetamine (Dexedrine) should not be used until other medications have failed, but they should not be withheld solely because of a patient's substance abuse history. Psychostimulants should be administered early in the day and monitored carefully because they cause insomnia. If prescribed to an outpatient, daily dispensing is recommended. If this is impractical, prescriptions should be written for limited quantities and compliance closely monitored.

■ Other side effects of psychostimulants include jitteriness, agitation, delusions, hallucinations, and anorexia, as well as abuse and dependence.

■ Monoamine oxidase (MAO) inhibitors should be avoided unless all other treatments fail. Use of these medications requires dietary restrictions and carries the potential for lethal hypertensive interactions with other drugs.

Bipolar disorder

■ When evaluating the substance abuser with mania, clinicians must consider that the disorder is caused by abuse of substances such as stimulants.

■ Lithium is as effective in substance-abusing patients with HIV/AIDS as in the general population in treating mania caused by bipolar disorder. It has no known abuse potential but must be monitored carefully because of side effects, which include dehydration, diarrhea, and altered mental state. Other adverse effects of lithium include tremor, excessive thirst, frequent urination, and weight gain.

■ The anticonvulsant medication carbamazepine (Tegretol) is also useful but it can cause severe neutropenia (bone marrow suppression). This may be dangerous when combined with AZT, which has a similar adverse effect.

■ Patients maintained on methadone and carbamazepine may induce liver enzymes that can metabolize methadone more rapidly than normal and lead to opiate withdrawal symptoms, which may necessitate higher doses of methadone.

■ Valproic acid or divalproex sodium (Depakote) is another alternative to lithium. It avoids the problems of carbamazepine and may be safer but is less proven as a mood stabilizer.

Figure 3-3 (continued)
Use of Medications for Psychiatric Disorders in HIV-Infected Substance Abusers

Psychosis/Severe Manic States

- Psychosis is frequently caused by substance abuse such as "crack" cocaine intoxication or alcohol withdrawal. Substance abuse should always be evaluated thoroughly before prescribing.

- Antipsychotic medications are nonaddictive and can be used effectively to treat both acute mania and psychosis. The lowest possible effective dosage should be used, with side effects closely monitored, and the patient should be frequently reevaluated. Abuse of antipsychotic medications, even by substance abusers, is rare.

- Antipsychotic medications include the older or "typical" agents such as haloperidol (Haldol), chlorpromazine, and many others, as well as the newer, "atypical" agents such as risperidone (Risperdal), olanzapine (Zyprexa), quetiapine (Seroquel), and clozapine (Clozaril). These medications are also occasionally used for the management of agitated confusional states, such as in late-stage dementia.

- Clozapine should probably be avoided in most HIV-infected patients because it can cause profound reduction of bone marrow and blood cell production in 1 to 2 percent of patients.

- Some patients develop extrapyramidal side effects (EPS)—involuntary muscle spasms, jerking, muscle stiffness, or tremor—from antipsychotic medications. Diphenhydramine (Benadryl) and other medications can be used to counter EPS, but these agents can produce anticholinergic side effects such as dry mouth, agitation, and confusional states. An alternative medication to treat EPS may be amantadine (Symmetrel).

- High-potency antipsychotic medications that have the fewest sedating or anticholinergic adverse effects, such as haloperidol, may have the most EPS side effects. EPS may be more severe in HIV-infected patients than in otherwise healthy patients with psychoses.

- Other adverse effects of antipsychotic medications include oversedation, low blood pressure, constipation, dry mouth, and blurry vision.

Abuse of Psychiatric Medications

In animal and human testing, most of the major classes of psychiatric medications have been shown *not* to have abuse potential. Studies have shown that neither animals nor humans will self-administer them and that humans will not rate their effects as pleasurable or euphoric. Examples include antipsychotic medications such as chlorpromazine, mood stabilizers such as lithium, and nonpsychostimulant antidepressants such as fluoxetine.

Clearly there are exceptions, and occasionally individuals do misuse even these medications, but on the whole the medications have no or very low abuse potential. However, two classes of psychiatric medications do have high abuse potential:

- Central nervous system depressant, antianxiety, and anti-insomnia medications such as diazepam, chlordiazepoxide, and others, as well as the barbiturates and other, older CNS depressants

- Psychostimulants such as amphetamine and methylphenidate

Figure 3-4 lists both abusable and nonabusable drugs. When working with any substance-abusing client, it is reasonable to expect that some misuse of legally prescribed controlled substances may take place.

Figure 3-4
Abuse Potential of Common Psychiatric Medications

Medication Class	High Abuse Potential	Moderate Abuse Potential ·	Low Abuse Potential
Sleep medications	Benzodiazepines: ■ Diazepam ■ Flurazepam ■ Chlordiazepoxide ■ Clonazepam (Klonopin) and others ■ Chloral hydrate ■ Barbiturates ■ Meprobamate	■ Diphenhydramine ■ Hydroxyzine (Vistaril) ■ TCAs	■ Trazodone (Desyrel)
Antianxiety	■ Benzodiazepines	None	■ TCAs ■ Buspirone
Antidepressants	■ Methylphenidate ■ Dextroamphetamine	None	■ Fluoxetine and others ■ SSRIs ■ TCAs ■ Bupropion ■ Venlafaxine (Effexor) ■ Nefazodone (Serzone) ■ Mirtazapine
Mood stabilizers	■ Clonazepam	None	■ Lithium carbonate ■ Carbamazepine ■ Sodium valproate (Depakote) ■ Gabapentin (Neurontin) ■ Phenytoin (Dilantin)
Antipsychotics	None	None	All, for example: ■ Chlorpromazine ■ Thioridazine ■ Haloperidol ■ Risperidone (Risperdal) ■ Olanzapine (Zyprexa)
Anti-Parkinsonian medications	None	■ Trihexyphenidyl (Artane) ■ Benztropine (Cogentin)	None

Medication Class	High Abuse Potential	Moderate Abuse Potential	Low Abuse Potential
Agents for treating substance abuse	■ Methadone ■ LAAM ■ Buprenorphine	■ Clonidine (Catapres) (This drug should be prescribed with caution since it can be used to self-administer for heroin withdrawal and can cause a rapid drop in blood pressure.)	■ Naltrexone (ReVia) ■ Disulfiram (Antabuse) ■ Bupropion (Zyban)

Figure 3-4 (continued)
Abuse Potential of Common Psychiatric Medications

A hierarchical approach to prescribing is recommended to minimize the potential for abuse. In this approach, the least abusable medications are prescribed first, and the most potentially abusable are used only when other agents have not been effective. Dispensing medication in small amounts helps limit overuse, misuse, or abuse of potentially abusable medications.

HIV-infected persons may be more sensitive to prescription medications as well as to drugs of abuse. When prescribing, clinicians should attempt to use the lowest effective dose to minimize side effects. With clients symptomatic with AIDS, it may be wise to start out with very low doses of the magnitude generally associated with geriatric psychiatry.

Suicide

Substance abusers are at increased risk of suicide (Tondo et al., 1999). Comorbidity is common among suicide victims, and substance abuse disorders are most frequently combined with depressive disorders (Berglund and Ojehagen, 1998). HIV-infected individuals may also be at risk of suicide, especially if they are suffering from a mood disorder. In a study of HIV-positive heterosexuals recently diagnosed

with HIV, anxiety, depression, and suicidal ideation were assessed. Depression was observed in 40 percent of study participants, anxiety in 36 percent, and serious suicidal intent in 14 percent (Chandra et al., 1998).

Studies have shown that both psychiatric and medical treatment can diminish rates of suicidal ideation among HIV-infected substance abusers. One study administered the Beck Hopelessness Scale (BHS) to 2,379 intravenous drug abusers who were not in treatment, unaware of their HIV status and seeking HIV testing and counseling. Results revealed that seropositivity was closely linked to self-reported depression and suicidal ideation (Steer et al., 1994). When substance abusers are diagnosed with HIV, their first reaction is often terror and panic. As the infected individual envisions a life with AIDS, suicidal ideation becomes more common. If a client is not acutely suicidal but wants to talk about suicide, the counselor should maintain genuine interest, assess the severity, obtain help if needed, and acknowledge the reality of the client's feelings and the severity of the situation. The counselor should not minimize the client's experiences because talking openly about suicide decreases isolation, fear, and tension, and may allow the client to move toward acceptance and commitment to life (Siegel and Meyer, 1999).

Suicidal ideation has been demonstrated to decrease with psychiatric counseling (Perry et al., 1990). When working with an HIV-infected substance abuser who has shown signs of suicidal ideation, the treatment provider should dispense medication in small amounts until the client's level of responsibility can be fully assessed.

Prescribers should be aware that some medications such as TCAs (e.g., amitriptyline) are especially likely to be lethal in overdose.

Side Effects

As HIV infection progresses, certain medications may cause adverse side effects in some clients.

- Medications that have anticholinergic effects block saliva flow, causing dry mouth. (For example, TCAs and antipsychotics can produce dry mouth and cause or exacerbate oral candidiasis and other mouth infections; the dry mouth also can result in a greater likelihood of dental caries.)
- Stimulation from antidepressants may trigger hyperactive or manic behavior, especially in the HIV-infected substance abuser who may already have mild central nervous system impairment from HIV.
- HIV-infected clients are more sensitive to movement disorder side effects such as extrapyramidal symptoms that can be caused by antipsychotic medications like haloperidol (Haldol). Therefore, the newer, atypical antipsychotic agents such as risperidone, olanzepine, and quetiapine may be preferable.
- Central nervous system depressants such as sedative-hypnotics should be used with caution because they may cause confusion, memory impairment, and depression.
- The atypical antipsychotic medication clozapine should not be used in HIV-infected patients because of its ability to cause agranulocytosis—a sudden, severe drop in white blood cell count.

Any sudden behavior change or new physical symptom in a client on medication may be medication related. With some medications such as lithium, the TCAs (e.g., amitriptyline), and certain antipsychotics (e.g., haloperidol), blood levels should be tested periodically to avoid drug toxicity.

Adverse Interactions

Clinicians must be aware of the potential for adverse interactions between HIV/AIDS treatment medications and psychiatric medications. HIV-infected clients often are prescribed complex medication regimens. Medications, either alone or in various combinations, may cause confusion and other psychiatric symptoms.

For example, a client may be prescribed fluoxetine for depression plus an antianxiety medication such as lorazepam and may also be taking AZT and the antibiotic trimethoprim-sulfamethoxazole (Septra), as well as other medications. In any individual client, it is difficult to predict the outcome of interactions among so many medications.

HIV/AIDS medications, such as the protease inhibitors, can potentially interfere with the metabolism both of psychiatric medications and of medications used in the treatment of substance abuse (e.g., methadone). Finally, they can interfere with the metabolism of abused substances—one example is the elevated levels of methylene dioxymethamphetamines (MDMA) that have been found to be associated with ritonavir use (Henry and Hill, 1998).

Because of the potential for adverse interactions among medications, it is essential that medical and psychiatric care providers communicate with each other when treating an HIV-infected substance abuse disorder client (see "Case Management" section in Chapter 6). Pharmacists also can help educate clients and reduce possible adverse effects of drug interactions; they are invaluable sources of information on what medications other health care providers may have prescribed to the client. If a client appears adversely affected by multiple medications, the alcohol and drug counselor must report the observed physical or behavioral change to the client's primary medical provider as soon as possible so the problem can be addressed. However, the counselor cannot contact either the primary care physician or the pharmacist unless the patient signs a consent form (see Chapter 9).

Methadone Maintenance Therapy

Methadone maintenance (or agonist) therapy is the most effective and widely available treatment for opioid abuse (U.S. General Accounting Office, 1998). It is the preferred method of treatment for HIV-infected opioid abusers because it substitutes an oral medication for an injected drug, and it involves regular attendance at a clinic that may offer access to medical care, psychiatric consultation and treatment, neuropsychological evaluation, and social services (Ball et al., 1988; Batki, 1988; Cooper, 1989). Furthermore, longer acting opioid substitutes appear to have a normalizing effect on the immune and endocrine systems, which are disrupted by irregular use of heroin or other abused opioids (Kreek, 1991). Overall, methadone maintenance therapy is associated with a reduced risk of contracting HIV/AIDS and may prevent infection of those patients not yet exposed to the virus (Baker et al., 1995; Iguchi, 1998; Lowinson et al., 1992; Metzger et al., 1993). For more detailed information about methadone maintenance therapy, refer to TIP 20, *Matching Treatment Needs to Patient Needs in Opioid Substitution Therapy* (CSAT, 1995f), and to TIP 22, *LAAM in the Treatment of Opiate Addiction* (CSAT, 1995g).

Mental Health and Substance Abuse Disorder Counseling

Counseling is an important part of treatment for all substance abusers, including those with comorbid psychiatric disorders. The goal of counseling is to help the HIV-infected substance abuser maintain health, achieve recovery from the substance abuse, build coping skills, and attain the best possible level of psychological functioning. Counseling may be done individually, in groups, or with clients' family members and significant others. (See Chapter 7 for more information about counseling HIV-infected clients with substance abuse.)

Individual Therapy

Individual therapy can be particularly helpful for a client who may not be ready to share intimate information with a group. Individual counseling allows clients to discuss subjects such as sexual behavior, fear of death, and other issues related to HIV infection, substance abuse disorders, or sexual identity. For some substance abusers, however, individual therapy may not be as potent as group intervention in reducing the sense of isolation, shame, and guilt that many clients feel because of HIV infection. One possible aim of individual therapy is to prepare clients to participate in group therapy.

Group Therapy

Most treatment programs working with HIV-infected substance abusers find that supportive group therapy can be highly beneficial. Groups can be structured in a variety of ways, but generally involve a dozen participants with one or two group leaders. Both heterogeneous and homogeneous groups can work well; however, there are occasional exceptions. For example,

HIV-infected substance abusers who are strongly self-identified as heterosexual may not feel comfortable in a group with openly gay members, and vice versa. Substance abusers in a group setting may be more restrained about exploring sexuality and sexual behavior.

In general, however, it is not absolutely necessary to segregate group members on the basis of sexual orientation or HIV/AIDS status. Good results can be achieved in a group that includes both HIV-infected and non–HIV-infected substance abusers, as has been shown in the Stimulant Treatment Outpatient Program at San Francisco General Hospital (Perez-Arce et al., 1993).

Stage-of-diagnosis model

A current model for structuring groups, based on the clients' stage of diagnosis, has been used successfully by Boston's Fenway Community Health Center. In this model, clients are grouped as follows:

- Those who have just learned about their HIV infection
- Those in the early stages of HIV infection
- Those in the early stages of AIDS

The first two groups focus on healthy lifestyles and improving quality of life. As the sessions progress, clients often exchange information about treatment. The latter type of group focuses more on adapting to illness, grief, and coming to terms with death and dying.

In addition to their therapeutic role, groups may play important roles in educating clients about risk reduction. Because it is important to promote behavior change among all substance abuse disorder clients, those who are not HIV infected should also have the opportunity to attend HIV/AIDS education groups, or should be provided HIV/AIDS education by their individual therapist.

Family Therapy

For some clients, "family" needs to be defined as broadly as possible. Some clients have traditional nuclear families. For other clients, family may include a nonmarital partner and additional significant others. Adult clients have the right to define their families and to decide whether to include the people they regard as family in the treatment process. For a socially isolated person, a friend from an AIDS service organization may fill the role of significant other.

Supporting clients in their recovery from substance abuse often is a principal goal of family therapy. Questions about partner or child abuse may also be addressed. In addition, family therapy may provide a useful opportunity to address issues of risk reduction for family members who are not (or not yet) HIV infected. This therapeutic setting is uniquely positioned to offer risk-reduction education to people who may not have been identified either as HIV-infected or as substance abusers.

Support Groups

Support groups fulfill a wide range of needs. They are useful in reducing anxiety and depression and can help with both the substance abuse recovery process and in HIV/AIDS treatment. They also have an educational function, helping clients gain knowledge and skills about the systems they must negotiate. Some support groups have a client advocacy role, helping link programs and lobbying for funding to fill gaps in services. No single organization can provide all the services needed by HIV-infected substance abusers with mental health problems. Substance abuse treatment programs should actively refer clients to appropriate outside support groups where their specialized needs can be met.

Structuring support groups

Among the factors that must be considered in structuring support groups are the need to protect client confidentiality and the possible stigmatizing effect of identifying a group for HIV-infected clients.

Among the issues to consider in establishing and maintaining support groups are language, ethnicity, gender, sexual orientation, type of substance abuse, stage of recovery from substance abuse, and stage of HIV infection. Occasionally, homogeneity is desirable and effective. Single-sex groups may be beneficial for both women and men in certain circumstances. Women who have suffered abuse may feel more able to divulge this information in a women-only group. Many HIV-positive women have not told their partners about their HIV/AIDS status, and some may be afraid of losing custody of their children if their status becomes known. Women who have been involved in the sex industry or in sex-for-drugs transactions may have difficulty speaking about these experiences in mixed settings and would benefit from participation in specialized single-sex groups. Single-sex groups are also beneficial for men who have difficulty discussing issues of sexuality, such as sexual abuse and incest, in a mixed-gender group.

Some clients have difficulty achieving full recovery from substance abuse without addressing issues related to sexual orientation. Homosexual and heterosexual clients may not always be comfortable with one another in groups. Ideally, if resources allow, specialized groups defined by both sexual orientation and gender should be offered.

Clients' perceptions and prejudices about the use of different substances are likely to surface in groups and affect the treatment process. For example, alcohol abusers may consider themselves less addicted than cocaine abusers and may be unwilling to admit that they also are abusing substances. In general, it is preferable to hold separate groups for alcohol abusers, heroin abusers, cocaine abusers, and so on.

An individual's stage of recovery may be as important as the type of substance abused. Although most substance abuse treatment programs stress abstinence, clients in early recovery who are also dealing with HIV infection may find total abstinence difficult to achieve. Many programs across the country use a risk-reduction model (see Chapter 4) when working with clients with substance abuse, recognizing that dealing with substance abuse, HIV/AIDS, and possible mental health issues often makes abstinence difficult. Figure 3-5 describes a group developed to assist HIV-infected substance abuse treatment clients.

Grief and Bereavement

In addition to facing the prospect of disability and death from AIDS, many HIV-infected substance abusers experience grief and bereavement as a result of the deaths of friends,

---

Figure 3-5

The San Francisco–UCSF AIDS Health Project's AIDS Substance Abuse Program

This group, sponsored by San Francisco General Hospital, is a popular support group for HIV-infected substance abusers who are ill or recently discharged from the hospital. Groups meet in a conference room adjacent to the main hospital cafeteria. Participants who are recovering from substance use discuss their experiences of withdrawal, and current abusers discuss the difficulties of discontinuing substance use. Members of the group also discuss whether abstinence should be the goal of all members of the group.

lovers, spouses, and other family members. There also is a need for grief and bereavement counseling for the client's family. For substance abuse treatment programs, there are at least three goals in addressing grief and bereavement:

■ Providing support and counseling for clients who are dying as well as for clients who are experiencing the deaths of significant others

■ Supporting staff members who are experiencing grief and stress as a result of working with dying clients

■ Establishing flexible program policies that accommodate the limitations of symptomatic HIV-infected clients

4 Primary and Secondary HIV Prevention

Primary HIV prevention reduces the incidence of transmission (e.g., fewer people become HIV infected), whereas secondary HIV prevention reduces the prevalence and severity of the disease through early detection and prompt intervention (e.g., fewer HIV-positive people progress to AIDS). For HIV-infected clients in substance abuse treatment, a comprehensive approach to HIV prevention must include three goals: (1) living substance free and sober, (2) slowing or halting the progression of HIV/AIDS, and (3) reducing HIV risktaking.

This third goal is crucial for the client in several ways:

- Different individuals may be infected with different strains of HIV. Because HIV mutates frequently, an individual can be infected with treatment-resistant forms of the virus. The possibility exists that treatment-resistant forms of the virus can be spread even to individuals who are already infected with HIV, and, if this is the case, further treatment options could be reduced. (See Chapter 3 for more information about resistance.)
- Behaviors that put an individual at risk for HIV will also put him at risk for other infections, such as hepatitis B or C, which can complicate treatment of HIV/AIDS.

- Clients do not want to transmit HIV to the people who are close to them.

In addition to the ways in which HIV prevention efforts directly help the client, the benefit to family and community is obvious. HIV prevention for those already infected is a key component of treatment for both the client and community.

Substance abuse treatment personnel may be among the few people the recovering abuser trusts. By taking the opportunity to advise each client on HIV risk reduction, whether that client is known to be HIV infected or not, the substance abuse treatment professional assists both the individual and all those connected to him. HIV has been spreading rapidly among substance abusers since the start of the pandemic but can be slowed if they are taught the skills to prevent transmission.

Risk reduction originally was called "harm-reduction counseling" by its creator, Edith Springer, in the late 1980s and was popularized by pioneering syringe exchange advocates David Purchase and Dan Bigg in the early 1990s. The term "harm reduction" was first associated with the approach of identifying and supporting "any positive change" by substance abusers toward less frequent substance use or abstinence. In this respect, the harm-reduction approach endorsed the social work adage of "meeting the client where he is."

In the mid-1990s, the term "harm reduction" was unfortunately associated with a brief and unsuccessful drug legalization/decriminalization movement. In an effort to distinguish the more specific service provision response from the larger, disparate political movement, advocates renamed the approach "risk reduction." The concept of risk reduction was further expanded to include both substance-related and sex behavior–related risks for HIV infection. Risk-reduction interventions have included media campaigns (Bortolotti et al., 1988; Power et al., 1988), syringe exchange programs (Des Jarlais et al., 1996; Watters et al., 1994), and substance abuse treatment (Ball et al., 1988; Booth et al., 1998; Hartgers et al., 1992; Iguchi et al., 1996).

HIV/AIDS Risk Assessment

Numerous risk assessment protocols exist and may be used with a minimum of training and familiarity (Chen et al., 1998). The goal of HIV/AIDS risk assessment should be to identify behaviors that place the client at risk for HIV infection. Figure 4-1 contains a brief HIV/AIDS risk assessment checklist that has been used successfully with a wide variety of populations at risk.

Figure 4-1
HIV/AIDS Risk Assessment Checklist

Within the past 3 to 6 months, have you

- Participated in unprotected vaginal intercourse?
- Participated in unprotected anal intercourse?
- Participated in unprotected oral sex?
- Had unprotected sex in exchange for money?
- Had unprotected sex in exchange for drugs?
- Had unprotected sex with more than three partners?
- Had unprotected sex with someone you think was an injection drug user?
- Had unprotected sex with someone you think was HIV infected?
- Had unprotected sex with someone you think had AIDS?

When you have sex

- Do you or your partner use condoms: _____ sometimes or _____ never?
- Do you use drugs before you have sex?
- Do you use drugs after you have sex?

When you use drugs

- Do you use syringes?
- Do you share syringes?
- Do you clean your works?
- Do you use crack cocaine or powder cocaine?
- Do you use several drugs at the same time?

Positive answers for half or more of the questions should indicate that the person is at *high* risk for HIV infection if current practices continue.

Sexual Practices Assessment

A comprehensive sexual practices history is important and should be taken early in counseling, although not necessarily at the first session. Clients must be reassured of the confidentiality of the information they provide.

Counselors should address the full range of potential risk behaviors in their questioning, including both syringe sharing and unsafe sex. They should take into account a wide range of sexual practices, including homosexual, bisexual, and heterosexual, as well as those of transgender clients. Condom use must be a special focus of counseling. The power issues over use/nonuse of condoms that can often occur in sexual relationships should be discussed as well.

After taking the client's history, the counselor can often proceed to HIV/AIDS education and then to risk reduction. A client who was diagnosed with HIV before seeing the counselor may already have discussed sensitive issues and risk reduction with someone else. Nonetheless, it is important that the substance abuse treatment counselor discuss these issues with the client as well.

Risk-Reduction Counseling

Changing risk behaviors such as substance abuse and unsafe sex requires more than a knowledge of why these are risky. Clients' attitudes and beliefs also must be addressed, as well as the beliefs and attitudes of their sexual partners. Substance abuse can lower inhibitions and increase impulsiveness, which may significantly contribute to risk behaviors.

In promoting risk reduction, the alcohol and drug counselor's goals are to

- Help the client understand the need for behavior change

- Provide psychological support for behavior change
- Assist the client in developing the appropriate skills to sustain the behavior change

Discussion of risk behaviors should take place in language that is culturally appropriate, clear, and understandable. Substance abuse treatment providers should know how to refer family members for HIV antibody testing and how to provide appropriate pre- and posttest counseling to clients. If onsite testing is not possible, referral should be available to an easily accessible site.

Risk-reduction counseling can be particularly difficult when a client is sent back to a nonsupportive community where high-risk substance abuse and sexual behaviors are not discouraged. Issues such as poverty and homelessness must be acknowledged and addressed when attempting to change high-risk behavior, and counseling should be provided for personal problems such as perceived powerlessness and low self-esteem. Practical assistance, such as providing emergency housing, is usually required before behavior change can occur.

Risk Reduction and Women

Encouraging risk-reduction practices in women can sometimes be problematic for treatment providers. HIV-infected women in substance abuse treatment are likely to be poorly educated about their sexual and reproductive health, financially dependent on a man, and consequently reluctant to challenge the status quo. A recent study examined the relationship between partner violence and sexual risk behaviors in a sample of predominantly Hispano/Latino and African American women. Nearly one half of participants reported having been abused by a partner or spouse in the past. It was discovered that abused women were five times more likely than unabused women to have reported a sexually transmitted disease (STD) and four times more likely to have engaged in sex with a risky sexual partner (El-Bassel et al., 1998).

Brief Intervention

One promising means of promoting risk reduction as well as treatment entry is known broadly as brief intervention. Brief interventions are a large class of interventions, all of which involve the use of approximately three sessions of assessment and motivational counseling intended to diminish substance abuse or promote treatment entry (Heather, 1995). Most brief intervention studies have focused on alcohol and nicotine use, but brief interventions are also effective for drug treatment programs (Miller, 1993; Schuster and Silverman, 1993). (For more information, see TIP 34, *Brief Interventions and Brief Therapies for Substance Abuse* [CSAT, 1999c], and TIP 35, *Enhancing Motivation for Change in Substance Abuse Treatment* [CSAT, 1999d].)

Sexual Risk Reduction

Sexual risk reduction is best approached in a stepwise manner. The greatest protection (and best step) is either to have one monogamous, HIV-negative partner or to abstain from sex. The next best step is to always use a latex condom if one is having sex with more than one partner, with a partner who is HIV positive, or with a partner who may not be monogamous. Male condoms are effective when used correctly, but female condoms, while showing some promise in preventing STDs, have not yet been scientifically established as effective in preventing transmission of HIV.

A condom can be cut open and used like a sheet for oral intercourse. Plastic kitchen wrap can also be used, except for the microwave type, which has tiny holes in it. Anal intercourse is safer if two condoms are used, and spermicides containing nonoxynol-9 appear to give additional protection. Only water-based lubricants (such as K-Y Jelly™ or Surgilube™) should be used because oil-based lubricants (such as petroleum jelly or vegetable oil) can cause a condom to deteriorate enough to allow HIV to pass through.

Providers should also remind clients that contraceptives such as Norplant and the birth control pill provide effective birth control when used correctly but provide no protection against HIV transmission. Clients should use condoms to protect themselves and others from HIV in addition to whatever birth control devices they may be using.

Another way to reduce risk is to avoid activities that cause trauma or bleeding (however, if clients engage in these activities, a latex condom should be used). Instances of trauma can include not only obvious bleeding but also microscopic abrasions produced by excessive teeth brushing just before oral sex, which could cause the gums to bleed. Anything that touches cut or irritated body tissue should be sterile, if possible. To date, there are no known cases of HIV transmission through kissing, but if both partners have cut or irritated areas on the lips or in the mouth, it is technically possible for the virus to be transmitted.

HIV sexual risk-reduction programs should be integrated into substance abuse treatment programs. Stall and colleagues found that among men who have sex with men in substance abuse treatment, substantial HIV risk reductions occurred after initiation of treatment but that lapses into unsafe sex were common during treatment (Stall et al., 1999). HIV sexual risk (e.g., unprotected anal sex) was most likely to occur among men who were riskier at intake, who continued to be more sexually active, and who were more likely to combine substance abuse and sexual behavior (Stall et al., 1999).

Paul and project staff from the New Village Program in San Francisco have developed an

HIV sexual risk-reduction program for substance abusers, especially for gay men (Paul, 1991a). Components of the "Clean and Sober and Safe" program may be useful to substance abuse treatment staff in general. Its group-format design allows it to be easily incorporated into group treatment settings to help substance abusers deal more effectively with situations that could lead to HIV risk. The format of the program incorporates many of the group principles used in substance abuse treatment settings, such as self-monitoring techniques, relapse prevention, building coping strategies, enhancing perceived self-efficacy, and developing necessary social support structures.

In general, Paul and colleagues recommend that the focus of these groups should be on "identifying high-risk situations for relapse into substance abuse and unsafe sex" and developing relapse prevention strategies to maintain abstinence and safer sex (Paul, 1991a). The same skills that clients learn when dealing with high-risk alcohol and drug situations can

be adapted for situations that present high risk for unsafe sex. Group members should be encouraged to talk about sex and relationship issues, as well as the intersection of these issues with alcohol and drug use. Discussions should occur within a "sex-positive" framework, in which sex is viewed as healthy and natural.

Adapted from the sexual risk-reduction program developed by Paul and colleagues, Figure 4-2 contains a topic outline that can be used in substance abuse treatment settings to reduce HIV sexual risk among HIV-infected persons (Paul, 1991a).

Sexual risk-reduction programs should provide clients with basic information about safer sex, as well as an array of alternative strategies and choices that are client controlled. For example, a client who engages in unprotected anal intercourse should be encouraged to reduce risk by either using a condom or switching to oral intercourse. Or a client who engages in unprotected oral sex might reduce risk by using a condom or

---

Figure 4-2
Sexual Risk-Reduction Topics

1. Identifying high-risk situations for substance abuse relapse
2. Identifying high-risk situations for unsafe sex (e.g., potential for having unsafe sex when high or when clean and sober)
3. Introducing relapse prevention planning (e.g., situation when relapse occurs, "slippery" situations, problemsolving, and planning)
4. Identifying riskiness of current sexual patterns
5. Teaching basic condom skills
6. Bringing up condoms with sexual partners (e.g., talking about condoms, role playing, identifying issues in talking about safer sex)
7. Choosing sexual partners (e.g., finding new partners, personal ads)
8. Taking steps to meet new people
9. Exploring the impact of AIDS on the community (e.g., "taking it 1 day at a time with HIV")
10. Reviewing skills
11. Building a social support system in recovery (e.g., getting support for safer sex)
12. Practicing social skills in sobriety

Source: Paul, 1991a.

switching to mutual masturbation. Such self-protection strategies should be encouraged and explored throughout the risk-reduction sessions.

Syringe-Sharing Risk Reduction

Risk reduction for injection drug use (IDU) is best approached strategically; for example, abstinence is the best step, no syringe use is the second best step, *not* sharing syringes is the third best step, using *only* clean syringes is the fourth best step, and so on. Successful drug treatment optimally will stop IDU and HIV risk. However, if abstinence is not working, the next best method is never to share IDU equipment with others and always to use clean equipment (including cookers, filters, water, and syringes). Some areas offer syringe exchange programs (SEPs) to assist in this effort, but if absolutely necessary a used syringe can be bleached (see Figure 4-3 for instructions on this). Another risk-reduction practice is not to allow others to contaminate drugs or equipment by putting a contaminated syringe into the prepared drug.

Syringe exchange programs

Under the terms of the Departments of Labor, Health and Human Services (DHHS), and Education, and the Related Agencies Appropriations Act, 1998, (42 U.S.C. §§300ee–300ff), Federal funds to support SEPs are conditioned on a determination by the DHHS Secretary that such programs reduce transmission of HIV and do not encourage use of illegal drugs.

In a 1997 report to Congress, the DHHS Secretary reported that a review of scientific research findings indicated that SEPs were an effective component of a comprehensive strategy to prevent HIV and other blood-borne infectious diseases in communities that included SEPs in their HIV prevention strategy. The Secretary also announced that research findings indicated that SEPs do not encourage use of illegal drugs (U.S. Department of Health and

Human Services, 1998). To date, the restriction on Federal funding has not been lifted.

DHHS has decided that the best course at this time is to have local communities that choose to implement their own programs use their own money to fund SEPs and to communicate available research results on the subject so that communities can construct the most successful programs possible to reduce transmission of HIV, while not encouraging illegal drug use (U.S. Department of Health and Human Services, 1998).

Three major expert reviews of the scientific literature on SEPs conclude that such programs can provide a pathway for linking injection drug users to other important services such as HIV risk-reduction counseling, substance abuse treatment, and support services (Lurie et al., 1994; Normand et al., 1995; U.S. General Accounting Office, 1993). Other studies strengthen the conclusion that SEPs do not encourage the use of illegal drugs (Brooner et al., 1998; National Institutes of Health, 1997a, b).

Prenatal and Perinatal HIV Prevention

A particularly important point at which to address HIV prevention is during pregnancy. From July 1997 to June 1998, women accounted for 22 percent of AIDS cases; of those, 30 percent were infected through substance abuse and 37 percent through heterosexual contact (CDC, 1998b). It is estimated that between 6,000 and 7,000 HIV-infected women give birth each year (Stoto et al., 1998). Without any treatment, the risk of an HIV-infected woman passing the infection to her child is between one chance in three and one in four. A child's chances of being infected during pregnancy and childbirth drops to less than 1 chance in 10 when the mother receives proper prenatal care and treatment (CDC, 1994).

In addition to preventing HIV transmission, prenatal care and treatment of the HIV-infected

Figure 4-3
Use of Bleach for Disinfection of Drug Injection Equipment

On April 19, 1993, the Centers for Disease Control and Prevention (CDC), the Center for Substance Abuse Treatment, and the National Institute on Drug Abuse issued a joint bulletin updating recommendations to prevent HIV transmission through the use of bleach to disinfect drug injection equipment. The bulletin particularly addresses persons who cannot or will not stop injecting drugs. This bulletin states that:

1. Bleach disinfection of needles and syringes continues to play an important role in reducing the risk of HIV transmission for injection drug users who reuse or share them.
2. Sterile, never-used needles and syringes are safer than bleach-disinfected, previously used needles and syringes.

The bulletin contains provisional recommendations for the use of bleach to disinfect needles and syringes (including the recommendation for using full-strength household bleach). CDC recommendations for disinfecting environmental surfaces contaminated with blood are unchanged.

Provisional Recommendations

There is currently insufficient laboratory and behavioral research to make definitive recommendations on the best procedures for bleach disinfection. However, the following steps will enhance the effectiveness of bleach disinfection of needles and syringes:

- Cleaning should be done twice—once immediately after use and again just before reuse of needles and syringes.
- Before using bleach, wash out the needle and syringe by filling them several times with clean water. (This will reduce the amount of blood and other debris in the syringe. Blood reduces the effectiveness of bleach.)
- Use full-strength liquid household bleach (not diluted bleach).
- Completely fill the needle and syringe with bleach several times. (Some suggest filling the syringe at least three times.)
- The longer the syringe is completely full of bleach, the more likely HIV will be inactivated. (Some suggest the syringe should be full of bleach for at least 30 seconds.)
- After using bleach, rinse the syringe and needle by filling several times with clean water. *Don't reuse water* used for initial prebleach washing; it may be contaminated.
- For every filling of the needle and syringe with prebleach wash water, bleach, and rinse water, fill the syringe to the top.
- Shaking and tapping the syringe are recommended when the syringe is filled with pre-bleach wash water, bleach, and rinse water. Shaking the syringe should improve the effectiveness of all steps.
- Taking the syringe apart (removing the plunger) may improve the cleaning/disinfection of parts (e.g., behind the plunger) that might not be reached by solutions in the syringe.

Staff of HIV prevention programs should review how the use of bleach is currently taught and promoted and how injection drug users are using bleach. The principles of bleach disinfection just described should be incorporated into guidance provided to them. Program staff, outreach staff, and drug users should work together to develop easily understood messages to communicate these steps.

Source: CDC et al., 1993.

woman will help her maintain her own health. Current recommendations are that a woman receive optimal HIV/AIDS treatment for herself during pregnancy (CDC, 1995). If a woman becomes pregnant and does not know whether she is infected with HIV, it is crucial that she be tested for HIV. Alcohol and drug counselors can help clients enter into prenatal care, be tested for HIV if they have not yet done so, and can encourage them to follow medical recommendations.

Zidovudine (AZT) (Retrovir)

Data indicate that AZT therapy has a key role in preventing perinatal transmission of HIV from mothers to infants. The Pediatric AIDS Clinical Trials Group Protocol 076, a multicenter, randomized, double-blind, placebo-controlled trial conducted by the National Institutes of Health AIDS Clinical Trials Group, found that only 8 percent of infants born to HIV-infected women treated with AZT were infected with HIV, compared with 26 percent of infants born to women treated with a placebo (CDC, 1994). A recent study evaluated the long-term effects of in utero exposure to AZT in 234 uninfected children who were born to women enrolled in the Protocol 076 program (Culnane et al., 1999). No adverse effects were observed in these children, who were followed for as long as 5.6 years, and the researchers advised further evaluations of children who were exposed to antiretroviral agents in utero or neonatally. At San Francisco General Hospital's program for pregnant women, there has not been an HIV-positive infant born in more than 2 years to mothers on Protocol 076.

Clinical experience with AZT has not revealed any fetal toxicity other than transient anemia, although theoretical risks remain. However, the benefits seem to outweigh the unproven risks. The Centers for Disease Control and Prevention (CDC) now recommend that pregnant HIV-infected women receive AZT therapy. More recent clinical trial data from Thailand using a simpler regimen (600 mg orally daily from 36 weeks' gestation to labor, then 300 mg every 3 hours until delivery) produced a 51 percent decrease in HIV transmission risk (Shaffer et al., 1999). Given the large number of childbearing women among clients in substance abuse treatment programs, these data indicate an immediate need for expanded HIV/AIDS counseling, testing, and education for women who are pregnant or likely to become so. Although antiretroviral combination therapy is more potent than AZT monotherapy, it is not necessarily more effective in preventing mother-to-infant HIV transmission. In some subgroups, viral load is closely associated with transmission risk, lending support to the move toward combination therapy. Studies of prototypic triple-therapy protocols for safety and tolerance have just begun.

Breast-feeding

Breast milk transmits HIV efficiently, which is one reason why so many children in developing countries are HIV positive. Breast-feeding is therefore contraindicated for HIV-positive women.

Neonatal HIV transmission through breast-feeding remains a problem, especially in countries where safe and affordable alternatives to breast milk are not available and antenatal HIV prevalence tends to be highest. The rate of acquisition of HIV through breast-feeding was 7.4 percent in a study of infants who had a negative virus test in the first 3 months of life and was 7.4 percent in one study and 9.6 percent in another study at 24 months. Oral AZT prophylaxis during pregnancy may produce children more at risk for acquiring HIV through breast-feeding. Also, it is possible that viral load rebounds in mothers after they stop taking AZT, which results in increased virus concentration in breast milk.

The World Health Organization (WHO) issued a recommendation that women with HIV should not breast-feed (World Health

Organization, 1998). The report recognized, however, that in some cultures women are stigmatized for failure to breast-feed and that in underdeveloped countries, breast-feeding may be the only way in which an infant can survive the first few months of life. This is a complex and delicate issue.

Cesarean delivery

Various studies that recently compared transmission rates between vaginal delivery and cesarean section demonstrate that elective cesarean section reduces the risk of vertical transmission of HIV from mother to child (European Mode of Delivery Collaboration, 1999). Elective cesarean sections were defined as those performed before onset of labor and rupture of membranes. According to a meta-analytic review of 15 research studies, after adjustment for factors such as receipt of antiretroviral therapy, maternal stage of disease, and infant birth weight, the risk of vertical transmission was decreased by roughly 50 percent with elective cesarean section (International Perinatal HIV Group, 1999).

Transmission of Resistant HIV

Transmission of forms of HIV that are resistant to one or another of the cluster of antiretroviral medications has already been well documented. However, whether it is possible to sexually transmit forms of HIV that are resistant to triple combination therapy remained an open question until recently; genetic analysis demonstrated the transmission of triple-combination resistant virus between a serodiscordant gay male couple (one HIV positive and one HIV negative) (Hecht et al., 1998b).

The implications of this finding are serious. Given the cross-resistance problems of many protease inhibitors, individuals newly infected with triple-combination–resistant forms of HIV may have few antiretroviral treatment options available to them. If it is possible to efficiently transmit triple-combination–resistant HIV

during unprotected sexual encounters, it follows that certain at-risk populations may return to the situation that existed before protease inhibitor treatments became available. Thus, primary and secondary AIDS prevention may turn out to be as important as the discovery of triple-combination treatment therapies themselves.

Infection Control Issues For Substance Abuse Treatment Programs

The AIDS pandemic poses a number of challenges for infection control policy and practice in substance abuse treatment programs. Effective institutional infection control is more relevant for preventing the transmission of tuberculosis than for preventing the spread of HIV, although the latter often has received a greater amount of attention.

Universal Precautions

Adherence to universal precautions for exposure to blood and bodily fluids—as recommended by the CDC, the National Institute of Occupational Safety and Health, and several other organizations—has been well established as the necessary standard of practice for all settings in which exposure to bodily fluids is a potential hazard. Substance abuse treatment programs should apply the same universal precautions that are in place in hospitals and other health care facilities (CDC, 1987b) (see Figure 4-4). Prompt referral of substance abuse treatment staff members who have been exposed to contaminated blood and bodily fluids is critical because antiviral therapy can be initiated within hours of exposure to reduce dramatically the risk of transmission.

Programs should seek guidance from local public health authorities or infection control staff of an affiliated institution on adhering to universal precautions. In settings such as

Figure 4-4

Universal Precautions for Substance Abuse Treatment Programs
Treating HIV-Infected Clients

Transmission of HIV is highly unlikely within institutions such as health care facilities, residential facilities, correctional facilities, residences, and substance abuse treatment programs when universal precautions are observed.

Because medical history and examination cannot reliably identify all HIV-infected patients, universal precautions should be used *consistently* with *all* patients.

1. Barrier Precautions

In any setting in which workers may come into contact with a patient's blood or bodily fluids, the following precautions should always be observed:

- Gloves should be worn when touching blood or bodily fluids, mucous membranes, or nonintact skin; handling items or surfaces soiled with blood or bodily fluids; or performing vascular access procedures such as venipuncture (inserting a syringe into a vein to draw blood or administer fluids).
- Gloves should be changed after each patient contact.
- Masks and protective eyewear should be worn during any procedure likely to expose mucous membranes of the mouth, nose, and eyes to droplets of blood or other bodily fluids.
- Gowns or aprons should be worn during procedures likely to generate splashes of blood or other bodily fluids.
- Hands and other skin surfaces should be washed immediately and thoroughly when contaminated with blood or other bodily fluids and whenever gloves are removed.

2. Use of Sharp Instruments

The following precautions should be taken to prevent injuries when using, cleaning, disposing of, or otherwise handling syringes, scalpels, and other sharp instruments:

- Do not recap syringes, bend or break them by hand, remove needles from disposable syringes, or otherwise handle them.
- Place disposable "sharps" in puncture-resistant disposal containers immediately after use.
- Place large-bore reusable syringes in puncture-resistant containers for reprocessing.

3. Other Precautions

- Ventilation devices such as mouthpieces and resuscitation bags should be available for use in areas where the need for resuscitation is predictable.
- Workers with exudative (oozing) lesions or weeping dermatitis should refrain from all direct patient care and from handling patient care equipment until their condition resolves.
- Pregnant workers should be especially familiar with, and should strictly adhere to, all of the above precautions.

Source: CDC, 1987b.

freestanding community-based treatment programs, safe disposal of infectious waste may require a deviation from standard waste disposal practices.

Postexposure Prophylaxis

The best way to reduce the risk of occupational HIV transmission is to prevent exposures. However, exposures occasionally occur, so every clinic should have a plan for postexposure prophylaxis (PEP). One consideration in postexposure management is to administer antiretroviral medications. The use of AZT as a PEP has been shown to be safe and associated with decreased risk for HIV infection (CDC, 1998e). Newer antiretroviral medications may be effective, but there is less experience with their use as PEP. The key to PEP is to initiate therapy immediately after the exposure. Some agencies keep PEP medications onsite so that they can administer them quickly if an exposure occurs. The San Francisco Department of Public Health is making combination therapy available to people who believe they have had an HIV exposure (within 72 hours). It must be noted, however, that because of side effects, very few individuals who attempt to follow the PEP regimen are able to stay on it for 30 days.

Rapid HIV Testing

Rapid HIV tests are becoming more available, and these tests will change how and when HIV prevention counseling is delivered. Clinical studies have shown that the sensitivity and specificity of rapid HIV tests are comparable to those of the enzyme immunoassays currently used. Because these tests can provide results in hours instead of days, counseling could increase from one session per client (risk assessment) to two sessions (risk assessment accompanied by test results) per client in a single day.

Counselors must understand the technical aspects of these screening tests and be able to assess each client's likelihood of being infected. Reactive rapid tests must still be confirmed by a supplemental test (either Western blot or immunofluorescence assay).

The CDC recommends that counseling before using rapid HIV tests should

- Ensure that the client is aware that rapid testing is being used and that he can receive test results during this visit.
- Include an explanation of a reactive screening test result and a statement about the necessity of waiting 1 to 2 weeks for the results of a confirmation test.
- Help the client identify the behaviors that place her at risk for HIV.
- Be used as an opportunity to help the client develop a realistic and incremental plan for reducing risk, regardless of her HIV test result (CDC, 1998h).

Several new, rapid HIV tests currently in use outside of the United States may soon be submitted for approval by the Food and Drug Administration. Many of these new tests require only a single step. When these tests become available, clinicians will have more options for delivering HIV testing and prevention counseling services.

5 Integrating Treatment Services

Substance abuse treatment is moving away from more intensive treatment programming toward less intensive, shorter term treatment; HIV/AIDS treatment also has shifted from intensive inpatient care to focus more on primary, clinic-based care. Providers are under pressure to perform with less money, less time, and more challenges. As a result, substance abuse treatment and HIV/AIDS treatment should reflect their interconnected relationship by coordinating as much as possible to maximize care for persons having both HIV/AIDS and substance abuse disorders. Substance abuse treatment programs and their personnel must stretch their dwindling resources by integrating the care they provide with that of other service providers.

HIV/AIDS Services in Substance Abuse Treatment

HIV prevention is an essential part of substance abuse treatment and relevant to any treatment setting. Addressing HIV/AIDS issues beyond prevention, however, is much more complicated. For the person who abuses substances and has HIV/AIDS, the complicated physical and mental health problems—such as tuberculosis (TB); hepatitis A, B, and C; sexually transmitted diseases (STDs) other than HIV/AIDS; dental problems; diabetes; poor nutrition; dementia; and depression—require that each substance abuse treatment setting

incorporate a holistic, integrated model of treatment. Treatment for the client with HIV/AIDS must be carefully reviewed. Important areas to examine are issues of confidentiality, quality of services to clients, complex treatments, staff training, client readiness, and use and allocation of limited resources.

Persons with HIV/AIDS and substance abuse disorders require more than the typical physical examination and TB test. The addition of nontraditional treatment components—such as nutritional counseling, exercise regimens, education about testicular self-examination (for men), breast exams (for women), and ways to lower cholesterol—will greatly enhance the mental and physical health of persons with HIV/AIDS. For persons with a long history of substance abuse, the possibility of mental health issues and psychiatric disorders should be explored. Many inpatient treatment and detoxification settings use a nurse to assist with physical withdrawal symptoms, medications, and occasional medical concerns. This type of care can be augmented by (1) incorporating some of the treatment components listed above, (2) using health educators and nutritionists, and (3) cross-training the treatment staff.

People with HIV/AIDS are in need of all levels of treatment for substance abuse disorders. In the early days of the HIV pandemic, individuals with HIV/AIDS did not have access to a full range of substance abuse treatment services; even today, some providers still do not offer all levels of care. Often, clients with HIV/AIDS present only their substance abuse for treatment. Their fear of disclosing HIV/AIDS status, their denial of having a substance abuse disorder, the lack of training of staff and clients, and homophobia make treatment of the "whole" person very difficult. Furthermore, the fact that HIV/AIDS case managers and health care providers are not adequately trained to screen and assess for either substance abuse disorders or psychiatric disorders and refer to appropriate treatment has limited the range of services for clients with HIV/AIDS who have substance abuse disorders.

Treatment of HIV/AIDS continues to become more complex and specialized. The resources and time needed to provide ongoing HIV/AIDS medical care are great. For the most part, it is unrealistic to expect these services to be provided within substance abuse treatment settings, but it is imperative that every substance abuse treatment program maintain a close relationship with HIV/AIDS medical care providers within its community and surrounding area. Drug and alcohol counselors and HIV/AIDS service providers must continue to develop their skills in assessing and establishing appropriate treatment plans that support the "whole" person. Medical providers and counselors can work together closely to support medical and substance abuse treatment and adherence to treatment goals. This includes establishing agency agreements and creating formal referral mechanisms.

Issues of Integrated Care

Early Intervention Settings

Early intervention often can be the first step in addressing HIV/AIDS issues in substance abuse treatment, or vice versa. The practice in early intervention for persons with substance abuse disorders has been to provide HIV pre- and posttest counseling to stop the spread of AIDS.

Today the emphasis is on testing, treatment, and followup. The latest medical research indicates that beginning combination therapy early in the pathogenesis of HIV/AIDS may enhance the health of the client over a long period (Hodgson, 1999). This will result in fewer opportunistic infections and, as revealed by the latest statistics from the Centers for Disease Control and Prevention (CDC), fewer people dying of HIV/AIDS-related illnesses (Vittinghoff et al., 1999). Now that there are known benefits to early treatment, counselors can feel justified in encouraging clients to be tested and then begin treatment (see Chapter 2 for information about treatment).

Another trend in early intervention is increased use of medical case management for persons with HIV/AIDS and of case management for those at high risk for becoming infected with HIV, specifically persons with substance abuse disorders. The complex regimens associated with HIV/AIDS care, along with the challenges of substance abuse treatment and aftercare, make it essential to include case managers as part of a substance abuse treatment program's responses. Many treatment centers and HIV/AIDS service organizations are receiving funding for case managers, who are sometimes called early interventionists. (See Chapter 6 for a more in-depth discussion of case management.) This service component targets those at high risk for HIV infection and provides long-term case management services focusing on risk reduction and supportive services. Risk reduction is defined with the client and based on the client's specific needs. This might mean, for example, that the case manager and client are focusing on other care needs such as dental care, mental health care, or finding stable housing. See Chapter 4 for discussion of risk reduction.

Once the client with HIV/AIDS is ready to obtain HIV-specific medical care, the case manager or early interventionist will focus on supporting medical adherence and maintenance of sobriety along with assisting with the psychosocial adjustments and the need for continued support and resources.

Early intervention also can be supported through the efforts of outreach workers or other community-based workers. Outreach workers have been an important part of HIV prevention work for many years. They have been involved in many high-risk communities and have learned much about the specific needs of high-risk clients. Outreach workers can have a great impact in helping people obtain substance abuse and HIV/AIDS treatment. Outreach workers also recognize that many people at high risk have ongoing medical, housing, and social problems and that neither HIV/AIDS nor substance abuse treatment may be the client's most pressing and immediate need.

Many clients from poorer, disenfranchised communities are dealing with basic survival needs (see Maslow's Hierarchy of Needs, in Maslow, 1970), such as food, escaping violence from an abusive partner, or keeping the electricity from being cut off. Early intervention within the context of the "culture of poverty" begins with tangible concrete service provision and establishment of trust and rapport. From this perspective—"starting where the client is"—the worker may spend time talking and getting to know the client while helping to find emergency assistance for the electricity bill and food. The worker will gradually shift from helping with the "here-and-now" challenges to developing a trusting relationship based on mutuality, which will allow the client and worker to eventually discuss long-term goals that may lead to sobriety, safer sex practices, and establishment of a more stable environment.

Obstacles to Integrated Care

Because of the many overlapping issues related to substance abuse and HIV/AIDS treatment and prevention, agencies providing both

services must coordinate their efforts to offer clients a full array of services. There are, however, significant barriers to complete integration of services. Some of these are:

- **Differences in priority.** A client entering either substance abuse treatment or HIV/AIDS treatment faces a myriad of required activities and treatments. Some of these activities may appear mutually exclusive, creating significant challenges in developing a treatment plan for clients seeking treatment in both areas.

- **Differences in philosophy.** Substance abuse treatment agencies often operate from an abstinence model. HIV/AIDS service and medical treatment organizations and public health professionals frequently use a risk-reduction model. This philosophical difference can create dramatic conflict in programs and approaches.

- **Differences in funding.** Public funding of prevention and treatment of substance abuse has generally focused on drug interdiction and prevention. Conversely, HIV/AIDS funding has focused on treatment and research. Although still inadequate, higher levels of social service funding are available for persons diagnosed with HIV/AIDS. Funding sources rarely recognize the challenges of coexisting disorders; however, some resources exist. Although funding amounts are difficult to obtain, both Title I and Title II of Ryan White allow for the funding of substance abuse treatment for HIV-positive individuals (see Chapter 10).

- **Differences in training.** Many substance abuse treatment providers are experts at detecting substance abuse disorders and developing treatment goals for substance-dependent clients but at the same time do not thoroughly address their clients' medical needs. Similarly, many public health providers do not address a client's possible substance abuse while dealing with the client's latest STD. Clearly there is a need for ongoing staff inservices and cross-training. The recently published CDC/CSAT cross-training curriculum, *HIV/AIDS, TB, and Infectious Diseases: The Alcohol and Other Drug Abuse Connection, A Practical Approach to Linking Clients to Treatment,* is an excellent resource for both mental health treatment providers and alcohol and drug counselors.

Any effort to develop integrated treatment for substance abuse disorders and HIV/AIDS, either within a single agency or through individual care plans, should include the following components:

- **Shared philosophy and priorities between the care providers in regard to the client.** The client must receive clear and consistent messages if he is to act as a full partner in his care.
- **A strong case management model.** One professional within the care system should be designated to work with the client as the lead case manager across all agencies. The case manager must be empowered to negotiate schedules and control resources to develop a care plan with the client. Within each client care team, only one provider should have the title of case manager. (For more information on case management, please refer to TIP 27, *Comprehensive Case Management for Substance Abuse Treatment* [CSAT, 1998b].)
- **Social services at the core of the treatment plan.** For many clients, the first priority is day-to-day survival. The individual's definition of survival may vary and may include housing, food, financial services, family maintenance, or work. Without addressing these basic client priorities, treatment cannot be successful.
- **All providers within HIV/AIDS and substance abuse treatment trained about the services available and requirements of the**

other setting. For example, several federally funded programs subsidize housing costs for persons with HIV/AIDS. These same services may not be available to an individual who is in recovery for substance abuse only. Availability of housing for an individual with coexisting disorders could be the determining factor in maintaining treatment adherence.

- **Cooperative eligibility determinations, which often are a key barrier to achieving integrated care.** Every agency establishes requirements for its own purposes, including varied documentation. It is essential that the client newly in recovery or recently diagnosed with HIV/AIDS be assisted in dealing with bureaucratic requirements that are often redundant. Workers from each agency must be willing to cross agency lines to cooperate with colleagues and advocate on behalf of the client.

Developing integrated services is rarely accomplished at the administrative level. Although solid, formal understandings and agreements are helpful, most success actually is achieved at the direct-care staff level. When working with two closely linked diagnoses that are also tied to other diseases such as TB, hepatitis, and mental disorders, the care provider cannot afford to think or work solely within the confines of his own agency or personal experience. Instead, the provider must build bridges to other providers that enable clients to address all of their needs.

Dealing With Ongoing Substance Abuse

Many HIV-infected substance abusers are unable to maintain total abstinence from substance abuse after the abrupt discontinuation at the start of treatment. In dealing with clients' ongoing substance abuse, treatment programs must find a balance between abstinence and public health approaches to substance abuse treatment.

Abstinence model

This approach traditionally uses confrontation, consistency of expectations, behavioral contracting, and limit-setting as treatment modalities, with the goal of achieving abstinence from all substance abuse. This approach might require termination from treatment if abstinence is not achieved.

Public health model

This approach, sometimes called the risk-reduction model, emphasizes incremental decreases in substance abuse or HIV risk behaviors as treatment goals and tries to keep clients in treatment even if complete abstinence is not achieved. The public health model sacrifices some of the consistency of expectations that is such an important part of abstinence-oriented treatment. Instead, it seeks to keep substance abusers in treatment and to reduce, if not eliminate, substance abuse- and HIV-related risk behaviors. Each increment of change is viewed as a success, which helps clients see that they can positively affect their lives. By contrast, a model that regards less than complete abstinence as failure may reinforce clients' feelings of helplessness and hopelessness at their inability to sustain behavior change.

If substance abuse is placed on a continuum from abstinence to severe abuse, any move toward moderation and lowered risk is a step in the right direction and not incongruous with a goal of abstinence as the ultimate goal of risk reduction (Marlatt et al., 1993). Moreover, research indicates that substance-abusing individuals who are employed and generally functioning well in society are unlikely to respond positively to some forms of traditional treatment that, for example, tell them that they have a primary disease of substance dependency and must abstain from all psychoactive substances for life (Miller, 1993).

Flexibility is needed with HIV-infected clients because of the importance to public health of keeping them in substance abuse treatment; they are likely to continue to put others at risk if they leave treatment and resume injection or other drug use. In order to reduce the spread of HIV, clinicians may need to work with these clients even if they continue to abuse substances.

Every substance abuse treatment program must establish a balance between the abstinence and public health approaches, based on the needs of the community it serves. For example, even a program that stresses abstinence may use a risk-reduction model to educate active injection drug users about safer sex and drug use practices, such as using condoms and sterilizing syringes with bleach.

Differential standards of care

One current example of a flexible approach to substance abuse treatment of HIV-infected clients is the differential standards of care approach used by the Opiate Treatment Outpatient Program at San Francisco General Hospital's Substance Abuse Services. This approach applies varying clinical expectations and levels of care to clients based on assessment of the clients' level of functioning in the areas of physical health, mental health, social support, and housing.

The treatment staff use a "standards of care" assessment tool to determine the level of severity of impairment among methadone treatment patients with HIV (see Appendix I for a copy of this tool.) Impairment is assessed along three domains of functioning—physical health, mental health, and social resources. The latter domain represents both social support and housing. Assessment of severity of impairment takes place during a team meeting in which substance abuse counselors, the program physician, nurses, and the program social worker offer input regarding each domain. Treatment decisions are subsequently made by consensus in accordance with this assessment. Clients with evidence of severe impairment are generally approached with lower expectations for treatment outcome (i.e., applying risk-reduction principles), and higher functioning clients are approached with higher expectations (e.g., maintaining substance-negative urine tests, attending self-help group activities).

Referral to and Coordination Of Linkages

Development of care networks

Counselors who work with HIV-positive individuals with substance abuse disorders should familiarize themselves with the local AIDS Service Organizations (ASOs) and substance abuse treatment services. Listed below are questions that all counselors who treat substance-abusing individuals with HIV/AIDS should be able to answer:

- What area physicians or clinics with experience in HIV/AIDS issues accept HIV-positive patients? Which ones accept Medicaid, Medicare, or specific insurance plans?
- What ASOs exist in the area?
- Are Ryan White Funds available in the area? If so, who administers them?
- Are Housing Opportunities for People with AIDS (HOPWA) funds available in the area and if so, who administers them?
- Does the State provide medical coverage for single adults who have no dependents, for indigent patients, or for undocumented workers?
- Where can an individual with HIV/AIDS obtain inpatient, residential, intensive outpatient, extended outpatient, or detoxification treatment for substance abuse disorders?
- Are area substance abuse treatment programs prepared to deal with a client's complicated HIV/AIDS treatment regimen?

- What forms of support are offered in the area to help with loss, death, and dying? Are there community mental health centers that can provide psychiatric evaluation, medication management, neuropsychological testing, or case managers with skill and sensitivity toward those with mental disorders?
- Are culturally appropriate local support groups available for persons living with HIV/AIDS and substance abuse disorders?
- What financial assistance is available to clients to pay for expensive HIV/AIDS treatment?
- What are the eligibility guidelines for the State's AIDS Drug Assistance Program (ADAP), and what drugs are covered by the program?

Creating medical referral networks or institutional linkages is essential and must be a top priority for anyone working with a person with HIV/AIDS. Counselors and case managers can often make the job of working with persons with substance abuse disorders easier for medical care providers by providing consultations, followup, and help acquire resources that affect the client's ability to obtain prescriptions, come to appointments, and so on. Service providers and agencies must coordinate with medical providers, including private doctors, public health clinics, and specialized HIV/AIDS facilities and treatment centers. (See Chapter 6, "Accessing and Obtaining Needed Services.") Providers should also explore the possibility of becoming members of their community's Ryan White Title II consortium of providers. There are usually two key areas in which providers can begin making contacts:

1. Local city, county, and State health departments. Every State has an HIV/AIDS or substance abuse treatment coordinator, or both (perhaps through the State department of mental health services

or substance abuse treatment services). These coordinators should be able to provide information about medical resources and special funding.

2. Regional and area teaching hospitals and medical schools. These programs often have special indigent care funding and specialized HIV/AIDS treatment programming and funding. They might also be research sites for HIV/AIDS clinical trials that could not only help clients access newer treatments but also provide high-quality, specialized HIV/AIDS care within their specific substance abuse treatment protocols.

When attempting to coordinate a service plan between several agencies or resources, counselors may encounter barriers, both expected and unexpected. Here are several issues that could arise:

■ The clinic or service provider from whom the counselor is attempting to obtain services may be too busy to talk. The counselor may have difficulty communicating the request directly to a person (rather than voice mail).

■ The service provider may consider HIV/AIDS a specialty condition and thus may be unable to provide the level of care the client needs.

■ Long waiting lists and applicant pools for services and resources may exist.

■ Other service providers may be judgmental or discourteous because the client is HIV positive or substance dependent.

■ Few or no services are available for the HIV-positive client living in rural or isolated areas.

■ "Turf" issues may cause providers to make inappropriate referrals or be resistant to serving a referred client.

Networking with other agencies is a valuable tool for the counselor who is attempting to coordinate a service plan for a client with HIV/AIDS and a substance abuse disorder. It is essential to find out what services are offered in the local and surrounding areas.

In addition to standard treatment services, less traditional therapeutic interventions or culturally based interventions may be available to clients. For instance, acupuncture is being used for detoxification and outpatient treatment for addictive behavior. Massage is a nurturing, hands-on therapy that can promote a positive attitude in the client. Yoga and breath training may be available to help a client stay focused on sobriety and a path toward health.

Holistic knowledge of living systems, both physical and mental (the mind–body connection), can be integrated into the treatment plan. Helping the client "tune into" the connections between thoughts, emotions, and physical health can facilitate treatment regimens.

The Internet can provide helpful treatment information and resources to the client. Many public libraries offer free Internet access. Local colleges usually have Internet access available to the public for free or for a small fee. If a remote area lacks resources but a client must live there, the counselor faces challenges in networking and resource coordination that are clearly different from those in urban settings.

When establishing a network of care coordination, the provider must consider the issue of confidentiality (see Chapter 9). Providers must be aware of State and Federal laws and professional codes of ethics, along with agency and community policies and agreements (see also Appendix E for sample codes of ethics). Confidentiality raises issues of consent, disclosure, and release of information. Because linkages and referrals for needed resources are part of the client's overall treatment plan, the client should not be surprised that other treatment providers will be contacted and that releases of information will be needed. The client might have fears about disclosure—

talking about this fear with the client is important. The counselor and client must develop a partnership that places the client in an active, empowered position so that she understands the value of connecting with other agencies. Eligibility for services at another agency may be based on need, and the agency may inquire about the client's condition to ascertain whether it pertains to the agency's services.

The counselor should also understand the difference between the terms "informed consent" and "consent." "Informed consent" refers to a client's consent to begin treatment after she understands her treatment options and the advantages and disadvantages of each option. "Consent" refers to the client's consent to allow confidential information to be disclosed as needed (see Chapter 9).

Case Finding

Case finding, or identification of individuals at higher risk for HIV infection, involves multiple levels of effort. Substance abusers may be located at public welfare agencies, emergency medical care facilities, other medical care settings, the criminal justice system, homeless shelters, STD clinics, churches, in the street, or in community settings. For example, hair and nail salons in regions with high numbers of injection drug users are common settings for locating women at risk. In traditional health care settings, case finding may consist of basic questions to determine risk-group membership (for more information on this topic, refer to TIP 24, *A Guide to Substance Abuse Services for Primary Care Clinicians* [CSAT, 1997]). In the criminal justice system, urine samples may be collected to identify substance abusers, and, again, basic screening questions regarding risk behaviors may be helpful.

Confidential HIV/AIDS counseling and testing (C&T) locations represent a major part of the screening effort, with as much as 25 percent

of the CDC HIV prevention budget going to C&T (Phillips and Coates, 1995). Unfortunately, many individuals at highest risk for HIV infection are unlikely to seek HIV testing for a number of reasons, including distrust of institutional settings, fear that the test results will not remain confidential, and fear that test results might be positive for HIV, thereby resulting in increased stigma, discrimination, and changed social relationships (Hull et al., 1988; Myers et al., 1993). The impact of C&T by itself on risk behaviors is unclear (Higgins et al., 1991; Wolitski et al., 1997).

Another means for locating this hidden population is through the use of community-based street outreach (Booth and Wiebel, 1992; Iguchi et al., 1992; Watters et al., 1990). A common form of community-based street outreach is the indigenous leader outreach model, which uses recovering substance abusers to locate and contact injection drug users. Indigenous outreach workers have the advantage of knowing the local substance-abusing community and the informal rules governing their behavior. These workers are therefore able to develop trusting relationships with active substance abusers, allowing them to more effectively intervene. However, this can occasionally trigger relapse in outreach workers; consequently, outreach programs should provide a forum in which workers can discuss the potential for relapse so that they will be prepared to revisit old issues while working with active substance abusers.

Early versions of this approach stressed HIV/AIDS prevention and the distribution of items to facilitate compliance with risk reduction, such as condoms, bleach, sterile water, or alcohol swabs. Injection drug users were encouraged to reduce AIDS-related risk along a hierarchy of behavioral options that emphasized taking some action, no matter how small, to reduce overall injection drug–related harm (see Chapter 4 for more information on risk reduction). Although outreach workers counseled abstinence and "getting off the needle," they recognized that in the real world, abstinence is not always immediately achievable and that a range of risk-reduction behaviors should be promoted (Wiebel et al., 1993). Once injection drug users took steps in the right direction, further steps were encouraged. One risk-reduction message is that injection drug users should always use new, sterile syringes when injecting (Normand et al., 1995). (See Chapter 4 for discussion of syringe exchange programs.)

Some outreach programs also used street outreach workers to distribute coupons redeemable for free treatment (Booth et al., 1998; Bux et al., 1993; Jackson et al., 1989; Sorensen et al., 1993). These interventions demonstrated that injection drug users will enter treatment in large numbers once barriers to treatment entry are diminished. In the case of the treatment coupons, financial barriers were lessened. Other investigators removed barriers, for example, by decreasing the typically long delay between first contact with a treatment program and the scheduled treatment intake. This "rapid intake" approach significantly increased the number of injection drug users entering treatment, without impact on rates of treatment retention (Dennis et al., 1994; Festinger et al., 1996; Woody et al., 1975).

Home-Based Services for Clients With End-Stage HIV/AIDS

Recent breakthroughs in treatment medications, which can potentially extend the life expectancy of someone with HIV/AIDS, have raised expectations that HIV/AIDS can be managed as a chronic disease instead of a terminal one. However, many substance abusers, even the most disciplined followers of the daily, multidosed medication regimen, are discovering that their bodies do not respond positively to these treatments. Many more people with

HIV/AIDS lack basic access to these medications because of an historical lack of access to health care services.

This lack of positive response and access to life-extending treatments causes many clients, their families, and their health care providers to examine end-of-life issues. Clients with end-stage HIV/AIDS present a challenge for counselors, who must create partnerships with other health care providers to integrate treatment services for these clients and who must deal with multiple stressors related to home-based caregiving.

Roles of health care team members

Such partnerships involve working with home health staff, hospice staff, and family caregivers. To define the relationship between the professional and the other health care team members, and to create goals and integrate treatment services, it is important to recognize the role of each member of the health care team.

Home health

The home health care team provides skilled nursing care for patients who are homebound. These services may also include social work, physical therapy, occupational therapy, respiratory therapy, and home health aides. Clients receiving Medicare benefits can receive home care services if they are homebound, have services provided under a plan of care, have only reasonable and necessary services reimbursed, require a skilled service, and require service only on a part-time or intermittent basis. Some coverage also is provided by Medicaid and private insurance policies (which may differ from State to State).

Hospice

The hospice care team provides all the same services as home health but with a focus on palliative or comfort care for the client. The physician's order must certify a life prognosis of fewer than 6 months. The hospice team members focus on spiritual, psychosocial, and emotional issues as well as the physical needs of the client. Coverage is provided by Medicare, Medicaid, and some insurance policies (this may differ somewhat from State to State).

Many in the health care field find it difficult to educate clients about home health and hospice services; Figure 5-1 should help distinguish between these two options.

Family caregivers

Whether home health or hospice services are used by the family at home, competent family members will likely be the primary caregivers for the client with end-stage HIV/AIDS and should not be supplanted by professional health care providers. It is helpful to define "family" broadly to include nontraditional families.

Family may include significant others—individuals who may be unrelated but have a close relationship with the client and provide for the client's physical, emotional, and spiritual well-being. Family caregivers can include same-sex partners, friends, and fellow support group members.

It is important for counselors to remember that family members who provide close support to the seriously ill client often need support themselves. Social service support for the family is a cornerstone in the provision of coordinated, comprehensive care to HIV-infected substance abuse disorder clients. Home-based services may be critical in enabling a family to remain together and may be more cost-effective than institutionalizing the ill family member.

Figure 5-1
Medicare and Medicaid Coverage of Home Health and Hospice Services

Services	Hospice	Home Health
Services even if client is not homebound	Yes	No
Skilled nursing care	Yes	Yes
Prescription medicines related to hospice diagnosis	Yes	No
Medical equipment/supplies	Yes	Yes
Home health aide	Yes	Limited
Social work services/grief counseling	Yes	Limited
Pastoral/spiritual counseling	Yes	No
Respiratory therapy	Yes	Yes
Short-term hospitalization for pain control and symptom management	Yes	No
Limited, intermittent, palliative radiation therapy	Yes	Yes
Lab and x-ray for palliative care	Yes	Yes
Bereavement counseling for family members	Yes	No
Support groups	Yes	No

Source: Adapted from handout created by Hospice Care Team, Inc.

Stressors in home-based caregiving
The counselor must be aware of the stressors that can make home-based service delivery more difficult.

Stigma of HIV/substance abuse
Many professional caregivers lack education and experience in working with homebound clients with HIV/AIDS and substance abuse disorders. Even though some home-based service providers employ staff with mental health/substance abuse experience, many do not, and it is important that the counselor intervene in providing coordinated home-based services.

Substance abuse in the home
The client may have a relapse, especially when faced with approaching end-of-life decisions. Both professional and family providers may be unable to continue to provide needed care when faced with a client/family member who has relapsed and who is not capable of following the plan of care. It is critical in these situations that the client and caregivers continue receiving substance abuse counseling and intervention in the home setting. However, providers should be aware that the home setting can present certain problems, including the possibility that other substance-abusing persons in the client's home are stealing or utilizing opioids intended for the client.

Economic needs
Even though home-based services are covered by some Federal, State, and private resources, additional stressors can affect the delivery of services. The loss of income from either the client or the family caregiver can create potential problems with housing, health insurance, nutrition, and medications. The counselor must be aware of how these conditions can disrupt the plan of care.

Emotional needs
As the client continues to need more interventions, the roles of family caregivers change, and health care professionals must be aware of the need to adapt to these changes. Family caregivers will need support in processing the anticipatory grief of losing their family members. After the client's death, help with funeral arrangements and further support of family members, who may also be dealing with their own addiction issues, may be needed.

Examples of Integrated Treatment

Provided below are examples of successful programs that have linked HIV/AIDS and mental health treatment. Also discussed are common elements of effective programs and future challenges to building effective treatment programs.

Active Referral Linkages for HIV/AIDS and Mental Health Treatment

Bailey Boushey
A successful program in Seattle, Bailey Boushey is a skilled nursing facility originally created for persons with AIDS (given the more recent changes in AIDS treatment, the facility's beds are sometimes used for other kinds of patients such as transplant or oncology patients). The facility's most relevant feature is its day health program, which provides services mostly to HIV/AIDS, mentally ill, and substance-abusing persons. Treatment includes the services of mental health professionals as well as substance abuse treatment specialists.

Montrose Center
Montrose Center, in Houston, Texas, has years of experience working with and strong linkages

to the Thomas Street HIV/AIDS Clinic, private doctors, and area substance abuse treatment programs. It includes intensive treatment services, outpatient support/therapy groups at various locations, and outreach programs. Its providers have a good reputation for working with dually and triply diagnosed clients (i.e., HIV/AIDS, mental health disorders, and substance abuse). The staff consists primarily of therapists with licensed professional counselors (LPCs) and masters-level social workers.

Hilltop Center

Hilltop Center, in Longview, Texas, is a new program offering inpatient treatment services for multiply diagnosed clients throughout Texas. The program has developed a strong linkage to traditional treatment programs, but also focuses on a variety of alternative models. Its providers have a positive relationship with funders and a strong commitment from the State drug and alcohol services department. This program also includes an evaluation component. The staff are well trained, motivated, and focused on the importance of preventing clients from "falling through the cracks."

The AIDS Health Project

The AIDS Health Project in San Francisco offers mental health services to HIV-infected clients with and without substance abuse disorders. It works in collaboration with Shanti and the San Francisco AIDS Foundation through the HIV Services Partnership. Shanti provides volunteers for practical and emotional support, and the AIDS Foundation provides case management housing in a treatment-centric model that includes treatment advocates to work one-on-one or in groups with clients struggling with HIV and substance abuse issues and/or mental health issues. The Project is committed to working toward a fully funded "treatment on demand" service for residents with substance abuse treatment challenges.

Opiate Treatment Outpatient Program

The Opiate Treatment Outpatient Program (OTOP) at San Francisco General Hospital treats nearly 160 HIV-positive patients as part of its 250-patient methadone treatment program. OTOP offers substance abuse treatment combined with onsite psychiatric care and HIV/AIDS primary care.

Common Elements of Effective Programs

The challenges to developing effective treatment programs that meet the needs of those who are dually and triply diagnosed continue to be substantial. Few programs across the United States have been able to maintain a high level of success along with the needed funding levels. The cost of these types of programs is a continuing challenge. Some programs are just now exploring new methods of treatment, although some began providing new services simply out of desperation and frustration.

Effective treatment programs, although they vary greatly, have common elements that contribute to their success. These traits, discussed below, include the program's treatment philosophy, outreach efforts, staff training, support groups, community linkages, and funding.

Treatment philosophy

The clear and repeated message from effective programs is that counselors must "start where the client is." Offering what the client wants is the key. It is essential that counselors shift from the rigid thinking that there is only one way for clients to become healthier and to recover. Effective programs have discovered that different treatment modalities are not mutually exclusive and can indeed coexist, particularly when it comes to risk reduction. Nontraditional treatment, neurotherapy, biofeedback, acu-detox, and other alternative therapies can be encouraged and integrated into clients' treatment programs.

Also, counselors and therapists in effective programs believe that labeling clients, confronting them too strongly or too often, and talking "at them" rather than "to them" are counterproductive approaches, create too much distance, and may be a major factor why many clients never return to programs. One clinic's approach to this problem is outlined in Figure 5-2.

Outreach efforts

Some effective programs send a newsletter to their dually diagnosed clients. The newsletter discusses topics that are supportive; for example, stress might be discussed, including how stress affects the immune system and can trigger relapse, and ways to reduce stress. The newsletter also can be distributed to every treatment program in the community, thus serving as an outreach tool. Although using a newsletter may sound simple, it is not a common practice.

Some treatment programs have brought in HIV/AIDS pre- and posttest counselors and educators to their treatment programs. These counselors are encouraged to run support or therapy groups for dually diagnosed clients. Because of stigmas and confidentiality, the roles of the HIV/AIDS counselors can vary; for example, one person may conduct the testing, another may serve as the educator, and a third may lead a support group, so that clients have less fear of disclosure of their HIV/AIDS status.

Staff cross-training

Effective treatment programs also are strong proponents of staff cross-training. One view is that substance abuse treatment providers should become experts in mental health and HIV/AIDS, and the HIV/AIDS providers should learn about substance abuse and mental health, and so on. Staff working with HIV-positive clients must pay vigilant attention to the constantly changing world of medications, side effects, and new discoveries. The main point is that the issues of HIV/AIDS, mental health, and substance abuse disorders coexist, and the only way to really effect long-term change is to combine treatments. The best integrated programs encourage continuing education for staff. Continuing education may include buying journal subscriptions, allowing staff time off for coursework, and providing frequent inservice training sessions. It is also important that programs hire highly trained, flexible, open-minded staff. To be successful, these staff must see beyond traditional substance abuse treatment modalities and be able to accept and affirm all cultures and lifestyles.

Figure 5-2

Listening to Clients

The Hilltop Center program in Longview, Texas, has clearly laid out the expectation that staff members must listen to clients from the beginning to gain a real understanding of where these clients are in their lives. Staff members are asked not to use labels or tag clients with what may be judgmental treatment jargon, such as

- "He's in denial and very resistant and hasn't hit rock bottom yet."
- "She's a borderline personality disorder."

Labels such as these do not help to develop an effective intervention and treatment plan or help the client and counselor to start working toward recovery.

Support groups

An effective treatment program will integrate support groups. For instance, a special group for HIV-positive substance abusers might integrate relapse prevention with adherence to combination therapy. The aim is to connect the milestones of HIV/AIDS disease with triggers for relapse, so that the group becomes relevant and provides the support needed.

Community linkages

One of the most important community linkages in successful programs is the relationship with the medical community and practicing physicians. This includes nurse practitioners, psychiatrists, internists, nutritionists, and others. Choosing medications, assessing medical status, and ruling out a diagnosis can be very challenging with dually or triply diagnosed clients. When service providers work closely with the medical care team to solve problems and formulate treatment plans, this allows clients and providers to be more proactive. Service providers may have to educate medical care providers about addictions and recovery. Working together is essential so that clients are not overmedicated or medicated in a way that jeopardizes their recovery.

Funding

The most successful programs that effectively treat HIV/AIDS, substance abuse, and mental health problems have learned how to obtain funds from a variety of funding streams. Successful programs apply for funding from sources such as the CDC, the Health Resources and Services Administration, the Substance Abuse and Mental Health Services Administration, and many local and State programs. Chapter 10 provides a more in-depth discussion about funding resources.

Current Challenges

Substantial challenges continue to face providers who wish to develop effective treatment programs that meet the needs of clients who are dually and triply diagnosed (HIV/AIDS, mental health, and substance abuse). Few programs across the United States have been able to develop highly successful programs and maintain the needed funding levels. For the most part, it is believed that these types of programs are quite costly.

When providers examine multiply diagnosed clients, they can see that these clients are a highly vulnerable group of people at great risk: risk for death, as well as risk for numerous medical problems and chronic illnesses, other infectious diseases, physical abuse, rape, poverty, starvation, and so on. They are also often the same clients who most easily "fall through the cracks" and challenge treatment providers' knowledge, skills, and patience. Efforts to create more effective programs that decrease the number of people "falling through the cracks" must be encouraged and these programs thoroughly evaluated in order to ensure that every client receives the best treatment possible.

6 Accessing and Obtaining Needed Services

The HIV-infected substance abuser can have multiple psychosocial and medical care needs that require extensive community resources. In areas where few or no resources exist, the treatment professional may have to be especially creative in working within existing systems. Because of the number of issues encountered in both substance abuse and HIV/AIDS, this chapter emphasizes the case management approach in dealing with this client population and encourages cooperation between mental health and HIV/AIDS service systems. Facts about general categories of resources are also provided to assist the substance abuse treatment professional with information on possible services.

The Use of Case Management To Coordinate Care

The term "case management" has been used to describe a wide range of interventions for a diverse number of populations. Mental health, aging, developmental disabilities, and primary care are just a few examples of systems that use a case management approach. For the purposes of this chapter, case management is the term used for coordinated care of the HIV-infected substance abuser and involves attempting to meet the multiple psychosocial and physical needs of individuals seeking assistance.

The purpose of case management is to ensure that all the needs of an HIV-infected substance abuser are recognized and met in a coordinated manner and that there are no gaps in, or duplication of, services provided by the many professionals who are involved in meeting the client's needs. When gaps do occur in services, this should not be because a need or resource was overlooked but because the resource was unavailable. In short, the purpose of case management is to make working with the client more efficient and more effective.

A case management approach recognizes that obtaining basic needs when an individual is actively using substances can be overwhelming and that substance-abusing behavior impairs a person's ability to gain access to a formalized system of services (Lidz et al., 1992). Drug abusers often have multiple, chronic problems beyond the need for substance abuse treatment alone, which require the coordination of services that case management provides (Bokos et al., 1992). The multiple problems often experienced by a substance abuser such as poor health, lack of housing, and a transient lifestyle can also inhibit seeking treatment (Cox et al., 1993). Not only does a case management approach provide realistic support for an individual's needs, but it has the potential to enhance the effectiveness of reatment by helping to manage the life stressors that can impede treatment progress (Graham and Timney, 1995).

Prevalence and Impact of Case Management Programs in Treatment

While there has clearly been a trend in substance abuse treatment programs toward integrating case management into the repertoire of interventions (Brindis and Theidon, 1997), there is still little information about the outcome of such interventions with substance abusers, especially those with HIV/AIDS (Brindis et al., 1995). Studies have suggested that case management may improve health care access and delivery of services to injection drug users and also may decrease a drug abuser's risks for HIV infection and thus lengthen survival time (McCoy et al., 1992). Case management also has been shown to help injection drug users gain access to treatment (Bokos et al., 1992).

A more recent study demonstrated that injection drug users receiving case management obtained substance abuse treatment more readily than injection drug users who were not and that case-managed clients remained in treatment for a longer period and showed better treatment outcomes than non–case-managed clients (Mejta et al., 1997). In a study of case management with chronic alcohol-dependent persons, case-managed clients increased their income, reduced the number of nights spent on the streets and in shelters, and increased the number of nights spent in their own housing. Certainly, more outcome data must be compiled before wide-ranging conclusions on the effectiveness of case management as an intervention can be assessed. Yet it is pertinent to note that in many situations, case management has been effective in helping substance abusers.

Case Management Models And Functions

There are various models of case management and an array of case management functions. Because case management is increasingly used within the treatment programs serving HIV-infected substance abusers, it is useful to review what case management may look like in its various configurations and what a case manager might do. TIP 27, *Comprehensive Case Management for Substance Abuse Treatment* (CSAT, 1998b), describes case management in a substance abuse treatment context: It describes different approaches to case management, elaborates on its functions, and includes a section on the special needs of clients with HIV/AIDS. Providers should refer to the various case management models illustrated in TIP 27 to assess their treatment program's ability to use case management approaches. In addition, providers should remember that the usual functions and activities associated with case management are more difficult in dealing with HIV-infected clients because of

- Clinicians' and clients' fear of contracting HIV
- The dual stigma of being a person with both a substance abuse disorder and HIV
- The progressive and debilitating nature of the disease
- The complex array of medical and pharmacological interventions used to treat HIV/AIDS
- The onerous financial consequences of the disease and its treatment
- The hopelessness—and concomitant lack of motivation for treatment—among the terminally ill

Part of the case manager's linking function in working with an HIV-positive client is to educate the network of service providers, including substance abuse treatment staff, to recognize the competing demands of staying sober and dealing with the social and physical consequences of HIV. However, treatment professionals are not trained to know everything about HIV/AIDS, so it is helpful to ask clients questions to ensure that they are accessing medical care and that they understand their treatment. Figure 6-1 lists suggested questions that counselors can ask during the assessment process.

HIV-Specific Issues Requiring Linkages With External Systems

Living with HIV/AIDS compounds the challenges already facing the client with a substance abuse disorder. Because the disease presents a host of medical complications and potential treatments, linking a substance abuse treatment program with HIV/AIDS resources and/or case management is essential. New information about HIV/AIDS emerges daily, and it is impossible for a client to stay abreast of current knowledge on his own. In addition, there are programs for persons with HIV that are not available to other populations. HIV/AIDS-related mental and physical health concerns are two specific areas that warrant

external linkages with an HIV/AIDS system. For more information on linkages, see Chapter 2, "Medical Treatment"; Chapter 3, "Mental Health Treatment"; and Chapter 5, "Integrating Treatment Services."

Using Case Management To Increase Access to Care

The Panel recommends using case management in dealing with the multiple problems presented by HIV/AIDS in combination with a substance abuse disorder. Case management promotes teamwork among the various care providers. For example, a linkage between the client's primary care provider, AIDS case manager, mental health provider, and substance abuse treatment provider can greatly benefit the client and improve care. On the other hand, when multiple service providers do not work together, clients can play one agency off another or access duplicative resources and subsidies. The client also may receive different messages from different providers who have conflicting goals for treatment. Sometimes the messages appear different because of differences in terminology. If providers work in coordination with other providers, they will gain a more accurate picture of the client's situation.

Figure 6-1
Helpful Questions To Ask When Assessing a Client's Needs

- Do you have a doctor?
- How often do you see your doctor?
- What do you see your doctor for?
- Are there other physical concerns bothering you that you don't discuss with your doctor? If so, what are they?
- Has your doctor prescribed medications of any kind for you to take?
- Could you give me the names of the medications? Or may I see the medications?
- Could you tell me what each medication is for and when you take it?
- Are you having any problems taking your medications?
- Are you satisfied with your medical care and with your doctor?

Examples of case management programs include the Linkage Program, in Worcester, Massachusetts, and AIDS Project Los Angeles Client Services Division (McCarthy et al., 1992; Sonsel et al., 1988). Clients of such programs are likely to receive more substance abuse treatment, health care, and other services (Schlenger et al., 1992). One means of ensuring that clients receive the services they need is through a multidisciplinary team.

Forming Multidisciplinary Teams

How can a provider begin to assemble a multidisciplinary team? There are several points to consider when forming an effective team, which are outlined in Figure 6-2.

Once a multidisciplinary team has been assembled, what are the signs that the team is not working effectively? Signs include the following: (1) the needs of the clients continue to be unmet; (2) there is uneven or unequal participation; (3) one person dominates the discussions; (4) members do not show up for meetings; or (5) there is not enough followup by group members on discussions made in the group setting. To help avoid these situations, the group should periodically assess itself to determine if there are any concerns or frustrations about the group. There also should be a periodic formal evaluation to allow members to more thoroughly review what is, and is not, working.

Treatment Professional as Advocate

In addition to serving as a monitor for the plan implementation, the treatment professional also serves as an advocate for the client. An advocate's role is to find resources, open doors, and represent the needs of the client to other individuals and organizations. While all individuals should be empowered to help themselves, it is often difficult for clients who are overwhelmed by substance abuse and

HIV/AIDS to meet their own needs by advocating for themselves.

Advocating does not mean "doing it all oneself," but rather ensuring that the work is done. As the treatment professional moves through the red tape of a State bureaucracy to obtain funding for a client, he needs to hold other people accountable. Examples of effective advocacy include asking for timelines, insisting on followthrough, and being clear about who is responsible once a request is made.

With HIV/AIDS, the advocate's role may be even more involved. The treatment professional may have to advocate for medical care for a client. This may mean obtaining funding for health care and medications and finding a medical team that understands HIV/AIDS. Advocating also means educating the treatment team about substance abuse issues, so that the client has access to a full spectrum of treatment options.

Resources for HIV-Infected Substance Abusers

Clients who have both a substance abuse disorder and HIV infection may require a number of specialized services as part of their overall treatment plan. Following is an overview of the primary resource needs clients may have. (See Appendix G for a list of State and Territorial health agencies and AIDS offices that can provide other resources.)

Housing

Housing for HIV-infected substance abusers is a major challenge for a number of reasons, including stigma and discrimination. HIV/AIDS seriously decreases many people's income, due to the inability to work and the cost of care. Without money, housing options are limited.

Figure 6-2
Forming a Multidisciplinary Team

1. Determine who the significant providers are in the client's network of care. Depending on the setting and area, there may be several candidates for the multidisciplinary team. When considering a biopsychosocial model, it is useful to have a representative from the client's medical, psychological, and social treatment providers. This could include a social worker, a physician, an alcohol and drug counselor, an HIV/AIDS case manager, and perhaps a representative from an agency (e.g., day health program) with whom the client has frequent contact. Additionally, consideration should be given to the cultural and linguistic makeup of the group.

2. The group can be a fixed one, in which members review the needs of several clients on an ongoing basis, or the group can form as needed for a specific client. Within fixed groups, members tend to be the same core set of providers, perhaps adding specific providers for a particular client's situation. The group that forms on an as-needed basis can be made up of different members each time.

3. When the group is brought together, members should first discuss the expectations of group members, the rules for how the group will interact, and how the group will structure the time. Time should be built in so that adaptations can be made as needed.

   ♦ **Expectations.** Group members should discuss what it is that they want to achieve. Does the group exist to provide brief information about the clients to ensure a basic level of communication, or does it exist to solve problems and provide consultation about each others' clients?

   ♦ **Rules.** Ground rules should be determined by the group members. Rules can include arrival and start times for meetings, keeping whatever is discussed in the group confidential, not interrupting when other group members are speaking, and not allowing one group member to dominate the discussion. Rules will vary depending on the purpose and structure of the group.

   ♦ **Structure.** Group structure should be discussed so that meetings can be the most productive and efficient for all the busy professionals involved. Questions should be asked, such as "How much time will be spent on each client?," "How will the group document its work?," "Will there be a facilitator and/or a timekeeper?," and "Who puts together the agenda?"

4. Establishing formalized linkages with other agencies is one means of building a team. Affiliation agreements, for example, between a public health department and a hospital that serves low-income pregnant women can allow for formalized sharing of client information as well as a partnership approach to serving the client. It is important to discuss issues such as identifying the roles and responsibilities of each party, the mode of collaboration, and who the participants will be. An affiliation agreement should be drawn up that includes a renewal date for the agreement, so that both parties have the opportunity to periodically reconsider the reason for affiliating.

5. In multisystem work, there can be several case managers. If possible, one "lead" case manager should be identified who has the responsibility to ensure that services are coordinated. This lead person can also bring together the various providers for ad hoc multidisciplinary meetings.

6. Confidentiality should be kept in mind when forming multidisciplinary teams. It is imperative that the group keep client information confidential, and it is necessary that the client agree to allow the treatment professional to share information with the other members of the group.

Difficulties also arise when trying to find housing for clients who are still actively using substances. Clinicians who believe in a harm-reduction model have particular difficulties finding recovery housing that is not based on an abstinence model. Most providers believe that it is nearly impossible to stabilize a client if that client cannot find adequate housing.

Counselors should be aware of a number of different housing options for people with HIV/AIDS; some of these are detailed below.

Services-enhanced, abstinence-based residential programs

Services provided to individuals in independent living residential programs—which are nearly all services-enhanced and abstinence-based—include substance abuse counseling, education regarding HIV/AIDS, mental health counseling, vocational rehabilitation, and support groups. These programs tend to be focused on helping an individual make the transition from active use to living without substances. These programs enforce rules against substance abuse, and a client's substance abuse may result in her dismissal from the program. Programs are designed to build the client's strengths so that she is able to succeed in recovery once she has left the facility.

Services-enhanced, risk-reduction residential programs

This is a vastly different approach from the abstinence-based model described above. While the services offered may be similar, they are offered to individuals who may still be using substances. The philosophy is to meet basic needs, while offering support and education to encourage the active abuser to reduce substance-abusing behaviors, or to quit entirely.

An example of this sort of housing is the Lyon Building in Seattle, Washington. This 64-unit facility serves substance abusers, the majority of whom are HIV positive, through a combination of support services. Staff at the facility know how to work with active abusers and do enforce clear rules for the residents' behavior. Although the Lyon Building uses a risk-reduction approach, each resident is still responsible for behaving in a manner that does not jeopardize other residents or harm the facility. If the rules are broken, the resident may be asked to leave the facility. This program has been welcomed by HIV/AIDS providers in the Seattle area as a means to house active abusers who could not be housed elsewhere because of poor rental histories or concerns about behaviors associated with active substance abuse.

Independent units managed by social service programs

Substance abuse treatment and HIV/AIDS agencies in some communities work to make a variety of different housing options available. The advantage of these units is that the agency can take the responsibility of securing the unit and maintaining the relationship with the housing provider. Thus, individuals who may have poor rental histories or criminal records can be given a unit through the social service agency arrangement and at the same time are given an opportunity to build a rental history. Some of the agencies may offer these units at a subsidized rate or may charge fair market value, depending on the resources of the agency. Specific services are usually not offered in the facility, but residents will have access to resources as clients with a specific agency. These units tend to be available on a time-limited basis, although in the HIV/AIDS community, where clients are now living longer, the initial premise of using these units in a temporary manner is being questioned. While clients are living longer, they may still not be in a position to earn their own living and afford adequate housing.

A client must have housing in order to receive needed social services. If the client has no stable housing, it is very difficult to maintain contact and design a plan of treatment for the client to follow. This is why so many programs have incorporated housing into the range of services they offer and why some housing providers are creating a niche for themselves in serving at-risk populations. Because of the costs and complexities in creating housing, housing providers must be aware of funding opportunities, local jurisdiction building requirements, and private/public sector possibilities.

There are specific housing funds allotted to both the HIV/AIDS community (e.g., Housing Opportunities for Persons with AIDS funds), and to the drug treatment community. In addition, innovative programs are using a combination of funds from mental health, drug treatment, and HIV/AIDS sources to create housing for dually diagnosed individuals.

Home-Based Services

A variety of home-based services are of use to clients with HIV/AIDS. These include home health care, chore services, and meal delivery.

Home health care

Home health care can be a useful resource for short-term or intermittent use. It is paid for by private insurance, Medicare, and Medicaid, but coverage varies. Clients must qualify as homebound (i.e., unable to go to a clinic to obtain services at a lesser cost). With the HIV/AIDS population, this rule has posed some problems because an individual may feel fine one day but be unable to leave home the next. Health care providers may have misperceptions about this population. There also are concerns about safety in certain neighborhoods, perceptions about lifestyles, and attitudes about substance abuse and HIV/AIDS that influence care. Education for home health workers should be undertaken to allow for fair and unbiased health care services.

Chore services

Chore services may either be professional or volunteer. Professional chore services provide in-home services such as cooking, cleaning, medication reminders, and transportation and are funded through private funds or through public programs. The availability of such services varies from State to State, and participants must pass specific eligibility requirements to obtain service. Chore service programs may have problems stemming from feelings concerning provider safety and comfort in working with an HIV-infected substance-abusing population.

Volunteer chore programs provide the same essential in-home services. Programs vary widely in how they train volunteers and the quality of services they provide, so the provider who makes the referral should know the program's limitations. Volunteer programs may not be able to offer an immediate response, and the volunteers may change, causing disruption in a client's life. Still, these programs often can help to fill gaps for service needs.

The HIV/AIDS community has been outstanding in its development of volunteer networks of care. As the pandemic moves more into substance-abusing populations, one issue in the community is the hesitation of long-time volunteers, as well as prospective new volunteers, about working with this population. The attitudinal training that has been provided to volunteers who work with gay men must also be provided to those volunteers working with HIV-infected clientele immersed in the drug culture.

Home-delivered meals

The "Meals on Wheels" model of in-home meal delivery, which has long been a resource for older homebound adults, has become available to the HIV/AIDS community. Meals are provided to those in need, but the service may require that participants' income not rise above a certain amount. The same safety and attitudinal concerns discussed in the in-home services sections above apply here. Another issue is ensuring that the meals reflect the tastes and nutritional needs of the clients. This requires that service providers understand current nutritional concepts while remaining flexible concerning the needs of the individual client. The case manager may have to advocate for changes in the menu to ensure that the client's needs are being met.

Homeless Shelters

Homeless shelters may be a necessary housing resource for providers who work with HIV-infected substance abusers. The strengths of shelters are the staff members, who usually possess a comfort level with disenfranchised populations, and the shelter's immediate accessibility and use as a short-term solution. HIV/AIDS service providers and substance abuse treatment workers are increasingly using homeless shelters as a place to provide education and to connect individuals to longer term, more stable resources.

The disadvantage of shelters is that the lack of available medical care exposes clients to other illnesses, especially tuberculosis (TB) and hepatitis. Shelters may also have limited hours of use. Many are open only at night and require people to leave in the morning, thus sending individuals back onto the street and making it difficult for a service provider to follow with needed services.

Adult Day Health

Adult day health is a useful resource for clients who need monitoring because of their health or mental state, or who face isolation. Adult day health is different from adult day care in that the former is treatment based, whereas the latter provides mostly socialization and support. Adult day health programs usually function

with a multidisciplinary team representing physical/occupational therapy, mental health, medical, and recreational therapy. The program provides a daily schedule of activities, therapies, meals and snacks, and interaction with other individuals who are experiencing similar concerns. Adult day health programs are funded by Medicaid, if the programs meet certain standards.

Finding and Funding Services

It is sometimes difficult for the HIV-infected substance abuser both to find and pay for needed services. The case manager can play an important role in helping find specific services and navigate the maze of public and private funding options.

Substance Abuse Treatment Services

Once an individual decides that she wants treatment for substance abuse, it is crucial that she be given immediate access to such treatment. Unfortunately, the substance abuse treatment community is underfunded and unable to provide adequate treatment services for all who need them. Access to treatment is particularly difficult for the working poor, who do not qualify for public programs, and chronic recidivists, who have exhausted available treatments but who still have a host of psychosocial and psychiatric needs that require intensive treatment.

Mental Health Treatment

The mental health system is also underfunded relative to the significant needs of HIV-infected substance abusers. Clients with serious mental health disorders do not always have access to the same avenues of support that are available to other substance abusers. The treatment provider should acknowledge the specific mental health issues that HIV-infected individuals often experience, so that identification of mental health concerns becomes part of the assessment process. Available mental health treatment options include support groups, volunteer peer counseling, and outpatient and inpatient therapy. (See Chapter 3 for assessment and pharmacological treatment of mental illness.)

Support groups

There are a number of different types of support groups available that operate on a community level—among them are Alcoholics Anonymous, Narcotics Anonymous, Women for Sobriety, Rational Recovery, and other self-help organizations. Chapter 4 provides a more thorough discussion of support groups.

Volunteer one-on-one emotional support

One-on-one emotional support, sometimes called peer counseling, involves the use of a trained volunteer to talk with the client and provide emotional support on an ongoing basis. This sort of counseling is not recommended for individuals with diagnosed mental health disorders. For some individuals who do not respond well to group interaction, or who cannot physically access a group, one-on-one support can be extremely useful. This peer counseling can complement support groups and therapy. The treatment provider should assess the quality of such programs and monitor for any inappropriate behavior on the part of the volunteer.

Outpatient mental health treatment

Many clients need more than volunteer, nonprofessional support, but their options can be rather limited. Managed care agencies, for example, may require clients to undergo more intense screening for admission to and continuation of services. Individuals who can pay privately have more options, although substance abusers with HIV/AIDS are not likely to have resources for these services. Both Medicare and Medicaid cover mental health treatment but require ongoing information regarding the intensity of need.

Some communities have created programs to address the need for outpatient mental health treatment. These programs maintain a list of counselors and therapists who have agreed to work with HIV-infected people at low or no cost. An AIDS case management program can provide information on the availability of such services.

Inpatient mental health treatment

If an individual is experiencing a severe mental health crisis, it may be necessary to find inpatient treatment. For example, if a client is suicidal or homicidal, or if his functioning is severely impaired, the situation is considered sufficiently *intensive* and *acute* to warrant an evaluation within an inpatient setting. In some cases, the client may have to be hospitalized involuntarily. Referrals for these services should use the words "intensive" and "acute." It is important that referring agencies be familiar with terminology from the *Diagnostic and Statistical Manual of Mental Disorders* (DSM-IV), 4th ed. (American Psychiatric Association, 1994) because managed care case managers need a diagnosis to begin assessing mental health service eligibility. Besides understanding the terminology, the provider should be able to articulate examples of the client's behavior, the duration and severity of the episode, and the impact on the client's daily functioning.

In addition, it is essential for the treatment provider to understand the intricacies of the local mental health system. The provider should know how to reach mental health professionals, understand the process for obtaining crisis services in the event of a mental health emergency, and learn what will qualify a client for different levels of service. For clients who are active substance abusers, providers may have some difficulty deciding whether behaviors are due to a mental health disorder, to substance abuse, to HIV/AIDS, or to side effects of medications. Good coordination between the substance abuse treatment specialist and the mental health provider can help with this determination.

Medical and Dental Care

In the HIV-infected population, clients can be divided into three categories: (1) those with no financial means who are considered disabled and can qualify for government assistance, (2) those with financial resources who have private disability or health insurance, and (3) those in the middle who cannot afford insurance but are not impoverished enough to qualify for government aid.

To help the working poor who cannot afford insurance, several States have created State-sponsored health plans or a Medicaid Expansion Program, which provides basic health care services to those who may not qualify for traditional Medicaid benefits. This program requires the payment of premiums and/or copayments but at rates lower than commercial plans; it also counters the increasing difficulty of obtaining individual health insurance. Most insurers favor group plans over individual plans, and while some States require insurers to provide individual plans, the cost often is prohibitive.

In some cases, social services agencies can assist patients in obtaining financial coverage for acute or emergency care. Individuals with AIDS who have a significant work history may be eligible for Social Security Disability Insurance (SSDI), which will provide Medicare benefits after 2 years. Individuals with AIDS may be eligible for Supplemental Security Income (SSI), which will also provide Medicaid coverage. Providers can also access Ryan White funds in some medical and dental cases. See TIP 29, *Substance Use Disorder Treatment for People With Physical and Cognitive Disabilities* (CSAT, 1998c),

for more information on funding options for people with disabilities (such as HIV/AIDS).

Community clinics are another option for care; they receive subsidies through Federal, State, and/or local agencies and can thus take uninsured or underinsured individuals. In addition, these clinics are staffed by individuals who know about the specific needs and concerns of low-income individuals and also may know of other community resources that could complement care.

Dental care is also important for clients and involves similar access issues. Some public funding can be obtained to help subsidize dental clinics and providers. Unfortunately, some dentists have demonstrated concern about treating HIV-infected persons because of the fear of infection. Stories of transmission occurring in dental offices have been misrepresented and have contributed to the unwillingness of providers to treat people with HIV/AIDS. However, in 1998 the U.S. Supreme Court held that under the terms of the Americans With Disabilities Act, HIV is considered a disability, making it therefore illegal for a dentist to refuse to provide care to an HIV-infected individual (*Bragdon v. Abbott*, 524 U.S. 624 [1998]).

As a provider of services, the substance abuse treatment specialist should know of medical and dental providers who will accept HIV-infected individuals, as well as the financial criteria required for obtaining care. Partnering and advocating with the public health department and community clinics may be required on a larger scale to obtain needed services.

HIV Drug Therapy

After a client has managed to obtain medical care, the next challenge is to find the means to pay for drug therapy. Persons with HIV can have multiple prescriptions, and drug costs may exceed $1,000 per month. Even individuals who have private insurance may have prohibitive copayments or restrictions on the drugs covered by the plan. Persons who rely on public insurance programs may also face such restrictions, and some public programs are moving toward a copayment system to reduce costs.

AIDS Drug Assistance Programs (ADAPs) have helped many persons with AIDS. These federally funded programs, administered by the States, have allowed persons with AIDS who are underinsured or have no insurance to obtain funding for AIDS-related drugs, including some prophylactic treatments. Unfortunately, the huge cost of combination therapy has significantly impacted the budgets of the ADAPs, and the number of clients relying on such services has increased. Several States have run out of funds before the end of their fiscal years, or have had restricted access to the funds. ADAPs have been curtailed in 23 States, and there are waiting lists for entry into the program in 9 States and specific waiting lists for protease inhibitors in 7 States. In 36 States, additional money has been added to the Federal amounts to meet the rising demand (U.S. Department of Health and Human Services [DHHS] and the Henry J. Kaiser Family Foundation, 1997). In addition, some States are expanding the program to benefit persons who are HIV positive but not yet diagnosed with AIDS in the hope that early intervention will lessen total cost.

Income and Other Financial Concerns

Financial assistance is a basic need, and obtaining resources for a client can be a challenging task. There are complex and constantly changing options for financial assistance available. Following is an overview of basic financial assistance programs. Eligibility criteria, duration of service, and amount of assistance available vary from State to State. Providers should be familiar with funding sources and should be aware of changes in these social programs.

Welfare

Welfare agencies are enforcing stricter eligibility criteria and imposing limits on the amount of time during which benefits are available. Welfare reform aims to provide enough assistance so that the individual can obtain training and move into employment. However, in reality this is not always possible. For example, States may now limit the amount of time allowed on welfare but not yet provide effective training programs to help welfare recipients become employable. Or, the training programs may not provide needed guidance in finding and maintaining a job. Or, the jobs available may not pay enough to cover child care or transportation expenses.

Welfare is available on a time-limited basis to single parents who are unemployed and to individuals whose disabilities render them unemployable. The treatment provider should help the client understand and navigate through the system of benefits, assist with the application process, explain what the limitations of the program are, and educate the client about how to maintain benefits for the period allowed. These programs usually include Medicaid coverage. For a fuller explanation of welfare reform, refer to the forthcoming TIP 38, *Integrating Substance Abuse Treatment and Vocational Services* (CSAT, in press [a]).

Unemployment Insurance

Unemployment insurance is useful for clients who have enough credits (quarters worked) to qualify. Unfortunately, many HIV-infected substance abusers do not have enough work credits to qualify. If unemployment insurance is an option, it is important that the provider discuss realistic next steps with the client. Is it the intention of the client to find another job? Is her HIV status such that applying for disability benefits might be necessary? Does the individual need vocational training to find a position that meets the needs of her situation? Because unemployment insurance is available for a limited time only, assisting the client in planning ahead can be helpful.

Disability Income

There are two types of disability income—private and public. Private disability insurance (which may be available through employers or paid privately) pays a percentage of one's salary as long as the individual remains disabled, or until the individual can find a position that may be physically possible to perform. It is important that the case manager realize that every individual disability policy is unique. The provider should encourage the client to review the policy and talk with the insurance provider about any questions.

Public disability insurance is available through Social Security (SSI and Medicare). Providers may become frustrated in working with clients whose perceived degree of disability is not enough to qualify for SSI or Medicaid. Many AIDS service organizations have financial or legal advocates who are experienced in the complexities of applying for benefits and who know how to appeal disability decisions. The treatment provider can work with these experts to strategize the appropriate next steps for the client who has been unsuccessful in obtaining disability benefits. It is important, when possible, to work with the client *before* she is rejected because it is easier to present the original case for disability than to try to overturn a negative decision. Providers should also note that although persons with HIV qualify as disabled, depending on their health, individuals whose primary "disability" is a substance abuse disorder do not qualify.

The concept of disability may also be changing for persons with AIDS. There have been some accounts of individuals whose cases have been reviewed and who have had their disability awards discontinued because of improved health. There also are accounts of more stringent screening of disability applications from persons with AIDS. As people with AIDS show improved health with new treatments, a presumption of disability may be more difficult to obtain or maintain.

Food Stamps

Food stamp programs have also been significantly revamped in some States with the advent of welfare reform and cost cutting. To qualify for food stamps, an individual must be in a low-income bracket; the amount of aid received will vary from State to State.

Vocational Rehabilitation

Longer term survival for persons with HIV has, in some cases, created a need for vocational rehabilitation. No longer facing a death sentence, persons with HIV who were unable to work are now looking to return to the work force. Organizations such as IAM CARES (International Association of Machinists Center for Administering Rehabilitation and Employment Services), which has provided traditional vocational rehabilitation services, are now targeting the HIV population with programs designed to promote reentry into the work force. For more information about vocational services for people with substance abuse disorders, see the forthcoming TIP, *Integrating Substance Abuse Treatment and Vocational Services* (CSAT, in press [a]).

Hospice Programs

Hospice programs try to provide a compassionate environment for those who are nearing death. Hospice programs are multidisciplinary, usually including a physician, nurse, social worker, and pastoral care provider to assist with the dying process. Hospice programs can be offered either in-home or in a facility setting. Many acute-care hospitals now have affiliations with hospice programs. Hospice programs are funded through Medicare, Medicaid, and private insurance, although there may be variability in the amount of care allowed or in how the hospice program allocates the funds allowed for hospice services.

Hospice services have not always been compatible with the needs of persons with HIV/AIDS because AIDS can be so erratic in its progression. There is not a predictable physical progression with AIDS, so it is difficult to know if a person will need hospice care. The advent of combination therapies has also made hospice services less necessary, as the disease becomes more chronic than terminal. Still, hospice care can be a positive experience for those in need and can be extremely supportive for family and other caregivers who are caring for a person with AIDS.

Suggestions on Finding Resources

Although some locations have all the resources discussed in this chapter, others have very few. Here are some ideas on what a provider can do if he is the only formal resource for the client with HIV:

- Mobilize friends, family, and the community for support. Church groups, for example, can help with day-to-day caregiving needs and respite. The provider may have to function as an educator within the community, especially concerning HIV/AIDS and substance abuse issues. Because of the degree of prejudice and the stigmas attached to both issues, the provider should take advantage of existing relationships within the community and build new relationships to manage community needs in these areas.

- Ask for support from other areas of the State. There may be professionals who represent more progressive services elsewhere who might be willing to come into a community and consult on ways to fund or create new resources. Public agencies that coordinate statewide HIV/AIDS care have a responsibility to ensure that all residents with HIV receive an equal level of services, and officials within such agencies may be able to assist with funds or resources. Where long distances are involved, it may be possible to establish relationships with experts who can be consulted by phone or e-mail.

- Counselors may need to suggest that the client relocate. To take advantage of options and receive the best care, a client may have to move closer to services. Clients will certainly find it difficult to leave family and friends behind, but if their health care is not adequate, relocation is a worthwhile option to consider.

7 Counseling Clients With HIV And Substance Abuse Disorders

The pandemics of substance abuse and HIV/AIDS are clearly moving along similar paths, and each continues to present unique, yet interrelated, challenges. First, both disorders are considered to be chronic—that is, lifelong diseases. Second, substance abuse is a primary risk behavior for HIV infection. Third, a diagnosis of HIV infection or related conditions can be a stressor for an individual already in recovery from a substance abuse disorder. However, the diagnosis of HIV infection may motivate a client to enter substance abuse treatment. Injection drug users who test positive for HIV are more likely to enter treatment than those who test negative (Bux et al., 1993; McCusker et al., 1994b). Also, studies have noted a reduction in risk-taking behaviors among injection drug users who test positive for HIV (Colon et al., 1996; MacGowan et al., 1997). The diagnoses of a substance abuse disorder and HIV/AIDS require extensive physical and mental health care and counseling in conjunction with extensive social services. To deal with the myriad issues surrounding substance abusers who are HIV positive, substance abuse treatment professionals must continually update their skills and knowledge as well as reexamine their own attitudes and biases.

Staff Training, Attitudes, And Issues

Before conducting any screening, assessment, or treatment planning, counselors should reassess their personal attitudes and experiences in working with HIV-infected substance abusers. This section discusses several ways in which counselors can accomplish this, including formal training within counselors' programs, examining personal attitudes (e.g., countertransference and homophobia), examining fears of infection, and avoiding burnout. It is important to reassess comfort levels with each client because each client will vary in demographic and cultural background. For instance, a service provider may feel comfortable working with a young Asian American male with a history of alcohol use, yet the same provider may not be at all comfortable with a pregnant Hispanic woman who is an active injection drug user and wishes to have her baby. Figure 7-1 provides an example of a comfort checklist for counselors to use as a routine self-evaluation.

Training

Staff members must have the proper training to screen, assess, and counsel clients. Achieving

> ## Figure 7-1
> ## Self-Inventory Comfort Scale
>
> Listed below are several situations in which a caregiver may find herself while working with a substance-abusing client. Rate your comfort level in response to each situation, with "1" being *least* comfortable and "5" being *most* comfortable.
>
> ___Conducting an assessment of a client's substance abuse history.
>
> ___Confronting a client who differs from your own race or ethnicity about his substance abuse.
>
> ___Working with a substance-abusing client who is gay or lesbian.
>
> ___Differentiating between depression, anxiety, delirium, psychosis, and substance abuse disorders.
>
> ___Demonstrating the proper way to disinfect drug injection equipment.
>
> ___Counseling an HIV-infected female client who is pregnant and actively using substances.
>
> ___Referring a substance-abusing client to a local syringe exchange program.
>
> ___Accompanying a client to an open meeting of Narcotics Anonymous (NA).
>
> ___Confronting a colleague on his suspected substance abuse.
>
> ___Advocating that an HIV-infected client with a history of substance abuse be placed on HIV combination therapy.
>
> ___Supporting a non–substance-abusing client with HIV/AIDS who is considering using marijuana to help curb nausea and increase appetite.
>
> ___Confronting a client who is actively putting others at risk.
>
> ___Confronting a client whom you believe is not adhering to a medication regimen but who claims to be.

staff competency is an ongoing process. The complexities related to people with HIV/AIDS and substance abuse disorders are constantly changing and do not allow staff members to defer learning or training or even to maintain a "status quo" attitude about their competency.

Examples of methods to help staff grow in the areas of assessment, screening, and treatment planning include the following (see also the section "Cultural Competency Issues" later in this chapter):

- *Model skills and competencies.* Less experienced staff can observe supervisors or more tenured staff who demonstrate desired qualities.
- *Peer training and feedback.* Peer teams can provide feedback through direct observation of staff members' interactions with clients, as well as review of staff members' client charts.

- *Case presentations.* Weekly or monthly group case presentations conducted by a different staff member each time can be effective for building skills and monitoring quality. Case simulation, in which each staff member has an opportunity to ask the "client" a question, is a highly useful training tool. At the end of the presentation, everyone attending can provide feedback about the activity.
- *Experiential skills-building exercises.* Many activities can be used to sensitize staff to the client's experiences. Activities can include encouraging staff members to go to a confidential and anonymous HIV/AIDS test site, or anonymously sit in the waiting room of the local food stamp office, HIV/AIDS clinic, or county jail. Staff must use different avenues to maintain a keen sensitivity to and awareness of the client's issues.

■ *Assessment instruments.* Use specific assessment tools, such as substance abuse and sexual history questionnaires (e.g., the Addiction Severity Index [ASI]).

■ *Formal conferences, training, consultations with clinicians.* Often agency budgets are tight, and the first expense to be cut is staff development. This is a major problem for many programs. Programs must establish that improvement and excellence are serious goals and that attending treatment-oriented conferences is a part of building staff competency and moving toward these goals.

Attitudes

It is important that counselors be aware of any of their own attitudes that might interfere with helping a client. By learning to put aside personal judgments and focus on client needs, staff members can build trust and rapport with the client. When a counselor can deal with a client in a sensitive, empathic manner, there is a much greater chance that both will have a positive and successful encounter.

Countertransference is a set of thoughts, feelings, and beliefs experienced by a service provider that occurs in response to the client. Although sometimes these beliefs and feelings are conscious, generally they are not. It is thus unrealistic to expect counselors, usually untrained in addressing unconscious mental processing, to be aware of countertransference. Regular clinical supervision, which should be integrated into the staffing of the program, can help raise their awareness. If such resources exist, counselors may, with caution, address this issue.

In order to deal with countertransference issues, counselors must be willing to examine their skills and attitudes. Working with clients who have HIV/AIDS and substance abuse disorders brings up issues for treatment staff that can be both physically and emotionally demanding. Counselors see a broad range of diverse clients from all walks of life. To work in both these fields, providers must learn to be comfortable in discussing topics they may never have talked about openly—sex, drug use, death, grief, and so on. To effect positive change, counselors also must be willing to seek additional specialized training and support.

Examining attitudes and skills

Countertransference can manifest itself in many different ways. The key to seeing countertransference issues is awareness and consciousness-raising. The commitment to "do no harm" to clients and their families, along with a desire to provide quality services, should be the driving forces for willingly examining these issues.

Following are some common countertransference issues for providers working with substance abusers who are HIV positive (adapted from National Association of Social Workers, 1997):

■ Fear of contagion
■ Fear of the unknown
■ Fear of death, dying, grief, and loss
■ Stigmatization (e.g., of people with mental health problems, "addicts," people who are HIV positive, homosexuals)
■ Powerlessness, helplessness, and loss of control
■ Shame and guilt
■ Homophobia
■ Anger, rage, and hostility
■ Frustration
■ Overidentification
■ Denial
■ Differences in culture, race, class, and lifestyle
■ Fantasies of professional omnipotence
■ Burnout
■ Measures of success and personal reward

Issues

Homophobia

To be aware of homophobic responses among treatment professionals and of their own countertransference issues, it is important that counselors understand how the client is handling his homosexuality. The counselor should understand the possible link between substance abuse and gay or lesbian identity formation. Substance abuse can be an easy relief, can provide acceptance, and, more important, can mirror the "comforting" dissociation developed in childhood. The "symptom-relieving" aspects of substance abuse help fight the effects of homophobia; substance abuse can allow "forbidden" behavior, allow social comfort in bars or other unfamiliar social settings and provide comfort just from the dissociative state itself. For example, some men have their first homosexual sexual experience while drinking or being drunk. This connection is a very powerful behavioral link—the pleasure and release of substance abuse with the pleasure and release of sex—and is very difficult to change or "unlink" later in life.

In regard to the issue of homophobia, it is also critical to understand how stereotypes affect the treatment options offered. The professional should take an inventory of these stereotypes to assess her homophobia potential and should be aware of the roles countertransference can play. The short assessment tool provided in Figure 7-2 can be used to examine where providers and clients alike might rank on a continuum of homophobic

---

Figure 7-2
Homophobia Questionnaire for Counselors and Clients

- Do you ever stop yourself from doing or saying certain things because someone might think you are gay or lesbian? What kinds of things?
- Do you ever intentionally do or say things so that people will think you're not gay/lesbian? What kinds of things?
- Do you think that lesbians or gays can influence others to become homosexual?
- Do you think someone could influence you to change your sexual orientation?
- If you are a parent, how would you (or do you) feel about having a lesbian daughter or gay son?
- How do you think you would feel if you discovered that one of your parents, a parent figure, or a brother or sister were gay or lesbian?
- Are there any jobs, positions, or professions that you think gays and lesbians should be barred from holding or entering? Which ones and why?
- Would you go to a physician whom you knew or believed to be gay or lesbian if he or she were a different gender from you? If he or she were the same gender as you? If not, why not?
- If someone you cared about said to you, "I think I'm lesbian or gay," would you suggest that the person see a therapist?
- Have you ever been to a gay or lesbian social club, party, bar, or sporting event? If not, why not?
- Would you wear a button that says, "How dare you assume that I'm heterosexual?" If not, why not?
- Can you think of three positive aspects of a lesbian or gay lifestyle? Can you think of three negative aspects of a heterosexual lifestyle?
- Have you ever laughed at or told a "queer" joke?

reactions. This tool is also useful in group supervision sessions or discussions with both gay/lesbian and heterosexual colleagues.

It is important that counselors have a working knowledge of some of the terminology and definitions pertaining to homophobia. Following is a brief list of terms and definitions.

- *Overt homophobia* includes violence, verbal abuse, and name-calling.
- *Institutional homophobia* describes the way in which governments, businesses, schools, churches, and other institutions and organizations treat people differently and less favorably based on their sexual orientation.
- *Cultural homophobia* includes social standards and norms requiring heterosexuality.
- *Internalized homophobia* is acceptance and integration by lesbians and gays of the negative attitudes expressed by society toward them.
- *Heterosexism* is the system of advantages bestowed on heterosexuals. It is the institutional form of homophobia that assumes all people are or should be heterosexual and therefore excludes the needs, concerns, and life experiences of lesbians, gays, and bisexuals.
- *Coming out* may possibly be the most important part of gay and lesbian development. This is the process, often lifelong, in which a person acknowledges, accepts, and in many cases appreciates his or her own lesbian, gay, bisexual, or transgender identity. This often involves sharing this information with others. Family members of gay and lesbian individuals go through a similar process.
- *Oppression* is the systematic subjugation of a particular social group by another group with access to social and political power, by withholding access to that power.
- *Lesbian/gay baiting* involves actions or words that imply or state that the presence of a gay

man or lesbian hurts or discredits a social system. The purpose is to hurt, demean, intimidate, or control, and to stop social change or acceptance of lesbians and gays within the social system.

These definitions can help the counselor become aware of the added layer of discrimination felt by gay men and lesbians in treatment for HIV/AIDS and a substance abuse disorder. Following is a list of some "Do's" to keep in mind when working with homosexual clients (adapted from Storms, 1994).

- Identify the lesbian/gay client's strengths and accept them as you find them.
- Listen empathically and refrain from making judgments about the client's lifestyle.
- Remain aware of the client's sexual orientation and the possible effects of this orientation on the client's experience and world-view.
- Explore the client's sexual practices with an eye toward internalized homophobia.
- Be aware of your own preference and mindful of possible homophobia or confusion in your own sexual identity.
- Be knowledgeable about compulsive sexual behavior and sexual practices in the lesbian/gay community.
- Ask your lesbian/gay clients what terms they prefer when discussing their sexual orientation and those of others.
- Encourage self-empowerment, consciousness-raising, and participation in the lesbian and gay community.
- Encourage your program to hire openly lesbian and gay counselors/therapists.
- Educate others about internalized homophobia and heterosexism. Be gay- and lesbian-affirming rather than just gay- and lesbian-tolerant.
- Stay abreast of current information on resources and display this information in your office. Attend seminars and

professional workshops about working with lesbian and gay clients.

Fear of infection

Fear of infection is one of the most challenging issues for counselors. It is essential that providers examine this issue without blaming or judging themselves and others. Most professionals who work with substance abusers and HIV-positive individuals have thought about becoming infected with HIV, hepatitis, or tuberculosis (TB) through their jobs (Sherman and Ouellette, 1999). Some fear that scientists are not aware of modes of infection or transmission that might put service providers and their families at greater risk of infection (Montgomery and Lewis, 1995). The key to dealing with this fear is to discuss it and vent the feelings with someone who is safe, trusted, and informed, *and* to practice universal precautions at all times.

Beyond this, it is essential for providers to have regular and frequent inservice training with updates on the latest research and data about transmission and treatment of HIV/AIDS, hepatitis, and TB.

Special considerations for counselors who treat HIV-infected clients

The challenges and stresses related to working with people with HIV/AIDS are in some ways unique. The fact that providers often deal with multiple and serial losses and see clients suffering on a daily basis clearly affects the providers' psychological health. In recent years, therapists have begun to examine and assess these service providers for symptoms of posttraumatic stress disorder (PTSD).

Burnout often is referred to as "bereavement overload." One definition characterizes burnout as lowered energy, enthusiasm, and idealism for doing one's job, that is, as a loss of concern for the people served and for the work (Hayter,

1999). Unlike fatigue, burnout does not resolve after a given amount of rest and recreation.

Burnout prevention and stress management techniques should be used both in the work setting and in counselors' personal lives. Working with HIV-infected substance abusers requires agencies and individuals to be more creative and flexible in finding new and different ways to support and nurture counselors to prevent burnout. Agencies that have taken on this challenge with integrity and commitment have seen highly effective staff function at optimal levels for many years.

Suggestions for ways in which agencies can take care of counselors at work include

- Assigning clearly specific duties
- Having clear boundaries on professional obligations
- Enlisting volunteer help from community organizations
- Allowing for "time out" activities
- Varying tasks and responsibilities
- Building in "mental health days"
- Providing for continuing education
- Holding staff retreats (with enjoyable activities planned)
- Holding discussion, process, and support groups
- Convening regular staff/team supervision meetings

In addition, it is important that agencies allocate time to discuss the deaths and losses faced by staff. This may mean supporting special memorial events at which those who have been lost to HIV/AIDS disease can be remembered. Agencies also can support staff through contracts with employee assistance program therapists and by providing an onsite therapeutic support group for staff members to attend as they wish.

Screening

Client-Specific Needs

A positive screen for HIV infection typically leads to a referral for formal assessment, usually to an HIV/AIDS case management service. Frequently, substance abuse treatment programs provide referrals to HIV/AIDS care services. Providers will want to identify substance abuse treatment programs and agencies with these networks. At a minimum, services should include the following client needs in priority order:

- Substance abuse treatment
- Medical care
- Housing
- Mental health care
- Nutritional care
- Dental care
- Ancillary services
- Support systems

Discussion of some of these needs appears below.

Interim substance abuse treatment for clients on waiting lists

Because of an insufficient number of substance abuse treatment slots, clients often must wait for treatment. Risk-reduction efforts can be made, however, while the client is waiting for substance abuse treatment.

If substance abuse treatment slots remain unavailable, alcohol and drug counselors should refer clients who need medical care to primary medical care services. Clients who display more acute symptoms or conditions should probably be referred to an emergency department. However, emergency department care typically is limited to wound care and provision of nutritional supplements. Clients who do not have acute symptoms or conditions but need medical care should be referred for primary medical care, either to their own physicians or to primary medical care clinics or services.

Primary medical care

Primary medical care should consist of a comprehensive physical exam, treatment for HIV/AIDS (e.g., combination therapy), and treatment for opportunistic infections. In particular, chronic substance use can result in significant weight loss, lack of appetite, poor digestion, substandard elimination, kidney and liver dysfunction, and weakened immune system functioning. See Chapter 2 for more information about medical care of clients with HIV/AIDS.

Mental health care

A diagnosis of mental illness may reflect the client's affective and mood responses to this medical judgment, may be a consequence of self-medication, or may reflect neurological complications of HIV/AIDS, as well as an underlying mental health disorder. Mental health care should consist of both a neuropsychiatric workup and full mental health status examinations (see Chapter 3). Service providers should be alert to and notify clients and psychiatrists that complications may arise from the use of prescription medication for mental health problems and interactions between drug residue in the body and medications for HIV/AIDS and opportunistic infections.

Nutritional care

Substance-abusing clients living with HIV/AIDS are typically mal- or undernourished because of street lifestyles, the effects of HIV disease, and the physical effects of substance abuse. This combination typically results in diminished appetite, weight loss (especially of lean muscle mass), poor hygiene, immune suppression, protein deficiencies, vitamin and mineral exhaustion, and anemia. In addition, providers should be aware that apparent lack of nutrition is not associated with digestive disease or parasites.

Good nutrition is a fundamental part of overall medical care. It improves strength, energy, longevity, and quality of life; increases muscle mass and body weight; decreases likelihood of hospitalization and length of stay; and slows progression of HIV to AIDS.

Without adequate nutrition, HIV/AIDS clients can easily develop malnutrition. Various causes of malnutrition and weight loss include

- Inadequate intake of food
- Anorexia
- Malabsorption of food
- Altered metabolism
- Food and drug interactions
- Androgen deficiency
- No cooking facilities
- Limited income
- Reliance on community food programs

With the onset of malnutrition, the client loses weight and experiences several body composition changes. *Starvation* results in loss of body fat and muscle. *Wasting syndrome* produces a loss of a serious percentage of body weight, with accompanying diarrhea and fever, and has been considered a defining symptom of AIDS since 1987. The degree of loss of lean body mass can indicate the length of time that the client has left to live.

Lipodystrophy syndrome

Lipodystrophy syndrome occurs in early end-stage AIDS and produces altered body composition and various hormonal and physiological changes. The cause of the syndrome and its relationship with HIV and protease inhibitors are unknown. Because of the disfiguring nature of some symptoms, lipodystrophy can be particularly distressing for women. Symptoms include

- Redistribution of body fat
- Increase in waist size
- Thinning of the arms and legs
- Increased facial wrinkling
- Weakness and muscle wasting
- Gastrointestinal symptoms
- Increased triglycerides and cholesterol
- Decreased testosterone levels
- Hypertension
- Diabetes

To determine body composition changes, provider staff should recommend that clients be measured on a bioelectrical impedance analysis machine. This noninvasive machine sends a weak electrical current through electrodes placed on the client's hands and feet to measure fluid volume, blood cell mass, extracellular mass, and level of body fat. Repeated every 3 to 6 months, this procedure can provide an accurate gauge of the client's biophysiological status.

Providers can treat weight loss and malnutrition by prescribing a nutritious, balanced diet with plenty of fluids and a daily multivitamin, if needed. Protein and calorie supplements are recommended if the client is losing weight. The client should avoid toxic substances such as alcohol, tobacco, and recreational drugs and should practice a daily routine of moderate exercise. Pharmaceutical interventions that may be required include appetite stimulants, thalidomide, and growth hormones.

Treatment staff should also discuss integrative therapies with the client. These can include herbs, acupuncture, meditation, massage, yoga, chiropractic, homeopathic medicine, megadosing, tai chi, qigong, and various religious practices.

Dental care

Substance-abusing clients typically have poor histories of routine dental care, which can lead to extreme physical pain and incapacitation. Persons living with HIV/AIDS usually require extensive dental care, up to and including tooth extraction, jawline reconstruction, and dental plate replacement.

Ancillary services

The steady increase in the number of women living with HIV/AIDS is creating a great demand for ancillary services such as child care, housing, and transportation. Families needing housing may face long waiting lists for Section 8 housing or may receive Section 8 certificates only to find few landlords willing to accept Section 8 housing payments. Another concern for substance abusers, whether currently using or in recovery, is the fact that most low-cost housing tends to be in areas known for high drug traffic and crime.

Disclosure Issues

Disclosure issues are difficult for all HIV-infected clients. For substance-abusing clients, these issues take on additional challenges. For example, disclosure of positive HIV status may lead to personal threats or harm to both client and family. A client's family may refuse to associate with him upon learning of his HIV/AIDS status. Particularly for clients whose culture reflects definition of self within a community or self in relation to a clan (as opposed to individual definition), separation from community can serve as a trigger for lapse or relapse into risky substance use and sex-related behaviors. Therefore, providers must use caution when notifying clients of test results and should comply with regulations to ensure that a client's confidentiality is preserved. Providers should refer to Chapter 9 for guidance in this area.

Also, during group therapy clients often feel an obligation to reveal their HIV status to the rest of the group. Counselors should caution clients about the impact of such disclosure and consider discouraging them from making it.

Clients who wish to disclose their HIV status generally do so in response to treatment themes of honesty and openness and are not completely aware of the consequences. Of course, in treatment settings where all patients are HIV positive, there is no need for this concern.

HIV/AIDS-Specific Substance Abuse Counseling Issues

There are many counseling issues specific to HIV/AIDS that providers should be familiar with when treating HIV-infected, substance-abusing clients.

Cultural Competency Issues

Culture is the integrated pattern of human behavior that includes thoughts, speech, actions, and artifacts. Culture depends on the capacity of humans for learning and transmitting knowledge to succeeding generations. It takes into account the customs, beliefs, social norms, and material traits of a racial, religious, or social group. With this type of definition, it is easy to see that there is indeed a culture of addiction, a culture of poverty, a gay culture, and even a recovery culture.

Cross and colleagues present a comprehensive discussion of culturally competent systems of care. Five essential elements contribute to cultural competence (Cross et al., 1989, pp. 19–21), which can briefly be described as follows:

1. **Valuing diversity.** Counselors value diversity when they accept that the people they serve come from very different backgrounds and may make different choices based on culture. Although all people share common basic needs, there are vast differences in how people go about meeting those needs. Accepting the fact that each culture finds some behaviors, actions,

or values more important or desirable than others helps workers interact more successfully with different people.

2. **Cultural self-assessment.** When counselors understand how systems of care are shaped by dominant cultures, it may be easier for them to assess how these systems interface with other cultures. Care providers can then choose actions that minimize cross-cultural barriers.

3. **Dynamics of difference.** When cultural systems interact, both representatives (e.g., care provider and client) may misjudge the other's actions based on history and learned expectations. Both will bring dynamics of difference—culturally prescribed patterns of communication, etiquette, and problemsolving, as well as underlying feelings about serving or being served by someone who is different. Incorporating an understanding of these dynamics and their origins into the system enhances chances for productive cross-cultural interventions.

4. **Institutionalization of cultural knowledge.** Workers must have accurate cultural knowledge and information or access to such information. They also must have available to them community contacts and consultants to answer culturally related questions.

5. **Adaptations to diversity.** The previous four elements build a context for a cross-culturally competent system of care and service. Both workers' and systems' approaches can be adapted to create a better fit between needs of people and services available. For instance, members of certain ethnic groups repeatedly receive negative messages from the media about their culture. Programs can be developed that incorporate alternative culturally enhancing experiences, develop problemsolving skills, and teach about the origins of stereotypes and prejudice. By creating and

implementing such programs, workers can begin to institutionalize cultural interventions as a legitimate helping approach.

Finally, becoming culturally competent is a developmental process for individual counselors.

> It is not something that happens because one reads a book, or attends a workshop, or happens to be a member of a minority group. It is a process born of a commitment to provide quality services to all and a willingness to risk. (Cross et al., 1989, p. 21)

Making culturally competent decisions

Treatment providers and counselors must examine two essential factors when working with culturally, racially, or ethnically different populations: the socioeconomic status of the client or group and the client's degree of acculturation. A distinction should be made when discussing a population as a whole and a particular segment of that population. For example, when treating an HIV-infected substance-abusing Hispanic woman, the counselor should focus on the woman as an individual and on the particular circumstances of this individual's life, rather than seeing her as an abstract representative of her culture or race. More often, poverty is the relevant issue to be discussed, rather than specific ethnic or racial factors (Centers for Disease Control and Prevention [CDC], 1998j).

The second factor, degree of acculturation, is important and should be part of the assessment process. How acculturated or assimilated are the family and client? What generation is this client? Assessing for this, and knowing that several generations with different values and levels of acculturation may all live in one household, can test the communication skills and counseling skills of the best service providers. When discussing acculturation/assimilation and values, counselors should keep in mind that, in general, the more years a family has lived in the United States, the less traditional their values tend to be. Thus a fourth-generation Chinese-American client may not speak Chinese or hold traditional Chinese values. Knowing the values and beliefs of a client is crucial if treatment is to be effective.

Providers must also help develop culturally competent systems of care. A part of this is making services accessible to and often used by the target risk populations. Culturally competent systems also recognize the importance of culture, cross-cultural

relationships, cultural differences, and the ability to meet culturally unique needs (Cross et al., 1989).

Aside from assessing cultural competence using the five elements discussed previously, it also is helpful to examine some ways in which providers can minimize cultural clashes and blocks that may exist when working with clients. The guidelines given in Figure 7-3 are adapted from a project conducted by the University of Hawaii AIDS Education Project.

One concern in providing culturally competent care is how to discuss values

Figure 7-3
Guidelines To Minimize Cultural Clashes

1. Plan to spend more time with clients holding values different from yours. The relationship is more complex, and it may take longer to establish trust.
2. Anticipate that past frustrations with insensitive or inappropriate providers may have made the client angry, suspicious, and resentful.
3. Acknowledge past frustrations.
4. Acknowledge the difference between your own experience and that of the client's.
5. Individualize (the clear message of all treatment planning)—a client is more than an "addict," an Asian, or a person with HIV/AIDS. Get to know the whole person.
6. Encourage disagreement and negotiation to ensure a workable plan.
7. Anticipate multiple needs: medical, legal, social, and psychological.
8. Be prepared to advocate for the client who may not have the resources, knowledge, or experience to negotiate the HIV/AIDS and substance abuse services systems.
9. Assist the client in getting other resources.
10. Involve friends and family. This can help ensure that the client receives other needed services.
11. Pay attention to communication: nonverbal, expressive style, and word usage and meaning.
12. Make use of providers from other cultures.
13. Learn the strengths of a culture. In Hispanic culture, for example, the value of "respeto," demonstrating appropriate social respect, can be used to support an intervention plan.
14. Expect differences in beliefs about

    ♦ Help-seeking behaviors
    ♦ Caretaking/caregiving
    ♦ Cause of disease/illness
    ♦ Sexuality/homosexuality
    ♦ Death and dying
    ♦ Making eye contact and touching

Source: University of Hawaii AIDS Education Project.

and differences around sex and sexuality. In many cultures, people avoid discussing sex because they find such discussions disrespectful. This is one reason why so many cultures avoid discussing homosexuality. A counselor should consider using a less direct approach when initiating discussion about issues related to sex and sexual orientation. Many providers believe that some of the public health problems faced in communities of color and the gay community are related to their inability to speak often and directly enough about safer sex practices, risky behaviors, and homosexuality. Even in the recovery culture and in many treatment settings, sex and sexuality are blatantly avoided. Service providers must acknowledge that they, too, in addition to their clients, are often uncomfortable talking about sexuality, sexual identity, and sexual orientation.

Providers also should be aware of the messages often given to communities of color and particularly women. The message, "stop having sex," often advocated by providers has been mixed with historical issues and fears of racial/ethnic genocide, thus making it difficult for most groups to give any credence to those expounding this method of reducing HIV/AIDS. The value of sex and procreation in many cultures makes it difficult for someone

from outside the client's culture, especially someone of a different gender, to tell people to not have sex or to have sex only with a condom.

Finally, it is important that the counselor recognize that much of what is asked of clients and their families is personal and private. Questions related to sex, dying, and substance abuse are not usual topics of conversation, and when asking these questions, the counselor crosses many boundaries. It often is considered disrespectful (and offensive to certain cultural values) to ask questions about these specific areas. One wise way to broach these subjects with clients, especially clients who are significantly older than the provider or from a more traditional culture, is to simply apologize

The most practical advice is for providers to (1) maintain an open mind, (2) use cultural consultants for training and support, and (3) when in doubt, defer to the concepts of health and stability over pathology and dysfunction.

Figure 7-4 presents the LEARN model developed by Berlin and Fowkes, an excellent cross-cultural communication tool that can be useful in all client encounters, especially with clients who are culturally different from the provider and who have HIV/AIDS and substance abuse disorders.

Figure 7-4
The LEARN Model

L—Listen with empathy and understanding. Ask the client, "What do you feel may be causing the problem? How does this affect you?"

E—Elicit cultural information, explain your perception of the problem, have a strategy, and convey it to the client.

A—Acknowledge and discuss differences and similarities. Find areas of agreement and point out areas of potential conflicts so they can be discussed, understood, and resolved.

R—Recommend action, treatment, and intervention. Incorporate cultural knowledge to enhance acceptability of the plan.

N—Negotiate agreements and differences. Develop a partnership with the client and the family.

Source: Berlin and Fowkes, 1983.

Special Populations

Gay, lesbian, bisexual, and transgender populations

Providers wishing to serve the needs of particular ethnic or cultural groups have learned that communities must be understood, respected, and consulted in order to make effective interventions; this also holds true when working with gay men, lesbians, and bisexual men and women. This population is defined not by traditionally understood cultural and ethnic minority criteria, but by having a sexual orientation that differs from that of the majority. Transgender people also form a unique population, often linked to gay men, lesbians, and bisexuals, although they differ from the majority by gender identification rather than sexual orientation.

Until recently, there has been no solid agreement about the amount of substances used or the incidence of substance abuse in the gay, lesbian, bisexual, or transgender populations. Most studies (Beatty, 1983; Diamond and Wilsnack, 1978; Lewis et al., 1982; Lohrenz et al., 1978; McKirman and Peterson, 1989; Mosbacher, 1988; Pillard, 1989; Saghir and Robins, 1973), reports (Fifield et al., 1975; Lesbian and Gay Substance Abuse Planning Group, 1991), reviews of surveys (Morales and Graves, 1983; Weinberg and Williams, 1974) and the experiences of most clinicians working with gay men and lesbians (Cabaj, 1989; Finnegan and McNally, 1987) have estimated an incidence of substance abuse of all types at approximately 30 percent, with ranges of 28 to 35 percent (contrasting with an incidence of 10 to 12 percent for the general population). The CDC's biannual report on HIV/AIDS clearly indicates a subgroup of gay and male bisexual injection drug users, and one of the routes of HIV infection for lesbians is via IDU.

A careful review of these reports, however, has demonstrated significant and persistent methodological problems, ranging from poor or absent control groups and nonrepresentative population samples (some studies gathered subjects only from gay and lesbian bars) to a failure to use uniform definitions of substance abuse or of homosexuality itself. Nevertheless, a recent study was conducted using data from the 1996 National Household Survey of Drug Abuse (NHSDA), a yearly population-based survey that applies standard epidemiological methods to determine the prevalence of substance use in the U.S. population. This study has concluded that homosexually active women are indeed more likely than heterosexually active women to evidence drug or alcohol dependency (Cochran and Mays, in press).

A sudden increase in the use of methamphetamine, known as "speed," "crystal," "ice," or "crank," by gay and bisexual men has become a matter of grave concern. A primary route of administration for this drug is injection. Combined with its disinhibiting and sexually stimulating effects, gay male injectors of methamphetamine are at extremely high risk for HIV exposure: The drug causes the abuser to suspend all judgment and leaves him often impotent but extremely sexually aroused and often an anal-receptive partner in sex (Gorman, 1996; Gorman et al., 1995).

Men who have sex with men (or MSMs—the CDC category used to report its data) may self-identify as gay (men with homosexual sexual orientations), bisexual (men who feel sexually drawn to both men and women), or heterosexual (men having sex with men as a purely physical act and not a reflection of innate sexual orientation). No matter what their sexual orientation, unprotected sexual contact puts MSMs at risk for HIV. In most reviews of gay men and safer sex practices, most men who were knowledgeable about safer sex failed to practice it while under the influence of some substance (Calzavara et al., 1993; Leigh, 1990; Leigh and Stall, 1993; Paul et al., 1994; Stall,

1987; Stall et al., 1986). Many men from minority backgrounds who have sex with other men do not self-identify as gay or bisexual, so interventions should be based not on sexual orientation, but on sexual behavior.

Some women who have sex with women continue to have sex with men. A number of these women may be injection drug users and share syringes; consequently, they are prone to HIV infection. Although it is unlikely that female-to-female transmission of the virus will occur, lesbians have been urged to use safer sex precautions, such as using dental dams during oral sex (White, 1997).

Lesbians present some specific issues that must be highlighted. Compared with gay men, they are more likely to have lower incomes (as do women in general when compared with men); are more likely to be parents (about one-third of lesbians are biological parents); face prejudice as women as well as for being gay, including the stronger reaction against and willingness to ignore females with substance abuse disorders; are more likely to come out later in life (about 28 years of age versus 18 years of age in men); and are more likely to have bisexual feelings or experiences, so that they are still at sexual risk for HIV infection as well as possible IDU risk (Banks and Gartrell, 1996; Bell et al., 1981; Bradford and Ryan, 1987; Mosbacher, 1993).

Gay youth also present treatment challenges. Special sensitivity and understanding are needed to work with youth of any background, especially youth who are gay or lesbian or from an ethnic minority background. Young gay males in particular may be subjected to harassment at home or school, and they are prone to alcohol use, dropping out of school, running away, and getting involved in sex for drugs or money (Ku et al., 1992; Rotheram-Borus et al., 1995; Savin-Williams, 1994). Many young gay male streetworkers abuse

amphetamines, "tweaking" to have a sexual experience, and may exchange sex for drugs.

In general, gay men, lesbians, bisexuals, and transgender people are wary of the medical establishment and may resist seeking health care, distrust the advice given, or question the treatment plan suggested if the provider displays evidence of homophobia or heterosexism.

Transgender individuals

Some substance abuse treatment clients are transgender. The following definitions have been provided to clarify the confusion some providers may feel when working with transgender clients (CSAT, in press [b]).

Transgender people are a diverse group of individuals who cross or transcend culturally defined categories of gender. They can include the following:

- Male-to-female (MTF) and female-to-male (FTM) *transsexuals*—those who desire or have had hormone therapy or sex reassignment surgery
- *Cross-dressers* or *transvestites*—those who desire to wear clothing associated with another sex
- *Transgenderists*—those who live in the gender role associated with another sex without desiring sex reassignment surgery
- *Bigender persons*—those who identify as both man and woman
- *Drag queens* and *kings*—usually gay men and lesbian women who "do drag" and dress up in, respectively, women's and men's clothing
- *Female* and *male impersonators*—males who impersonate women and females who impersonate men, usually for entertainment

Gender identification is different from sexual orientation. *Gender identity* refers to a person's basic conviction of being male, female, or transgender. *Sexual orientation* refers to sexual attraction to others (men, women, or transgender persons). For example, many cross-dressers are heterosexual men who have active sexual relationships with women. Many homosexual men, although historically considered effeminate, identify strongly as men and appear very masculine.

Substance use plays a significant role in the high HIV prevalence in MTF transgender individuals (Longshore et al., 1993, 1998). One study that investigated 519 transgender individuals in San Francisco found high rates of substance abuse among both MTF and FTM individuals (Clements et al., 1998). The study reported that 55 percent of the MTF sample indicated they had been in substance abuse treatment at some time during their lifetime. The study also found that HIV prevalence was significantly higher among MTF individuals (35 percent) than FTM individuals (2 percent), and among the MTF individuals, HIV prevalence for African Americans was 61 percent. Although the HIV prevalence rate was low in the FTM individuals, they commonly reported engaging in many of the same HIV risk behaviors as the MTF individuals (Clements et al., 1998). Counseling transgender individuals who are HIV positive and in substance abuse treatment can involve many different issues. Some of these issues are obvious: lack of family and social supports, isolation, low self-esteem, and internalized transphobia, to name a few. Some issues are not so obvious; for example, transgender clients currently undergoing hormone therapy often experience emotional and physical changes that can make treatment for substance abuse more difficult and relapse more likely. Although medically managed hormone treatment should not be interrupted, both the clinician and client must be aware that estrogen and testosterone therapies are mind- and mood-altering substances, particularly when incorrectly taken. Improper administration of estrogen mimics the premenstrual symptoms of nontranssexual women, which can have a deleterious effect on recovery (CSAT, in press [b]). These premenstrual symptoms can trigger or exacerbate Post Acute Withdrawal Syndrome, which is believed to be the leading cause of relapse.

Additional relapse triggers or clinical issues may include the following: (1) inability to find, engage in, or maintain gainful employment due to employer prejudice against transgender individuals; (2) lack of formal education or training because the client was forced to leave school or home before completing his or her education; (3) the fact that HIV-positive transgender clients may be denied sex reassignment surgery due to their HIV status, even if they are asymptomatic and healthy; and (4) the general lack of substance-free role models and widespread social support for transgender individuals.

Clinicians, particularly those in rural areas, may have had little experience in treating transgender clients. Figure 7-5 lists some guidelines that clinicians may find helpful in working with this population. Some resources providers may also find helpful include the Lambda Center in Washington, D.C. (202-965-8434), which provides behavioral healthcare programs for transgender clients and others with HIV/AIDS and substance abuse problems, and the Center Gender Identity Project in New York City (212-620-7310), which provides HIV/AIDS and substance abuse counseling and referral services exclusively for transgender clients.

Women

The needs of women have always represented a unique challenge to health care and substance abuse treatment systems. Traditionally, these challenges have not been well met and are being exacerbated by the growing number of substance-abusing women infected with HIV. The diseases of substance abuse and HIV/AIDS

Figure 7-5	
Guidelines for Working With Transgender Clients	
Do	**Don't**
■ Use the pronouns based on their *self-identity* when speaking to or about transgender individuals. ■ Obtain clinical supervision if you have reservations about working with transgender individuals. ■ Allow transgender clients to continue the use of hormones when prescribed; advocate for the transgender client who is using "street" or illegally prescribed hormones to receive immediate medical care and legally prescribed hormones. ■ Ensure that all clinic staff receive training on transgender issues. ■ Ascertain a transgender client's sexual orientation before treating him or her. ■ Allow transgender clients to use appropriate bathrooms and showers based on their *gender self-identity and gender role.* ■ Require all clients and staff to create and maintain a hospitable environment for all transgender clients. Post a nondiscrimination policy, including sexual orientation and gender identity, in the waiting room.	■ Call someone who identifies as female "he" or "him," or someone who identifies as male "she" or "her." ■ Make transphobic comments to other staff or clients. ■ Ask the transgender client to choose between hormone therapy or substance abuse treatment. ■ Leave it to the transgender client to educate clinic staff. ■ Assume all transgender individuals are gay. ■ Force transgender clients identifying as male to use female facilities; likewise, don't force those identifying as female to use male facilities.

present differently in women than in men and progress at different rates for a variety of reasons, including the fact that women usually present later in the HIV/AIDS disease process than men.

Gender-specific services for women should include the following:

■ Medical and substance abuse treatment that is accessible, available, and incorporates
  ♦ General health (including reproductive health) and wellness across the life span
  ♦ Mental health counseling (particularly for PTSD)
  ♦ Parenting skills and support
  ♦ Family-focused support

  ♦ Relationship issues
  ♦ Trauma/abuse support
  ♦ Educational/vocational services
  ♦ Legal services
  ♦ Sexuality and sexual orientation issues
  ♦ Eating disorder support
  ♦ Women-only support groups
■ Empowerment—that is, holistic programming that emphasizes the development of a partnership with a female service provider, one in which there are mutual respect and many opportunities for positive role modeling
■ Transportation services
■ Child care, both onsite and supervised

- Woman-sensitive women working with women
- Long-term case management services that extend to the client and her family

A woman's identity as caregiver/caretaker must be recognized as an extremely powerful factor in how she accesses care and treatment and how successful she is in her recovery and health maintenance. There is no question that this identity/role can explain why a woman seeks treatment ("for the kids") or why she leaves treatment ("to get home to my husband/partner/kids"). This is also a factor in a woman's sense of guilt and shame from becoming HIV infected—a societal stigma that only "bad girls" get HIV or are addicts or alcoholics, and the stigma of being an unfit mother if she has lost custody of her children.

Providers must be open and prepared to discuss safer sex and drug and alcohol abuse from a risk-reduction perspective. They must be well informed about and comfortable in discussing sexuality. Risk reduction is an ongoing type of intervention that goes beyond assertiveness training and teaching women how to put condoms on men. It recognizes the need to "start where the client is" and use appropriate interventions, which may help a woman reduce her risk of getting reinfected or of infecting a partner. This includes instructing female injection drug users about how to use bleach to "clean their works," how to use a female condom, or how to use a vaginal spermicide foam (not the safest risk-reduction method, however) to lower their risk of HIV infection when having intercourse. It also involves making referrals to substance abuse treatment and instruction for male partners on how to use a condom correctly.

Reproductive decisionmaking

Reproductive decisionmaking is an important area for providers to examine with both female and male clients. Providers must be prepared to discuss pregnancy and family planning with respect and without judgment. This is a difficult task for providers and clients; counselors may have many judgments about "right" and "wrong" and many opportunities for countertransference. One way providers can interact with clients is to help them openly and honestly consider various factors when making reproductive decisions. Figure 7-6 is adapted from an article written by Rebecca Dennison, director of a women's health advocacy organization based in San Francisco, who is HIV positive and considered these issues with her husband in her own reproductive decisionmaking.

The questions listed in Figure 7-6 are extremely helpful, but it is also important to remember that many clients have never made reproductive decisions. Their substance abuse problems have been at the forefront of their lives for so long that they may find it difficult, even in recovery, to "own" their decisionmaking responsibilities. One way to provide support in this area, and help build coping skills, is to encourage women to talk with other women—to become part of a support group that is based on empowerment and women helping women. Counselors should see reproductive decisionmaking as a very high priority and move toward this goal in small, incremental steps.

At present, no one knows exactly how to predict which mothers will transmit HIV to their infants. Although there is some speculation that a mother's viral load, measured through viral load assays, may indicate whether her infant becomes HIV infected. Much is still unknown, and controversies abound, but providers must understand and respect the importance of self-determination and the right of women to make their own decisions. Ultimately, it is the woman's choice.

Figure 7-6

Reproductive Decisionmaking Questions

- Statistics and information are constantly changing. The latest research from NIH still supports the Pediatric AIDS Clinical Trials Group Protocol 076 study, which indicated that about 8 percent of women treated with AZT during pregnancy and delivery transmitted HIV to their infants. It is unclear to date what the long-term health ramifications are for children who received AZT in utero and at birth. Are you willing to run the risk of having a child who is infected or has been affected by medications used to counter HIV infection?

- Are you able and willing to love and care for a baby, whether or not it is infected?

- How will pregnancy affect your health? In women with high T-cell counts, pregnancy has not been shown to make HIV/AIDS progress, but less is known about women who have AIDS or symptomatic HIV disease.

- Do you have the support of a partner, family members, or friends who can help care for a child?

- Who will care for your child if you become sick or die? Will there be people who will teach your child about his culture, help your child remember you, and raise your child according to your values?

- In what ways (good or bad) will having a baby change your life?

- What are the reasons that you want (or do not want) to have a child?

- Do you have children now? How are things with them?

- Do you feel pressured by others (partners, family, friends, your religion, cultural values) to have (or not have) a child?

- Do you have a family physician or obstetrician who knows about HIV/AIDS and who can give you the health care that you need?

- Do you have enough information to make an informed decision? If not, find someone who can give you information and who will not insist on telling you what to do.

- Are you willing and able to go without substances for at least 9 months? Do you know how their use will affect your unborn child?

Source: Dennison, 1998, p. 7.

Today, HIV-positive women are looking at the prospect of pregnancy differently than they did in 1989. HIV-positive women who think about becoming pregnant have access to information about viral load testing and the possibility of artificial insemination. Also, HIV-positive women can consider a natural rhythm method, identifying fertile days and limiting unprotected intercourse to those times to decrease their partner's risk of HIV infection. There is no question that even today, facing pregnancy while HIV positive, examining the options related to terminating or continuing a pregnancy, deciding about medications, examining the woman's health and the infant's health, and addressing the long-term implications are all complex issues.

It is essential that providers examine these issues with clients within the context of a biopsychosocial framework. Counselors and health care providers must work together, along with the female client, to stay aware of the latest research and information regarding HIV/AIDS treatment. It is also important to remember that data and information on HIV/AIDS are constantly changing and that the "facts" provided to clients today may be very different tomorrow.

Parents who are HIV positive

More and more resources have been developed for single- and two-parent households in which one or both parents are HIV positive and/or the children are HIV positive. There must be a continued awareness of the needs of these families.

These families experience the need for a variety of services, both child-centered and adult-centered. Concerns about guardianship for children after the parent is unable or unavailable to care for them must be a major focus for the parent and the service provider. Unfortunately, many clients who have long histories of substance abuse may have "burned many bridges," and the family support they need for permanency planning and establishing an appropriate guardian for their children is no longer available. All too often, there is only a tired, abused, and used grandparent who is dealing with chronic ailments, limited resources, and little emotional energy to raise more children.

If a child also is HIV positive, there will be special needs that the parent may not be able to address while facing her own issues. The already demanding dynamics of childhood, school, and growing up become more challenging for an HIV-infected child and parent. Even if the child is not HIV positive, the demands of parenting can prove rigorous for single parents with HIV/AIDS. Although the parent experiences the relief of knowing the child is all right, the poignant realization that he may not live to see that child grow up can still be painful.

The HIV-infected single parent with a substance abuse disorder is at risk of losing custody of her minor children if convicted of drug possession or substance abuse. If family members disapprove of the single parent's lifestyle, they may seek custody of the active substance abuser's minor children. The counselor may facilitate a plan encouraging the single parent toward goals that support the parenting relationship. This enables the recovery process to take place while the parent and child are working out their own version of permanency planning.

It is difficult for a child to witness the effects of a substance abuse disorder on a parent; surely the difficulty increases enormously when the child is told that the parent has HIV/AIDS. Children whose parents are in recovery from substance abuse disorders or who are maintaining some stability despite periodic substance abuse may experience some changes in their relationships with their parents.

There are support groups and programs for children whose parents are affected by HIV. Although not available in all communities, these groups offer children a chance to talk about their fears regarding their parents' health, learn more about the disease, and socialize with others who are facing these problems. At the same time, the programs can provide the parent with some respite time. In addition, groups like Al-Anon and Alateen can provide children with support and education about the recovery process.

If service providers work in a large urban area, chances are there will be an AIDS Service Organization (ASO) listed in the phone book. This agency is likely to have lists of support groups of all kinds. Single parents with substance abuse disorders who are HIV positive should also have a support group.

Hispanics

The Hispanic population in the United States is diverse, composed of a wide range of racial, indigenous, and ethnic groups. The following are important statistics related to the U.S. Hispanic population that affect how outreach, prevention, and treatment planning should be conducted:

■ Hispanics have the highest labor force participation rate of all groups.

- Hispanic men have the highest fertility rate of all groups across all ages.
- Hispanic men have the lowest divorce rate of all groups.
- Hispanic men are on average younger than other men in the United States (with median age of 26.2 years).
- Hispanic women seek detoxification and treatment for substance abuse disorders in lower numbers than women from any other ethnic/cultural group.
- 90 percent of Hispanics are Catholic.
- 36 percent of Hispanic children live below the poverty level.
- There is a clear increase in substance abuse as Hispanics become more acculturated (i.e., in second and third generations, and so on).
- Hispanics are overrepresented among HIV/AIDS cases for men, women, and children.
- Hispanics as a group may include aliens who are undocumented or carry immigrant visas (green cards) and who avoid contact with the health care system because they fear possible deportation.

Within the context of acculturation and socioeconomic status, providers should be aware of specific cultural issues that can support interventions and improve a provider's ability to engage Hispanic clients, such as the role of the family, the values of interdependence, respect, and "personalismo" (i.e., importance of personal contact). Understanding these concepts will help establish rapport and trust.

The Hispanic family is generally extended and has many members. A Hispanic client's support system may be composed of siblings, godparents, aunts, and uncles who are all very involved with the client. The family as a whole is of great importance, and often what is best for the family will override what is best for one of its members. Because the family is so important to most Hispanics, children are highly valued. This makes it easier to see how some Hispanic

women who are HIV positive grieve deeply about the decision not to have children and may feel unfulfilled and inadequate as a result. This also sheds some light on the challenges of involving Hispanics in substance abuse treatment. Leaving their children behind while in treatment or turning guardianship over to a State agency may be unacceptable and create more conflict.

Often, families are aware of homosexual family members, but usually this is not discussed openly. The reality is that many Hispanic men who prefer sex with other men do marry and have children. This partly explains why Hispanics are at such high risk for HIV/AIDS. If the man has married and fathered a child, he has been congruent with the values relating to family; if he then goes out with men, or even with other women, this behavior may be tolerated as long as he continues to provide for his family. Figure 7-7 offers additional considerations for working with Hispanics.

African Americans

As is the case with members of other minority groups, the health and social repercussions of substance abuse problems are magnified in the lives of African Americans (CSAT, 1999b). In terms of past-year prevalence rates of illicit drug use, the 1998 NHSDA (SAMHSA, 1999) found that the rate for African Americans (8.2 percent) was somewhat higher than for whites (6.1 percent) and Hispanics (6.1 percent). In addition, HIV/AIDS disproportionately affects African Americans, and from July 1998 through June 1999, injection drug use accounted for 26 percent of AIDS cases among African American males and 26 percent of cases among African American females (CDC, 1999b). (See Chapter 1 for more information about the epidemiology of the AIDS pandemic.)

African American women in particular have special needs. Minority women represent the fastest-growing segment of the U.S. HIV/AIDS

Figure 7-7
Case Study: Heterosexual Minority Men Living With HIV

One recent study recruited 18 HIV-positive, heterosexual, minority men from an outpatient HIV/AIDS clinic in upstate New York and a community-based AIDS service organization in New York City to explore the experience of heterosexual minority men living with HIV. Findings revealed that the experience of surviving HIV infection encompassed several stages.

The participants in this study identified the choices they made in adolescence that led them down a hazardous pattern of behavior as the majority became involved in substance abuse or other illicit activities. With the diagnosis of HIV infection came a "falling off" stage, in which the participants went "over the edge" and initially were afraid to die but then realized that they were okay but vulnerable.

The next stage was "hanging on," in which study participants attempted to reassert control, reevaluated priorities, and developed a new perspective on life and health. In the "pulling up" stage, participants realized that the rescue team included self, God, family, and friends, with self-rescue taking place on emotional, physical, and spiritual levels.

As the participants reached the "turning around" stage, they began to accept responsibility for their health, focused on their abilities rather than their limitations, and began to see themselves as "living with HIV" rather than "dying from HIV."

Source: Sherman and Kirton, 1998.

---

pandemic. One study (Kalichman and Stevenson, 1997) examined the psychological and social factors related to HIV risk among 153 African American inner-city women. The women completed measures of HIV risk history, sexual and substance use behaviors, perceived risk for HIV infection, self-efficacy to reduce risk (i.e., the belief that one can effectively perform specific behaviors), and perceived social norms supporting risk reduction. Fifty-five percent of the women reported at least one factor that had placed them at known risk for HIV infection. Results showed that HIV risk history was associated with a self-perceived risk for HIV infection and low self-efficacy to perform risk-reducing actions, suggesting that HIV risk-reduction interventions targeting inner-city women should focus on skills training approaches to build self-efficacy and empower women to adopt risk-reducing practices (Kalichman and Stevenson, 1997).

Many African Americans have a deep-seated mistrust of the health system. This dates back to the pre–Civil War period when, because they were considered property and had no legal right to refuse, slaves were sometimes used in medical experiments (Gamble, 1997). A collective memory thus exists among the African American community of their exploitation by the medical establishment (Gamble, 1997). More recently, the syphilis study performed at Tuskegee University from 1932 to 1972, during which 400 African American men infected with syphilis were deliberately denied life-saving treatment, has fostered in some African Americans the belief that contact with health care institutions will automatically expose them to racist administrators and policies. Several articles point to the Tuskegee study as a significant factor in the low participation of African Americans in clinical trials and organ donation efforts and in the reluctance of many African Americans to seek routine preventive care (*AIDS Weekly Plus*, 1995; Karkabi, 1994; Thomas and Quinn, 1991). As one AIDS educator said, "so many African American people that I work with do not trust hospitals or any of the other community health care service providers because of that Tuskegee experiment. It is like ... if they did it once, then they will do it again" (Thomas and Quinn, 1991).

A study (Longshore et al., 1992) that compared the use and perceptions of substance abuse treatment services among African American, Hispanic, and white substance-abusing arrestees confirmed that African American substance abusers were more likely than white substance abusers to hold unfavorable views of treatment. Another study (Gary, 1985) examined the attitudes of African Americans in a northeastern city toward mental health treatment and found that only 34 percent of the sample felt positively toward community mental health centers. The study also revealed that women and married persons demonstrated more positive attitudes than did men and unmarried persons and that participants with a high tolerance of substance abuse possessed more negative attitudes than did others.

Counselors should be aware that the issues of slavery and institutional racism are constant and prevalent facts in the lives of many African Americans and should be addressed early in treatment so they are acknowledged, validated, and brought into the treatment process (CSAT, 1999a). In order to provide effective substance abuse treatment for African American clients, providers need to take into account the social, economic, political, and cultural contexts of their lives (Pena and Koss-Chioino, 1992).

Spirituality is very important for many African Americans. The relationship between an individual and the faith community is a critical source of strength that can help prepare clients to succeed in substance abuse treatment. In addition, many African Americans have strong social networks. They may have friends or a pastor with whom they might share information they would not share with a substance abuse counselor. These confidants

might act as "co-therapists" for the client. It can be helpful for clients if counselors can identify and integrate clients' co-therapists into their substance abuse treatment plans (keeping in mind clients' rights to confidentiality and the need for signed consent forms—see Chapter 9 for more information). Along these lines, for African Americans with substance use disorders and HIV/AIDS, support groups of friends may be more likely to be helpful and less undermining than support groups of families. This is perhaps due to the lingering stigma of the ways in which HIV/AIDS is acquired—both intravenous drug use and homosexual activity are still highly stigmatized acts within many African American communities. Thus, activating family supports may be difficult, and providers should encourage clients to participate in support groups composed of their peers.

Asian Americans

Asians and Pacific Islanders are a culturally and linguistically diverse people from the Asian continent and the Pacific Islands. In the United States, they include nearly 40 different nationalities, 50 different ethnic groups, and more than 100 languages and dialects. Asians and Pacific Islanders comprised 4 percent of the total U.S. population in 1999. From July 1998 through June 1999, they accounted for 0.7 percent of all adult and adolescent HIV cases (these include only persons reported with HIV infection who have not developed AIDS), and 0.4 percent of adult and adolescent AIDS cases. Of the total AIDS cases reported for this population through December 1998, 89 percent were in men; 79 percent of those were reported in men who have sex with men (CDC, 1999b). Among women, nearly half the cases (48 percent) are associated with sex with an infected or high-risk partner, and 17 percent are reported from IDU (CDC, 1999b).

The increasing size and diversity of the Asian and Pacific Islander population make it difficult to discuss group norms regarding substance abuse. Norms for alcohol and tobacco use vary by culture and there appear to be no norms governing the consumption of narcotics or other substances.

Service providers also should shed the notion of the "model minority," which often typecasts Asians and Pacific Islanders and limits treatment access. Often, Asians and Pacific Islanders believe the model minority myth and feel isolated when they test positive or report substance abuse disorders. They may also feel they have let down their families and communities.

Despite differences in cultural norms and mores among Asians and Pacific Islanders, cross-cultural beliefs in the importance of group and collective identity, service, and responsibility suggest the use of treatment strategies that incorporate biological or constructed families and communities rather than a focus on individual behavior change. Moreover, treatments that emphasize nonverbal or indirect communication skills, not confrontation, may be more culturally appropriate and more effective. Most American treatment modalities rely heavily on verbal therapies that require direct verbal emotional expression and a high level of personal disclosure. Many substance abuse treatment programs favor a confrontational approach, and many HIV/AIDS programs favor support groups and psychotherapy. These treatment approaches, unless modified for Asian and Pacific Islander clients, are often unsuccessful because they violate Asian and Pacific Islander cultural norms. By American standards, Asians and Pacific Islanders tend to communicate more indirectly, often by telling stories and discussing what happened to themselves and others. Their feelings and opinions are implied rather than directly stated. Asians and Pacific Islanders are also less likely to provide direct verbal expression of their feelings by using "I"

statements than are members of other groups. Providers should expect to reveal personal information about themselves if they want clients to disclose their own problems. Asians and Pacific Islanders may prefer to keep strong feelings under control so that they will not become disruptive. Caring is often demonstrated by physical support such as by giving money, cooking favorite foods, or giving advice rather than by verbal expression or physical affection.

A problemsolving approach rather than an intrapsychic one is more effective with Asian and Pacific Islander clients. Problemsolving enables a counselor to provide information, educational materials, and referrals without probing for more personal information and pushing a client to express feelings. For Asian and Pacific Islander clients with somatic complaints, suggest relaxation and breathing techniques, meditation, qigong, yoga, massage, acupuncture, tai chi, or biofeedback. It is generally not helpful to discuss underlying feelings because it is not only culturally unacceptable, but many Asian and Pacific Islander clients do not see the emotional–physical connection. In problemsolving, providers should actively give suggestions and if necessary, be directive rather than let Asian and Pacific Islander clients struggle to figure out what options are available to them.

Asking personal questions about substance abuse and sexual risk factors, especially early in the helping relationship, could be viewed as intrusive and disrespectful. Asian and Pacific Islander clients may not answer truthfully, if at all, and may not return. It is best to start with the least intrusive or nonthreatening questions during the intake and explain why the information is needed. If clients seem uncomfortable with certain questions, ask them at a later date.

Making an effort to connect with clients outside actual treatment appointments when they come to the agency for other activities or via followup calls is also helpful. Asian and Pacific Islander clients may not initiate contact when they have a problem because of cultural tendencies to minimize problems to reduce stigma and because they do not want to be intrusive and bothersome. In all interactions, it is helpful to minimize the stigma Asian and Pacific Islander clients attach to their HIV/AIDS status and substance abuse disorders. Counselors should not refer to themselves as HIV/AIDS, mental health, or alcohol and drug counselors unless they know the client is comfortable with this. These titles imply the client has an unacceptable condition and can increase stigma. Clients may be more receptive to treatment for HIV/AIDS and substance abuse issues if they are combined with other, less stigmatized health issues.

Group interventions can be effective if everyone speaks the same language well enough and if the group is centered around an unstigmatized activity, social gathering, or education session. Providing refreshments also facilitates bonding. Asian and Pacific Islander participants will look to a facilitator to provide direction and guidance. Rather than be assertive in talking, Asian and Pacific Islander clients will more likely wait for a space to open up for them to speak and consequently will rarely have the opportunity to do so when in a group with predominately non–Asians and Pacific Islanders. Should this happen, the group leader needs to facilitate opportunities for Asian and Pacific Islander clients to participate.

Native Americans

Native Americans and Alaskan Natives comprised 0.9 percent of the total U.S. population in 1999. From July 1998 through June 1999, they accounted for 0.4 percent of all adult and adolescent HIV cases reported (these include only persons reported with HIV infection who have not developed AIDS) and 0.6 percent of adult and adolescent AIDS cases. The largest percentage of HIV and AIDS cases in women was from heterosexual contact (39 percent and 23 percent, respectively). The largest percentage of HIV and AIDS cases in men was reported in men who have sex with men (43 percent and 47 percent, respectively).

The CDC found that Native Americans have high rates of STDs and substance abuse, which in turn raise their risk of HIV/AIDS. They also lack access to diagnosis and treatment. Gay men and substance abusers run the highest risk of HIV/AIDS among Native Americans and Alaskan Natives, just as they do among white Americans.

The combination of high rates of cofactors for HIV/AIDS, limited access to health care, lack of information and education about HIV/AIDS issues, substantial numbers of Native Americans who are already infected with HIV, and the flow of Native Americans between urban centers and reservations all lead to an HIV/AIDS crisis for Native American communities.

Limited treatment services for HIV-infected substance abusers exist on and outside tribal lands. In 1991, the American Indian Community House, which ministers to the health, social service, and cultural needs of Native Americans in the New York City area, created the HIV/AIDS Project, the first Native American program east of the Mississippi River to provide culturally sensitive legal services, HIV/AIDS treatment information, emergency assistance, and prevention education. The Friendship House Association of American Indians in San Francisco provides another example of treatment (drop-in centers). This program provides comprehensive treatment to Native Americans living with HIV/AIDS as well as treatment for substance dependency. Services target the gay, lesbian, and bisexual communities. HIV/AIDS is presently underreported for Native Americans and is based on the high incidence of sexually transmitted diseases (STDs) in general, and thus substance abuse treatment centers will be faced with more and more HIV-infected Native Americans.

Clients involved with the criminal justice system

Many persons with substance abuse disorders receive treatment only after arrest and are offered treatment as a diversionary service or receive treatment while they are in jail or prison. The racial and class patterns characterizing arrest, adjudication, and sentencing in the United States skew more white Americans (regardless of social class or income) to treatment trajectories and more persons of color to jail or prison trajectories. Access to treatment within the criminal justice system is thus highly associated with ethnicity and social class. Only a handful of correctional facilities in the United States have instituted some type of therapeutic community treatment program in prison with a parallel transitional program for new parolees (for more information on these programs, refer to TIP 30, *Continuity of Offender Treatment for Substance Use Disorders From Institution to Community*, [CSAT, 1998d]). Unfortunately, many HIV-infected individuals who are in treatment for HIV find it impossible to remain on their medication schedules after being arrested because their medications are often confiscated for days at a time.

The population in prisons and jails tripled between 1987 and 1997. Overcrowding and understaffing are common in prison facilities and can increase inmates' risk of contracting HIV. In 1992, HIV/AIDS cases for people in State and Federal prisons reached 195 per 100,000 compared with 18 per 100,000 for the general U.S. population.

Risky behaviors that lead to HIV infection are not eliminated when a person is imprisoned but may actually increase in frequency and availability. This occurs for several reasons. First, drug offenses count for the single largest number of Federal and State crimes for which

people are arrested and incarcerated. In 1996, 79 percent of State inmates reported at least one use of illicit drugs during their lifetime. Therefore, high rates of HIV infection are not surprising in a population so closely characterized by heavy substance abuse involvement. In addition, many people enter jail or prison already infected with HIV. A 1993 study of 46 correctional facilities found people entering these facilities had an average infection rate of 1.7 percent. In some facilities, however, rates for women were as high as 21 percent and 15 percent for men. Among injection drug users, rates ranged from less than 1 percent to 43 percent.

Injection drug users face particular risk in prison settings as clean syringes are all but impossible to secure. Although syringes are not officially available, they can be acquired through illicit prison markets at exorbitant prices ($34 in one Canadian facility) or through risky exchange of syringes for unprotected sex. Syringes are typically not new or sterile. As a result, injection drug users have as their only recourse used or shared syringes, which increases their chances of HIV infection. Tattooing is also common practice among prisoners and is another source of HIV infection. To date, there have been at least two documented cases of HIV/AIDS related to tattooing with unsterile needles in a correctional facility.

Only six prison systems in the United States distribute condoms: Mississippi, New York City, Philadelphia, San Francisco, Vermont, and the District of Columbia. Distribution strategies range from receipt of a single condom per medical visit to receipt of multiple condoms during HIV/AIDS education workshops. Furthermore, condom distribution programs send mixed messages because sexual activity in some facilities is illegal and a punishable offense. In other facilities, correctional medical and social service staff may advocate condom availability while administration and security officers oppose it.

Sixteen prison systems mandate HIV testing, and although 77 percent make testing available to inmates on request, few inmates request it for several reasons. First, confidentiality of results is not guaranteed. Second, mandatory testing may result in the segregation of those who test positive from those who test negative or who do not test. Third, prisoners do not wish to acknowledge activities that could subject them to further sanctions. Fourth, confidentiality on discharge is eliminated because the Federal Bureau of Prisons requires HIV testing for all inmates on their release. HIV-positive inmates are asked to directly notify sex partners and significant others of the results. However, the Bureau of Prisons handles only a small percentage of inmates, and its policy is not the norm.

Treatment for HIV-positive inmates is often inadequate when available. Primary medical care may be limited to *Pneumocystis carinii* pneumonia prophylaxis and HIV monotherapy. Combination therapy may not be available or accessible to inmates, given the cost of medications, limited storage, refrigeration requirements for some medicines, and the strict adherence regimen required by combination therapy, which would require round-the-clock monitoring and assistance by typically unwilling and suspicious security staff.

Although there are large numbers of substance abusers within correctional facilities, less than 15 percent participate in treatment programs. This is partly because of lack of program availability and the common type of program offered (i.e., 12-Step, abstinence-based.) A 1991 study reported that only 1 percent of inmates with moderate to severe substance abuse disorders received appropriate treatment. Many of these treatment programs advocate sexual abstinence during recovery. Often, these programs offer no or little information about

safer sex practices or advocacy around changing sexual behaviors. When persons with substance abuse disorders in treatment relapse, as is often the case, they may also engage in risky sexual behaviors. They are most likely to engage in risky sexual behaviors with sexual partners from similar treatment networks. These partners may include people who have used syringes, traded sex for money or drugs, or been victims of trauma. All of these populations are likely to have higher rates of HIV infection, making transmission likely.

Inmates who do complete or participate in treatment programs often rapidly relapse on discharge. For inmates who do complete treatment, there are often no aftercare programs to help them remain substance free. A 1995 study of Hispanic inmates in California State prisons found that 51 percent reported having sex within the first 12 hours after release, and 11 percent reported injection of drugs during the first day after release.

Adolescents

Adolescents are another group that is experiencing an increase in incidence and prevalence of HIV. Since 1994, findings from the Monitoring the Future surveys have revealed a dramatic and sustained increase in consumption of licit and illicit drugs among adolescents—this after nearly two decades of sustained decrease in drug consumption. Studies also note that teens are having sex earlier than ever before, often with multiple partners and inconsistent use of condoms, putting them at greater risk for HIV/AIDS. Beyond this, young people find themselves marginalized in U.S. society; this is especially true for young gay and bisexual youth, sexually active young women, and young people of color.

According to the CDC, AIDS is the fifth leading cause of death for Americans between the ages of 25 and 44 (CDC, 1999f). At greatest risk are young, disadvantaged females, particularly African American females, who are being infected with HIV at younger ages and higher rates than their male counterparts (CDC, 1998j). Because of the long and variable time between HIV infection and AIDS, surveillance of HIV infection provides a clearer picture of the pandemic in young people than surveillance of AIDS cases. From the States for which HIV is a reportable condition, young people ages 13 to 24 accounted for a much greater proportion of HIV than AIDS cases (17 percent versus 4 percent). Of these HIV infections, 38 percent were reported among young females, and 56 percent were among African Americans (CDC, 1999b).

Adolescents may benefit from treatment that is developmentally appropriate and peer oriented. Addressing educational needs may be particularly important as well as involving family members in the planning of treatment and therapy.

Substance abuse among adolescents is frequently associated with depression, eating disorders, and sexual abuse history. Histories of familial sexual and substance abuse are predictive of serious adolescent substance involvement and subsequent treatment needs. For a discussion on adolescents and substance abuse disorders, see TIP 31, *Screening and Assessing Adolescents for Substance Use Disorders* (CSAT, 1999a), and TIP 32, *Treatment of Adolescents With Substance Use Disorders*, (CSAT, 1999b).

Older adults

The last few years have witnessed greater increases in the number of HIV/AIDS cases among middle-aged and older individuals than in those under 40 years of age. Through June 1999, people over the age of 50 account for 11 percent of cumulative AIDS cases and 5 percent of cumulative HIV cases in the United States. Women comprise a greater percentage of all AIDS cases as age increases, ranging from 13 percent of AIDS cases among people aged 50–59,

15 percent of AIDS cases among those aged 60–69, and 21 percent of those 65 and over. For women with HIV, 22 percent of this group is in the 50–59 age bracket; 24 percent is aged 60–64; and 31 percent aged 65 and older. The rate of HIV infection in older women reflects the greater incidence of surgeries (such as hysterectomy) that require blood transfusions.

Although many of these AIDS cases are the result of HIV infection at a younger age, many people become infected after age 50. Rates of HIV infection among older adults are difficult to ascertain because very few people over 50 years of age routinely test for HIV. Because older adults are diagnosed with HIV/AIDS at advanced stages, older adults are less amenable to treatment, become sicker, and die faster than their under-50 counterparts. In addition, retroviral treatments and opportunistic infection prophylaxis may interact with medications the older person is taking to treat other preexisting chronic illnesses and conditions. Also, the vast majority of medication studies are done on much younger subjects. There is little research on the metabolism of anti-HIV drugs in older adults.

There is, as well, little research on the substance-abusing behavior of older adults, and very few substance abuse treatment programs address the needs of older adult substance abusers (see TIP 26, *Substance Abuse Among Older Adults* [CSAT, 1998a]). Unfortunately, many medical professionals do not consider older patients to be at risk for either substance abuse (with the exception of alcohol use) or HIV infection. A study in Texas found that most doctors never asked patients older than 50 years questions about substance abuse or HIV/AIDS or discussed risk factor reduction. Doctors were much more likely to rarely or never ask patients over 50 about HIV/AIDS risk factors (40 percent) than to rarely or never ask patients under 30 (7 percent). Older persons may not be comfortable disclosing their sexual behaviors or substance abuse to others, since their generation or culture may not encourage such disclosures. This can make finding treatment programs and support programs especially difficult.

Certainly, there is a need to educate service providers about the sex- and substance-related behaviors of older persons. At the very least, service providers should conduct thorough sex and substance abuse risk assessments with their patients over 50, and challenge all assumptions that older people do not engage in these activities or will not discuss them.

Sex industry workers

Among sex workers, street prostitutes are the most vulnerable to HIV infection, given the coexisting features of poverty, homelessness, history of childhood sexual abuse, and alcohol and drug dependence. Comparatively, male and female sex workers who work in massage parlors, escort services, their own apartments, or brothels rather than on the street are far less likely to be at risk for infection, less likely to depend on substances, and more likely to control sexual transactions and insist on condom use.

Seroprevalence rates among sex workers vary dramatically. A 1990 study of nearly 1,400 sex workers in six U.S. cities yielded a seroprevalence rate of 12 percent, ranging from 0 to 47 percent as a function of the city and the level of injection substance abuse. Most alarming was the high association of injection substance abuse and HIV infection rate.

Among female sex workers, IDU continues to be the major cause of HIV infection. Female injection drug users who trade sex for money or drugs are more likely to share syringes than injection drug users who do not exchange sex for money or drugs. Drug use also increases the likelihood of sex work and risky sex. Studies of crack cocaine abusers in three urban neighborhoods found that 68 percent of the women who were regular crack smokers exchanged sex for drugs or money. Of those, 30

percent had not used a condom in 30 days. Recent research has also demonstrated an association between HIV infection, heavy crack use, and unprotected fellatio. This is likely due to the combination of poor dental hygiene, damage to the mouth from hot crack stems or pipes, high frequency of fellatio, and inconsistent or marginal condom use. Street-based sex workers may agree to unprotected sex if clients offer more money, if workers themselves are desperate for money to buy drugs, or if activity has been slow.

HIV treatment challenges may occur given the sex workers' more immediate needs for drugs, food, and housing. These needs overshadow future concerns about living with HIV/AIDS. Beyond this, sex workers with HIV/AIDS may continue to work routinely for the purpose of exchanging sex for drugs or money. Sex workers thus run risks of spreading HIV/AIDS as well as reinfection of HIV and the acquisition and transmission of other diseases such as hepatitis and STDs.

There are many examples of effective treatment programs for sex workers with substance abuse disorders, including the California Prostitutes Education Project (CAL-PEP); Sisters Helping Each Other in Chicago, Illinois; Second Chance in Toledo, Ohio; the Threshold Project in Seattle, Washington; Alternatives for Girls in Detroit, Michigan; and the On the Streets Mobile Unit-Options Program in New York City. Most of these programs use former sex workers as outreach staff, use a risk-reduction model of care, and establish linkages with organizations in the treatment continuum.

Homeless people

Homeless people suffer higher rates of many diseases, including HIV/AIDS and substance abuse disorders, than the general population. No national statistics exist, but studies within major U.S. cities are illustrative. In a 1990 survey of homeless adults in St. Louis, Missouri, 40 percent of men and 23 percent of women reported substance abuse, and 62 percent of men and 17 percent of women reported alcohol abuse. Another 1993 study of homeless adults in Mississippi revealed that 70 percent of respondents engaged in at least one of the following high-risk behaviors: unprotected sex with multiple partners, injection substance abuse, sex with an infected partner, and exchanging unprotected sex for drugs or money. Of these respondents, nearly half reported two risk factors, and 25 percent reported three or four risk factors. Homeless people—especially women and youth—may engage in risky behaviors for survival reasons.

Developing New Substance Abuse Treatment Goals

Altering admission requirements

A "one-size-fits-all" abstinence-based approach to admission effectively serves only a small number of clients. Insisting that clients detoxify and remain substance free prior to admission to substance abuse treatment programs assumes a homogeneity of substance abuse and substance abuse behavior that does not exist.

Providers should realize that some clients use substances as a way to control mood, monitor affect, and adhere to a schedule of activity. Drug use as a life management strategy may seem dysfunctional but is not necessarily a personal deficit. Eliminating substance abuse without understanding the context and role it plays in the lives of clients may, in counter-intuitive fashion, increase the chances of lapse and relapse among clients. Stopping substance abuse without substitutes or proxies for its socially constructed meaning is fraught with risk.

Removing substances of abuse without acknowledgment of the psychological benefits perceived by abusers is also laden with risk. Providers should appreciate (without necessarily agreeing) that many people use

substances because they like the way substances make them feel. Many substance abusers find replacement of this feeling extremely difficult, if not impossible, to obtain. Breaking, changing, or altering a chronic cycle of substance abuse is difficult under optimal circumstances where clients have social, psychological, and material supports and services. Changing chronic cycles of substance abuse without these supports and services is not impossible but very nearly so.

Programs should include a harm-reduction treatment track that can accommodate the retention in treatment of clients who are active substance abusers but willing to control their substance use (i.e., agreeing not to consume substances on the premises and agreeing not to participate in programs when under the influence). Admission requirements might be altered depending on level of care, motivation and coping resources of client, and treatment agency and philosophy.

This program flexibility is crucial to improving treatment outcomes. Because HIV is a pandemic that has spread across the globe over the past two decades and remains a public health crisis of epic proportions, an "abstinence-only approach" will not be effective. The goal for treatment programs that serve HIV-infected substance abusers must be to initiate treatment—HAART, if available—for these individuals as soon as possible. Awareness of and education in HIV-related issues can help treatment providers recognize potential barriers to effective treatment, such as homophobia and irrational fears of infection, that can occur in both counselors and clients.

What programs should try to achieve in treating the HIV-infected substance abuser is a base of clients who are as healthy as available treatment can make them. A client who has stabilized his illness has a better chance of decreasing his substance use than one who has not.

Continuum of Care: Different Treatment Strategies for Different Levels of Care

Detoxification

Most of the client work during this stage of care is directed to surviving the physical and psychological traumas of separation from addictive substances. The degree and range of trauma will vary greatly depending on the substance used. Often clients will benefit from an initial placement in a 12-Step program to begin the long process of breaking through denial, consciousness raising, and discussing feelings.

Medical supervision during this process is critical. Detoxification of HIV-infected clients presents considerations not usually encountered in other clients. Many HIV-infected clients either are on, or will soon be on, a complicated schedule of medications to which strict adherence is necessary. These clients may also suffer from medical conditions that have occurred as a result of the disease, which can interfere with the detoxification process. Thus, while the counselor focuses on the client's psychosocial issues, it is imperative that an experienced physician monitor her closely and supervise treatment during this process.

Inpatient and residential treatment

Care strategies during inpatient treatment consist of consciousness raising, contemplation of behavior and personal changes around risky behaviors, and developing plans for action. It is recommended further that clients begin to discuss the problems of relapse and interaction of competing problems from sex and drug domains.

Individual therapy is often used to clarify comments and observations raised by clients who participate in group therapy, which in turn usually reinforces personal gains achieved in individual sessions. Group therapy is optimal for consciousness raising and convincing clients

to move toward a more consistent level of safe behaviors. During this initial period, efforts should be made simply to get the client to begin thinking about safer behaviors and activities.

Individual therapy strategies

Clients may raise several issues in therapy that then become clinical issues. Following are common issues that clients raise during the inpatient treatment process along with suggested responses from the counselor during individual therapy:

- Feeling the problem (of HIV infection or living with AIDS) has not "hit them" yet. The counselor can provide the client with education about risky behaviors, living with AIDS, and so on. Presenting the client with future scenarios and life trajectories if behaviors remain unchanged may be helpful. Sharing success stories about positive changes in peers may also be a helpful strategy.

- Expressing the need to make their own decisions and choices regarding care, treatment, and their lives. Counselors should underscore the fact that clients must decide what is in their best interests, taking care to define "their best interests" within the client's definition of self as either an individual, a provider, a parent or caregiver, a member of a family or community, or a combination thereof. Counselors should balance this by letting clients know that no one has all the answers to their problems, and reassure clients that their feelings are valid, not unusual, and realistic. Changing one's life is hard work.

- Knowing how to change behavior, yet not making these changes. The counselor should support client efforts to reduce risk behaviors but educate the client as to why risk remains. Exploring what the client is willing to consider changing provides an outline of possible actions. Working together with the client on strategies to resolve barriers to change in small steps may be a useful tactic as well.

- Giving up hope for change or feeling overwhelmed by problems. Workers should reassure clients that their feelings are typical and that change is hard. Telling clients about positive role models who have successfully changed after facing many difficulties along the way is another useful approach.

Service providers should know that this initial phase of client change is the longest and most difficult for many clients. It is not uncommon for clients to spend a lot of time in inpatient treatment weighing the pros and cons of their behavior. Clients may have invested much energy in intentionally not thinking about the problem. Thinking about the problem may release painful issues (real or perceived) for clients that they have not allowed themselves to reflect on. Service providers should be acutely aware of the power of denial for many substance-abusing clients living with HIV/AIDS.

It is often difficult for the client to anticipate potential problems, interactions, and pitfalls, particularly those that will be faced in the external community. The counselor must help the client examine the barriers that may arise and develop strong responsive coping skills and activities. A weak plan of action can lead to quick lapses and relapses. This level of client activity (preparing for action) is characterized by switches in both personal external cues for behaviors and the ways in which clients perceive and cope with internal situations. This is a time for counselors to develop specific plans and identify individuals in a person's social environment who may provide support or information to the client upon discharge.

The idea of self-liberation can be used to influence a client to choose to act in a specific manner or believe in his ability to change. Clients can benefit from thinking about what

may change once the new behavior(s) have begun so they can be prepared for those changes. Questions similar to the following can be used to facilitate self-liberation:

- Is this what you want to do? Are you prepared for the risks involved?
- What are your reasons for changing your behavior?
- When do you want to make your change?
- What problems do you think you may face in the future?
- Whom have you discussed this with?
- How do you feel the environment is going to affect your change?
- Are there any support groups you could join in the area? Would you like to join any?

Group therapy strategies

The gains made in individual treatment can be consolidated in well-designed and well-facilitated group therapy. Consciousness-raising techniques may help when talking with a client who seems to lack basic information about behaviors or topics, such as HIV transmission. Questions such as the following can determine how much consciousness raising is needed:

- What are your concerns about HIV/AIDS?
- What do you think about "cleaning your works" in order to protect yourself?

Dramatic relief strategies can be used when talking with a client who knows something about topics like HIV/AIDS but still engages in unsafe behavior. Questions such as the following are helpful in determining the level of dramatic relief strategies:

- Do you feel you are at risk for HIV/AIDS?
- Do you worry about getting an STD?

Group therapy also can be used to present role models (peers) who have successfully addressed many of the issues clients in inpatient treatment may face. Peer programs can provide support for substance recovery and other psychosocial services. There are many resources in the community for these interventions; all a program must provide is a meeting place. It is helpful if the peer group facilitator has some training, even if this consists solely of the orientation that all substance abuse treatment program volunteers receive. Because they are not led by professionals, peer groups may be limited in what they can achieve. However, the absence of professional involvement may give peer groups greater credibility with hard-to-reach clients.

Self-reevaluation (or self-reflection) and environmental reevaluation are good activities to use in group settings during inpatient treatment when clients might be motivated to change behavior. Self-reevaluation occurs when clients think about their behavior, and environmental reevaluation occurs when they think about the impact of their behavior on others. A counselor can initiate self-reevaluation by asking questions such as the following:

■ How would you feel about bleaching all the time?
■ Are there times you are willing to take risks by not using a condom? Why or why not?
■ How often do you think about HIV/AIDS?
■ Do you ever worry about getting something from your partner? What do you worry about? Why do you worry?
■ Do you ever worry about giving something to your partner? What do you worry about? Why do you worry?

Environmental reevaluation can be facilitated with questions such as the following:

■ How does your partner (partners) feel about using condoms?
■ How would your partner (partners) feel if condoms were used?
■ Do people close to you ever talk about your addiction? What do they say?
■ Do people close to you ever talk about HIV/AIDS? What do they say?

■ How does your addiction affect people who are close to you?

Group therapy in inpatient settings can be very helpful in setting the stage for actual behavior change. It is challenging for clients who have started to change behavior within a structured setting to continue the change when they return to the less structured environment from which they came. This environment may not necessarily support newly acquired lifestyle changes.

Stage of HIV infection

Segregating groups by stage of HIV infection presents difficulties, but not doing so can also be problematic. Clients who are HIV positive but asymptomatic and attending a support group for the first time may be uncomfortable when encountering clients in the late stages of AIDS. Such a meeting may force them to confront fears about their own mortality before they are ready to do so.

Because treatment programs have limited resources, separating groups by stage of HIV infection may be impractical. Programs able to support separate groups may wish to use the three-group model, with groups consisting of

■ Clients newly aware of their positive HIV status
■ Those who are asymptomatic or mildly symptomatic
■ Those with more advanced disease

The interplay between substance abuse disorders and HIV infection in groups can be complicated. As clients move further into substance abuse recovery, they may be getting progressively more ill from HIV disease. In a mixed group, healthier clients may provide support to sicker ones.

In a group consisting solely of clients symptomatic with AIDS, members are vulnerable to becoming involved in a process of continual grieving. Sometimes groups have to discontinue for a period of time when too many members become sick or die. For this reason, it may be helpful to establish support groups for time-limited periods.

Outpatient treatment

Outpatient treatment consolidates the gains made in the detoxification and inpatient and residential treatment levels of care. Typically, clients may still need to think about change or begin to plan for change on their discharge frominpatient or residential treatment. On entering outpatient treatment, clients may have actually begun some behavior change, but the novelty of the change can lead to relapse as the client moves away from the controlled and structured environment.

Clients in outpatient treatment usually need support from at least one other person who cares about them. This can be a time when clients are vulnerable because as they change, others around them may change in response. Friends and significant others may feel threatened, abandoned, jealous, or angry and may try to sabotage the client's efforts. This puts tremendous pressure on clients because they are experiencing new feelings and new, difficult ways of life. Although many of these life changes may be positive, they are also unfamiliar for many clients.

During outpatient treatment, group therapy could focus on the use of successful peers in modeling helpful but difficult strategies such as stimulus control and counterconditioning. Individual therapy will involve helping the client balance and coordinate recovery with other issues, such as assessing client responses and concerns with case management, care coordination, and child and family issues when relevant.

Stimulus control and counterconditioning are two strategies clients may find helpful. Stimulus control helps clients restructure their environment so they can avoid circumstances that elicit problem behaviors. There are three methods for managing tempting stimuli:

- Develop a plan for managing the situation.
- Manage the situation so the temptation does not occur. For instance, a person who knows alcohol puts her at risk for unsafe sex will not drink when sex may occur.
- Restructure the environment so that stimuli for more positive events occur and so clients remain aware of people, places, and things that cause relapse.

In developing stimulus control strategies, consider developing questions such as the following:

- What are the situations where you may be at risk of not using a condom?
- How can you avoid them?
- How do you stay safe when you have sex?
- Where do you keep your condoms?
- What are the situations in which you find yourself using substances?
- Do you keep your own "works" with you?
- When are you tempted not to bleach?

Counterconditioning involves exchanging risky behaviors with less risky alternatives in situations that are not amenable to stimulus control. To develop counterconditioning strategies, questions such as the following can be used:

- If you found yourself in a situation where you were tempted to have sex without a condom, how could you deal with it so that you could have safer sex?
- How would you deal with a situation where you insisted on having safer sex and your partner got angry?

A major risk during outpatient treatment is the involvement of the client in sexual networks and sexual mixing. Many clients in treatment may select sexual partners from similar networks (recovery programs, 12-Step meetings, and so on). These partners might include persons who have used syringes, traded sex for drugs or money, been victims of trauma, or been incarcerated. All of these populations may have higher rates of HIV infection, making transmission more likely, and clients should be counseled about these risks.

Drop-in centers

Drop-in centers are an excellent way to engage homeless people in treatment. These centers offer a needed service for substance-abusing individuals who are homeless. As individuals start dropping in, they begin to interact with staff and form trusting relationships, which builds a necessary foundation for beginning treatment. The use of maintenance strategies characterizes treatment in drop-in centers. At this phase, service providers must work to prevent relapse and bring together the gains achieved during inpatient and outpatient treatment. During this time, clients may have learned to adjust their new behavior to the environment in which they live, and the behavior has perhaps become habitual.

Also during this time, many clients relapse and may return to earlier treatment levels and milestones. As discussed elsewhere, there are many factors leading to client relapse. Situations such as breaking off relationships, starting new ones, severe temptation, or lack of environmental support may contribute to relapse. In addition, the client can easily choose not to try again due to the negative feelings associated with relapse such as shame, embarrassment, guilt, failure, regret, anger, or denial.

Service providers may work with clients so that they can realize that their past successes indicate better chances of success in the future. They should underscore the fact that clients have learned new ways of coping with old behaviors and have developed supportive relationships. Service providers may find the use of reinforcement management a helpful strategy that can be facilitated in either individual or group level modes. Reinforcement management helps clients develop internal and external reinforcers and rewards that increase the chance of new behaviors continuing.

Workers can also reassure clients that relapse encounters are part of an ongoing process. Helping clients determine what caused the slip can be useful in helping them develop strategies to avoid lapses in the future. Workers can also work with clients to help them learn more about themselves, their environment, and their addiction and risky behaviors.

Questions similar to the following can help determine if clients need better or more reinforcement management:

- Do you feel good about your new behavior?
- What kind of things do you tell yourself, knowing you are practicing safer sex?
- What kind of things do you tell yourself, knowing you are controlling your substance abuse?

Counseling Terminally Ill Clients

The counseling of ill and dying clients should be supportive and nonconfrontational, addressing issues relevant to the client's illness at a pace determined by the client. However, clients are not the only ones to be affected by the approach of death; counselors too may need assistance in dealing with clients' deaths. This section addresses the issues of denial, planning for death, pain management, unfinished business, and bereavement. A five-stage bereavement and loss model, based on Elisabeth Kübler-Ross' book *On Death and Dying*, also is presented.

Denial

Denial about a client's HIV/AIDS diagnosis can be experienced by both clients and counselors. Denial is a natural response and should be confronted only if it causes harm; for example, when a client in denial about his illness delays in making arrangements for medical and nursing care or procuring assistance with daily living activities. Counseling can play an important role in helping clients accept their illness and the eventual need for home health or hospice care.

Denial can also affect counselors. For example, because of the advances being made in the medical treatment of HIV/AIDS, a counselor may be in denial that a client will die of AIDS. Counselors must recognize and confront their own denial issues so that they are able to discuss death and dying and realistically explore these issues with their clients. Programs need to have inservice education and proper supervision for counselors who work with terminally ill clients. Proper supervision will help the counselor confront her denial and help lessen her stress.

Planning for death

It is often difficult for a counselor to know how or when to talk to a client about planning for death. It is optimal, if possible, to begin a discussion of the client's future, including death, before the client is extremely ill. Questions that often lead the counselor into a discussion of death and dying, and also are centered on contingency planning, include, "if you were to become too ill to care for yourself any longer, what would you do, who would help, where would you go?" The counselor and client should also consider where the client would like to die because different arrangements may be required.

Counselors who will be working with clients at the end stages of AIDS should examine their own beliefs about death and dying. In addition to this, counselors may need to learn about the physical and biological process of dying so that it can be explained to clients. It is also important to keep in mind that clients' perspectives on death and dying are deeply rooted in their personal histories, religious practices, ethnic customs, family traditions, and community standards.

Many clients fear dying alone or in pain, or of losing control of their bodily functions, and thus having to rely on others for care. If clients want to talk about this personal and often frightening experience, the counselor should listen and help the client locate answers to any questions concerning the process of dying. Counselors should ask their clients how much they want to know and make sure that clients know what to expect physically. Understanding the process and planning the details within their power can give clients a sense of control.

In addition, clients may ask counselors to share their own beliefs about death and dying. Minimal sharing can be reassuring, but counselors should focus on the clients' perspectives, beliefs, and needs. As counselors listen, valuable information and insight into possible resources and support needed by clients will come to light.

Pain management

Pain management is often a difficult struggle with those who are in the end stages of AIDS. The issue of pain is complex because many medical conditions related to a client's HIV/AIDS can cause her pain. Clinicians may be concerned that pain medications may reinforce an addiction. Also, clients who have achieved abstinence from drugs may not wish to use medications for pain relief. Another concern of clients is the appropriateness of pain management when it might hasten death. If a client raises this issue, the counselor should be prepared to discuss it, however, the counselor does not initiate discussion on this topic. If the topic arises, clients should be encouraged to discuss pain management issues with their physicians and, if appropriate, their significant others. Pain management is discussed (i.e., from a medical perspective) in Chapter 2.

Unfinished business

One important area that counselors should explore with their clients is "unfinished business." For example, a counselor might suggest that a client make a will. But there may remain other issues to be addressed. Should a client consider making an advance directive or a living will? Will the client want to appoint a health care proxy? Should he consider granting power of attorney to a significant other? Should he appoint a guardian for his children? Are there family issues that he wants to address?

Some counselors express a desire to be there at the time of a client's death, or a client may request that someone be there until death. Counselors and health care providers may also spend more time counseling the client's significant others or support people during this time than they spend counseling the client. Here again, a little information can go a long way to reduce fear and anxiety in clients and their significant others.

Bereavement

Bereavement is a particular problem for programs with large numbers of HIV-infected clients. Bereavement can affect clients (who may grieve at the deaths of other clients, friends, or loved ones from HIV/AIDS); clients' significant others; and counselors who work with dying clients. The following strategies may be helpful in supporting those clients who are dealing with bereavement.

- Acknowledge the reality of the bereavement in supportive individual counseling.
- Encourage the expression of grief both verbally and nonverbally (e.g., art therapy, expressive movement, psychodrama).
- Provide group support for clients and their significant others who are experiencing grief and bereavement.
- Acknowledge deaths with memorial services, flowers, photographs, and participation in commemorative projects such as The NAMES Project Foundation's AIDS Memorial Quilt, which attempts to include the names of everyone who has died of AIDS.

Kübler-Ross bereavement and loss model

One of the best and most often referred to models of bereavement and loss comes from physician and psychiatrist Elisabeth Kübler-Ross. In her book, *On Death and Dying*, she provides a five-stage theory that has become common language when dealing with death and dying. Her model of bereavement is essentially a series of defense mechanisms, or coping strategies, that are used by an individual confronted by death. These stages can also be observed as individuals are confronted with other traumatic circumstances or information, such as a positive HIV test, an HIV/AIDS diagnosis, or the death of a friend or peer. The five stages are denial, anger, bargaining, depression, and acceptance.

Individual interpretations of and responses to death and dying vary greatly, not only between people, but between cultures and religions. Yet, as this model eloquently describes, adjusting to death is a process, not an event that occurs seamlessly and in a logical sequential order.

The coping strategies and stages described below are not a recipe for health. Acceptance may not be the goal for everyone. Emotional processing is made more challenging when survival needs such as shelter, food, and medical care are not being met. Many clients are used to surviving with "street smarts" and not by psychoanalytical parameters and discussions about childhood. This model is included merely to help providers understand and relate to their experiences and their clients' experiences.

Denial

This is a time of terror management, an effort to psychologically buy some time while adjusting to the information or situation. It is here that people can feel the most isolated and the most suspicious and doubtful of the information that they are receiving. Denial is a natural and healthy response. It is not necessarily something that counselors must feel compelled to confront and rid clients of at the earliest possible moment. Allowing clients to have denial can be challenging, and for the caregivers and support staff it can be anxiety producing, but it is important to remember that above all else, this is the client's experience. Denial is not always negative. The times that denial must be confronted are when it causes a danger to self or others.

Anger

This stage emerges as the person accepts the diagnosis and begins to strike out. The most common targets for this anger are the people closest and safest to him, especially caregivers and service providers. Anger can also be a test. The person facing death may want to know who can be counted on as the end nears. This can sometimes be indirectly demonstrated by the client who may test the counselor's tolerance of anger; if the anger can be tolerated, perhaps the counselor can be trusted to tolerate the client's death and feelings of fear.

Bargaining

Bargaining is the stage at which the individual commits to an uncommonly generous or humanitarian act with the belief that she will be spared or miraculously cured if deemed "good enough." The goal is a miraculous correction of the wrongs she has done, or possibly to buy some valuable time for treatment or dealing with end-of-life issues. The obvious danger is that most are not "cured" in that sense of the word, so what can happen is a loss of belief or faith.

Depression

Depression represents a loss of denial, and an acknowledgment that the information is accurate and the situation and its consequences are unavoidable. As with clinical depression, the depth and severity depends on the specifics of the situation, mitigating factors, available resources, and the individual. This stage is marked by surrender to sadness; it is appropriate and adaptive. It is a time to collect resources and energies so that more processing can occur at a later time.

Acceptance

This is the stage in which some come to terms with their situation and feel a welcomed release from struggle and strife. Option formation and reality-based planning, given the circumstances, become the focus. Acceptance occurs when there is agreement between the physical body, the emotional heart, and the cognitive mind, that death will eventually be the outcome.

No code or do-not-resuscitate orders

The responsibilities for determining when, how, and under what circumstances to evoke or effect no code or do-not-resuscitate (DNR) orders are properly the role of the family, or those with power of attorney, and the physician. The order itself comes from the physician or from the client through the physician. Although alcohol and drug counselors do not initiate discussion of this topic, they should be aware of these terms and what they mean so that they can help prepare and inform the client and his family of these options.

No code and DNR are terms used while a client is receiving care at an inpatient facility to identify a client who does not wish to receive medical intervention to save his life. For example, if a client has a DNR order and his heart stopped, he would not receive electric shock or cardiopulmonary resuscitation. It is the framing of these decisions and the terms used to help clients understand them that make all the difference. A counselor can help clients and their families talk about these concerns by first normalizing the process. That is, to present issues as no codes or DNRs, wills, and guardianship of minor children as decisions each person or family must come to grips with—whether they are ill or not, HIV positive or not. Counselors can approach and begin to discuss these issues within a context of "hoping for the best and planning for the worst." The discussion, then, is not related to being terminally ill, but rather to choosing, taking control, and making difficult, responsible decisions.

It also is helpful for the client or the family to discuss with the physician changing the goal of medical treatment. For example, at some point in the treatment process, when death is imminent and further aggressive medical intervention will be futile, the goal of treatment could be changed to "comfort care" from "no code."

Some States also permit a person who has been discharged from a hospital to home to have a DNR, which can be tacked to the door. The drawback of home DNRs is when a client dies and emergency medical personnel arrive, in most places they are required to try to revive the client. A counselor should be familiar with State laws about home DNRs so that a client who wants to die at home can be given the best information about this option.

Health care providers and counselors must maintain a sense of how their communication efforts are affecting the people they are trying to help. A specific and practical example of this is in discussions around no code or DNR orders. As health care providers discuss treatment options with clients and their significant others and the possibility of changing the goal of treatment to comfort care, one distinction that can be helpful for some people is the difference between "life support" and "death prolonging."

The current standard of care as defined by the Joint Commission on Accreditation of Healthcare Organizations (JCAHO) states that providers should develop a framework for decisionmaking in situations that may require

the withholding of resuscitative services or the foregoing or withdrawing of life-sustaining treatment. Decisionmaking in such cases should reflect the following priorities (JCAHO, 1999):

- Enhancing the client's comfort and dignity by addressing treatment of primary and secondary symptoms
- Effectively managing pain
- Responding to the client's and his family's psychosocial, spiritual, and cultural needs

Many believe that decisions about medical treatment should not be based on "heroic" or "extraordinary" measures, or on medical complexity. They should be based on the potential outcomes and the benefits and burdens to clients and their support systems. An open and honest dialogue with the client, followed by a similar meeting with the entire care team, can facilitate decisions and move people to a place of comfort and resolution. Many States allow an individual to designate someone to serve as their "Durable Power of Attorney" for health care. Staff and clients should know what the State's regulations are.

Assisting Clients in Preparing Their Children for the Loss of a Parent

It is estimated that the number of children orphaned by HIV/AIDS will increase by 200 percent in the next 20 years. Parents living with HIV/AIDS face a multitude of issues in preparing both seropositive and seronegative children for the loss of their parents. Fortunately, the child care system is developing credible guidelines on working with children with parents living with HIV/AIDS. In addition, placing a focus on providing for the future care and maintenance of the children can serve as a cause for personal motivation and empowerment. Pragmatically, clients should be assisted in preparing their children for the loss of parents in the following areas:

■ **Legal guardianship**. Workers should help clients identify significant others or friends within the client system who could serve as legal guardians for their children. By stressing that children without legal guardianship become wards of the State, clients sometimes find the motivation to search for and secure guardians for their children. Workers should understand that the search for guardians for children of clients with substance abuse and HIV/AIDS-related issues can be difficult because clients often have exhausted their support system of family and friends well before involvement in formal treatment systems or programs.

■ **Standby guardianship**. A standby guardian is someone who agrees to stand ready to assume guardianship (legal responsibility) for a minor when the parent of that child dies or becomes incapacitated. A parent will use the procedure when there is significant risk that he will die or become incapacitated within a certain period of time (e.g., in New York, this period is 2 years). The parent must usually petition a court for the appointment of a specific individual to be the standby guardian. The standby guardian can assume responsibility when the parent becomes incapacitated and then relinquish it when and if the parent recovers. The standby guardian's authority is effective when she receives notification of the parent's incapacity or death.

■ **Leaving a legacy of living memories**. An approach often used in agencies is working with parents to create living legacies for their children. For instance, families may be encouraged to make videotapes or audiotapes of themselves for their children. The National Hospice Organization has an excellent library of grief and bereavement materials, including some very good age-appropriate materials for children.

■ **Dealing with survivor guilt**. The issue of survivor guilt is relevant for all family members but particularly so for the infected parent whose infant dies first. The problem of guilt must be brought forth, discussed, and processed so that clients can take a more proactive approach to their other problems.

HIV and Risk of Relapse

Declining health as a result of HIV disease is a recognized risk factor for relapse into substance abuse. Physical and psychological stresses associated with HIV disease include pain, decreased functional ability, fatigue, and weakness, as well as fear, anxiety, grief, and possibly increased isolation and separation from loved ones, all of which increase individuals' risk of resuming substance abuse.

HIV/AIDS milestones are significant for the client, her significant others, and her support network. Counselors often can anticipate crisis, upset, or a readiness for change when a client reaches an HIV/AIDS milestone. Counselors who know and understand these milestones have an opportunity to prepare clients through the development of coping skills and strategies. It is a time of great opportunity for change (becoming clean and sober) or for relapsing. Milestones can create the impetus for a new way and learning new behaviors, or they can serve as an impetus for clients to act in self-destructive or harmful ways.

Following are some of the milestones of HIV infection that counselors should learn to recognize.

■ Taking an HIV test
■ Receiving positive or negative HIV test results
■ Experiencing the first symptoms
■ Experiencing the first opportunistic infection
■ Experiencing the first AIDS-related hospitalization
■ Being diagnosed with AIDS

- Losing a friend, or significant other who dies from AIDS
- Beginning the medication regimen
- Experiencing little or no response to various medication regimens
- Decreasing CD4+ T cell count or increasing viral load

Alcohol and drug counselors may wish to suggest the following strategies to clients who are at risk of relapse because of HIV-related stress:

- Individual counseling
- Participation in a peer support group
- Medical attention to relieve physical discomfort and alleviate anxiety
- Relaxation and stress management techniques
- Recreational activities

Dealing with client relapse

The most successful relapse counseling is nonjudgmental. However, clients should understand that preventing relapse is their responsibility. If a client relapses into a risk behavior for substance abuse or HIV, the counselor's role is to help the client to understand the conditions that caused the behavior to occur and to identify alternative behaviors that could have been substituted to prevent the relapse. Relapse should be viewed as a learning experience and part of the recovery process. Clients should not be dismissed from substance abuse treatment or HIV/AIDS support groups because of a relapse. Rather, peer pressure may be constructively used to help clients acknowledge the reasons for and the consequences of their actions.

However, if the client's relapse includes the risk of nonadherence to HIV medications, these medications should be stopped entirely to prevent the emergence of resistance. Once the client is recommitted to therapy, the regimen should be reevaluated.

Case Studies

Case Study 1

Frankie is a 21-year-old, self-admitted gay man. He has been injecting "crystal meth" off and on for 3 years. He has also been a chronic marijuana and alcohol abuser since he was 12 years old. He uses these substances particularly when he can't afford the "rig" and other drugs. He has sold his body for drugs but claims that he only has sex with "nice businessmen types." Frankie is new to the area and has been in town for about 9 months. He says his family does not approve of his lifestyle, so they made him leave home. He is in phone contact with his sister occasionally but only to let her know that he is "alive." Frankie lives in shelters and on the streets with other homeless adults and youth.

Frankie decides to enroll in an outpatient program because he has been hassled by the police lately and he went on a bad run using something called "fry" (marijuana soaked in formaldehyde, then smoked). He ended up in the emergency psychiatric unit at the county hospital and the staff there suggested that he seek some help. In addition, Frankie does know about HIV/AIDS and STDs and is concerned about his sexual behavior.

Issues for the alcohol and drug abuse counselor

Referral and linkages

Frankie will need referrals for counseling and possibly testing for HIV and STDs if the facility does not provide these services. Referrals and linkages can be obtained by getting Frankie's written consent if the facility is communicating with another organization about services for its clients. However, if an outside agency is providing services to the facility, then a Qualified Service Organizational Agreement (QSOA) (see Chapter 9 for more information about QSOAs) or Release of Information form will be required in order for the substance abuse treatment facility to be compliant with confidentiality laws. Frankie will also need a risk assessment to help him determine just what his risks are and risk-reduction counseling regardless of his decision about any medical testing.

Special population/cultural competency

The fact that Frankie is gay could be a concern if the treatment facility has not dealt with members of the gay population or has difficulty in dealing with this population. It will be important that Frankie is assigned to a counselor who is nonjudgmental and has had some experience with young gay men.

Relapse

With Frankie, it may not be an issue of relapse as much as getting Frankie to discontinue or cut down his use. He is currently motivated for treatment but this "scare" may not last. A risk reduction model may work best with Frankie as this appears to be his first attempt at treatment and total abstinence may be unrealistic. This should be explored further with Frankie.

Denial/anger

Although Frankie may not have shown any of these emotions yet, they probably should be explored with him (as well as others, such as depression, grief, loss) specifically as it relates to his family and their treatment of him, as well as his having to survive on the streets.

Medical complications

There may be a need to further examine Frankie if he does not stop using fry or other substances. The medical complications to the heart, kidneys, lungs, and brain would be worse if he has HIV/AIDS or any other STDs. Because he has been on the streets, he probably has not seen a doctor for anything until he ended up in the emergency room.

Case Study 2

Tina is a 29-year-old African American female. She has been using marijuana and alcohol since she was a teenager and progressed to using cocaine by her early 20s. Tina reports snorting cocaine for a couple of years when working as a dancer. She then discovered crack, which has been her drug of choice for the last 6 years.

Tina has been in and out of jail several times over the past few years, usually on prostitution charges. While in jail, she always tests for STDs and HIV/AIDS. She has repeatedly tested positive for chlamydia and has received treatment numerous times. Despite the treatments for the STD, she continues to test positive. During her most recent incarceration she was diagnosed with pelvic inflammatory disease, had an abnormal Pap smear, and tested positive for HIV. Other than being a little underweight she looks good and states that she feels fine with the exception of some abdominal pain.

Tina is very excited about her "new life" with her boyfriend, by whom she has been trying to become pregnant. Having HIV/AIDS does not seem to be a major concern for Tina because she knows that there is medication out there for the disease. She reports that she was already getting off drugs before the bust because she wants to get married and have a baby now that she's found the right man. She reports her main support to be her boyfriend of 2 months. She does have a couple of female friends but does not consider them close.

She has been court ordered to go to substance abuse treatment. She has made several treatment attempts before and states she doesn't understand why she has to go to treatment now when she was already planning to stop her drug use voluntarily. She is now being admitted to a 30-day inpatient treatment program; otherwise, she faces going to jail for a minimum of 1 year.

Issues for the alcohol and drug abuse counselor

Relapse

This is the main area of concern. Tina has a long history of substance abuse. She reports little to no social support for her recovery. The nature of crack addiction suggests that a 30-day inpatient setting will "only be the beginning" of the treatment episode. The connection and consequences of high-risk activities need to be discussed and risk-reduction practices demonstrated and rehearsed. It appears that Tina is clearly in denial about her addiction and diseases and does not understand treatment and recovery. This may be exhibited through her either becoming a "compliant client" just to get along or a defiant, angry client because she doesn't think she needs treatment.

Medical

Tina has a number of medical issues that must be addressed and further explored. Tests and treatment for recurrent STDs, pelvic inflammatory disease, abnormal Pap smear, and HIV/AIDS are needed. With further exploration cervical cancer may be revealed, which could, in turn, give her an AIDS diagnosis. A pregnancy test may also be needed. The counselor needs to remember that it is Tina's decision about the issue of pregnancy. A counselor should watch for the issues relating to HIV/AIDS and pregnancy that can arise.

Referrals and linkages

Tina will need medical referrals. She has so many issues in this area she would benefit by having an HIV/AIDS case manager to assist her in linking with and coordinating appointments, medication, and so on. She may also need all the "standard" services such as housing, transportation, and clothing.

Compliance

There could be some compliance issues with this client. This is indicated by the good possibility that she was not taking her STD medication as directed and her statement that she doesn't understand why she has to go to treatment. This belief should be explored further because it could be a lack of information/education and not a compliance issue at all.

8 Ethical Issues

Ethics is a term that can imply lofty, philosophical discussions, far removed from the everyday world. In reality, workers in the substance abuse treatment field are constantly faced with ethical dilemmas on an individual as well as a societal level. Ethics is an intellectual approach to moral issues, a philosophical framework from which to critically evaluate the choices and actions people take to deal with various aspects of daily living (National Association of Social Workers [NASW], 1997).

Working in the substance abuse treatment field presents dilemmas relating to personal beliefs, judgments, and values. The history of how society views persons with addictions is fraught with emotion, misperceptions, and biases that have affected the care of drug abusers. For example, it is not unusual in a health care setting for a patient to be perceived negatively just by being labeled a drug abuser (Carroll, 1995). Because of the highly charged emotional nature of the substance abuse treatment field, providers should possess the tools to explore ethical dilemmas objectively. By doing so, and by examining their own reactions to the situation, providers can proceed with the most ethical course of action. (See Appendix E for the Federal and State codes of ethics for programs treating HIV-infected substance-abusing clients.) Chapter 9 discusses the legal constraints, obligations, and options that provide the framework within which ethical issues must be decided.

Ethical Issues for Treatment Providers

The Ethics of HIV/AIDS

Taking the most ethical course of action becomes even more complex when HIV/AIDS is thrown into the mix of concerns that the client may present. HIV/AIDS has its own unique ethical issues. Because HIV can be transmitted through sexual activity and by sharing drug equipment, it evokes significant personal feelings and judgments in the general public, as well as in health and social service providers. Advocates for persons with HIV have fought for years to maintain confidentiality, avoid mandatory reporting, and ensure access to care for those with the disease. Because of the labels "drug abuser" or "homosexual" and the fear of a backlash toward people with HIV, advocates have been pushing strongly toward preventing discrimination. This has led to creating safeguards to protect these individuals from discrimination in health care, employment, housing, and other services.

Ethics on Micro and Macro Levels

Ethical issues are both personal (micro) and societal (macro) in nature. There is an ongoing struggle between legislating morality for the "public good" and fighting to retain an individual's right to autonomy. It is the intense emotional nature of such concerns that takes an issue from a personal level to a societal level.

Syringe exchange programs (SEPs) are a good example of such ethical dilemmas. While the Secretary of the U.S. Department of Health and Human Services announced in 1998 that a review of scientific reports indicated that SEPs can be an effective component of a comprehensive strategy to prevent HIV, the restriction on Federal funding for SEPs has not been lifted. At issue is whether giving out clean syringes may sanction or encourage illegal drug use (see Chapter 4 for more information).

Alcohol and drug counselors may find that their time is spent not only sorting out client-level ethical dilemmas, but also dealing with societal-level dilemmas. This could involve advocating for legislation that protects the rights of clients or adapting to the impacts of a policy that will further restrict a provider's ability to intervene effectively with a client group.

Balancing Personal and Professional Standards

Alcohol and drug counselors must balance what is right for them personally with what may be right based on professional standards. Substance abuse treatment professionals who are social workers, for example, should be familiar with the NASW Code of Ethics and may have to reconcile personal beliefs with the profession's code. There also may be agency standards that conflict with an individual's personal beliefs. In either case, there is a constant need to weigh what may "feel right" personally with the standards and policies of the environment and profession.

Perhaps the most difficult dilemma occurs when there are conflicts between the clinicians's values and the client's behaviors. Professionals know that if a client threatens suicide or homicide, there is a duty to report. But most of the daily concerns that arise are not so simple. Ethical issues come up in numerous, seemingly insignificant ways. Did the client understand what the release of information stated, or did

she rush so that the provider could make the next appointment? Did the clinician listen to what the client said about her culture, and how the treatment plan would not work because it was not created in a culturally competent manner? Was information about the client shared with another helping agency, even though she did not give a release to that particular agency? These are the kinds of issues that arise every day, affecting client care and reflecting on one's status as a clinician, as well as on the agency's reputation.

The Need for Staff Training

Issues relating to ethics rarely are covered in orientation sessions or continuing education activities within agencies. Perhaps this is because these issues can be so personal and there are no right or wrong answers in many of the case examples. Yet, the intense nature of the job and the problemsolving required in the daily work of a substance abuse treatment professional require that further training about ethics be provided. This section can be a starting point for ongoing discussions among those treating persons with HIV in substance abuse treatment programs.

Basic Ethical Principles

The study of ethics has produced an abundance of writings, and many standards and principles have been brought forth. However, there are five general principles that provide a firm basis from which to explore the ethical concerns that arise daily in the substance abuse treatment and HIV/AIDS fields (Kitchener, 1985). These are reviewed below.

Justice

The principle of justice assumes impartiality and equality. It means that a clinician will treat all clients equally and give everyone their due portion of services. This principle applies to the individual client as well as on the larger societal level. Yet, given human nature, how possible is it really to treat everyone equally? Can it be honestly said that a clinician does not have "favorite" clients? Are there clients with whom a clinician instinctively wants to limit contact? Are there agency policies or informal agency practices that limit access to a program? Counselors may find that their comfort level is being challenged as increasing numbers of substance abusers with HIV/AIDS comprise their caseloads. Although they may have felt entirely comfortable working with someone who has a substance abuse disorder, they may not understand, or feel awkward working with, someone with HIV/AIDS.

While it is normal to have bias, it is important to know when and how it affects one's ability to practice within the principle of justice, so that no client is discriminated against or denied access to treatment that other clients have. This requires an understanding of countertransference—one's conscious and unconscious reactions to what the client may present in treatment. It also requires knowing when to ask for consultation with a supervisor, so that personal issues do not stand in the way of working with clients.

Although it may be difficult for a provider to treat everyone exactly the same, there are safeguards that agencies and providers can institute to ensure an equitable level of service. Standards can call for every new client to receive an intake interview within 24 hours, or the agency may work toward clarifying its criteria for services so that they are weighed more heavily on objective information rather than on the personal impressions of a substance abuse treatment worker. These sorts of policies can help ensure a general level of fairness, regardless of a worker's personal feelings.

Autonomy

The principle of autonomy assumes that individuals have the right to decide how to live their own lives, as long as their actions do not interfere with the welfare of others. This principle respects the unconditional worth of the individual and promotes the concepts of self-governance, self-determination, and self-rule. In working with HIV-infected substance abusers, the substance abuse treatment counselor can play a key role in determining if the client is competent to make his own decisions and establishing whether or not the client has the information needed to make a personal choice.

The issue of competence can be one of the most difficult ethical issues when working with this population. Persons with HIV/AIDS can be affected by numerous neuropsychiatric, metabolic, nutritional, and psychological concerns that can affect their judgment. Substance abusers also can experience poor judgment due either to active substance use or to the results of long-term use. In cases of incompetence, it is not fair to the client to allow for full autonomy in decisionmaking as the client could unwittingly harm himself. Yet it is not always clear whether the person is truly incompetent, and the process of proving incompetence can be burdensome and time consuming.

Competency issues are rarely clear cut. There are several factors that can temporarily make a client seem incompetent. A client may seem unable to make independent decisions one day, and then the next day be quite lucid. In reviewing a client's ability to maintain autonomy, consider not only the initial impression, but the duration and severity of the behavior, as well as reports by other persons in the client's life. Consultation with other medical or psychiatric professionals, reports by the client's support system, and a strong baseline assessment can help clarify the presence of mental state changes.

If it appears that a client may be experiencing a loss of mental functioning that is unrelated to a medication-based problem, the question of the client's competency must be addressed. Competency can be complete or partial in nature. The client may demonstrate full competency in some areas of her life and only partial competency in others. For instance, she may be quite capable of caring for herself physically but may no longer be able to make sound financial decisions. In this particular case, she may have to sign a power of attorney to allow someone else to deal with her financial affairs. (However, the client must be of sound mind before she can legally sign such an authorization; if the client is not of sound mind, provider staff should petition the court for appointment of a guardian to make such a decision.)

Before the client became incompetent, she may have signed other legal instruments, like a living will or health care proxy, and these may come into effect if the client appears to be incapable of attending to her own physical or medical care. Finally, if the client appears seriously incompetent, provider staff should petition the court to appoint a guardian.

The other issue involved in autonomous decisionmaking is whether the individual has the necessary information to make a sound decision. This is where bias and personal values on the part of the substance abuse treatment professional can cloud the issue. For example, a clinician strongly believes in combination therapy for persons with HIV and takes on a Native American client whose doctor is suggesting more aggressive treatment. The client wants to know about alternative therapies. Can the clinician set aside personal beliefs and provide an objective array of information without biasing the client's decision?

In many cases, it may be extremely difficult not to "push" the client toward a decision by emphasizing certain information. If nothing else, the biases should be acknowledged to the client. A client will then be able to listen to what the worker is saying, knowing that there is a bias, and be able to respect the worker for acknowledging bias up front. In addition, the client may be more open to asking about the combination therapies at another stage in treatment because he was not "pushed" early on.

Beneficence

Beneficence assumes a responsibility to improve and enhance the welfare of others, or more simply put, to "do good" for others. But what does "doing good" really mean? What may be doing good in the eyes of the substance abuse treatment counselor may be seen as doing harm in the eyes of the client. The counselor needs to consider whether it is the client's agenda or his own agenda. The counselor's or agency's culture also may conflict with the client's. The role of the family, medical practices, and lifestyle issues all affect treatment, and these can differ greatly, depending on the various social norms of all those involved.

The issue of paternalism also must be considered. For example, a clinician might feel justified in telling a physician that the client is not a candidate for the complex regimen of combination therapy. The reasons for doing this may be justified to the clinician because the client is still using drugs and there is concern about the client's ability to take the medications. However, is the clinician's assumption that the client cannot comply based on fact or on personal perceptions and attitudes about drug abusers? In fact, some drug abusers live incredibly organized lives in order to maintain their addiction. Has the clinician discussed the regimen with the client, and has the client had the opportunity to advocate for herself? The clinician must take the client's point of view and cultural context into account before determining what "doing good" truly means.

Nonmaleficence

Similar to beneficence, nonmaleficence means "to do no harm." This principle often has been highlighted when discussing client exploitation, such as sexual contact or financial exploitation. Both of these examples are active means of doing harm to a client. However, doing harm also can be more subtle, especially given the complex population of HIV-infected substance abusers. An example of conflicting interpretations of this principle is in the debate over abstinence versus risk reduction approaches to drug treatment. Advocates of abstinence may claim that a risk reduction approach harms a client by enabling his addiction, keeping the client from truly "hitting bottom" and seeking help. Risk reduction advocates argue that the abstinence-based model harms the client because it does not allow for compassion or for meeting the basic needs of individuals who are in the throes of addiction. Advocates for risk reduction may claim that the abstinence-based model actually prohibits recovery because it does not take into account that recovery is a process, rather than a rigid philosophy. This is one ethical dilemma that truly reflects the passionate nature of personal values and beliefs.

Another example, on a micro level, is termination or transfer of clients. In both the HIV/AIDS and substance abuse treatment fields, there is a high degree of staff burnout. As an individual clinician becomes increasingly stretched, her ability to be flexible with clients and to treat them as individuals diminishes. In some situations, a client who breaks a rule or shows up late may suffer the wrath of a clinician only because he is the third client to show up late that day, and this is the last time the clinician is going to deal with a lack of respect.

Thus, the client may be terminated or transferred to another clinician. This may be a fairly common experience, but what does it mean to the client? Will it harm the development of future relationships? What if the client knows of other clients who were late that day but who were not transferred or terminated? What impression does that give the client about her own self-worth?

Clinicians must be sure that they are not acting like parents to clients and making the clients feel like bad children. If rules regarding transfers and terminations are not clear from the start and followed through consistently, then the clinician is violating the principle of nonmaleficence.

Fidelity

The principle of fidelity requires telling the truth and keeping promises. Fidelity is a fairly simple concept that can be violated easily. When a substance abuse treatment counselor takes on a client, there is an implicit contract with the client. The contract assumes that the counselor will work to resolve the client's concerns and that information will be shared in a truthful manner between the counselor and the client. By having the client sign consent forms, the counselor is promising that the information provided will remain confidential to anyone who is not listed on the form. The client agrees to follow the agency's rules. (Of course, confidentiality must be extended to the client whether or not he obeys program rules.) How frequently is the first session taken up with the more interesting issues, and the paperwork given to the client quickly at the end?

If a clinician is going to keep promises, he must be clear up front about when the promises may have to be broken. If the client is suicidal or homicidal, for example, confidentiality may be breached. If the client speaks of child abuse, the contract will be breached. If the client breaks certain agency rules, the relationship between the clinician and the client may be terminated. It is important that the clinician is extremely clear about the limitations to fidelity so there are no surprises later on. (See the "Confidentiality" section later in this chapter and Chapter 9 for specific details about the legal issues involved.)

Another issue of fidelity is the counselor's focus on the primary client. If the counselor is involved with a complicated family system, it can be difficult to remember who the client is, especially at times of conflict. In working with clients who have questionable competency, it can be convenient to let someone else speak for the client. But it is the counselor's responsibility to ensure that until the competency issue is resolved, she will have to represent the primary client and act according to the client's wishes.

Ethical Issues in Working With HIV-Infected Substance Abusers

There are several specific ethical issues that predominate in the substance abuse and HIV/AIDS treatment fields that warrant more focused attention. These issues are discussed below in a social and ethical context; further information on the legal aspects of these issues is provided in Chapter 9.

Duty To Treat

The duty to treat, from an ethical perspective, is especially relevant when working with disenfranchised populations. A clinician involved with homeless, chronic alcohol-dependent individuals may find it difficult to access adequate medical care for a client with HIV. Or it may not be easy to find a dentist willing to work with an HIV-infected client. Substance abuse treatment professionals may have to take on an advocacy role within their community to educate and campaign for care.

At the same time, it is important that the counselor and the counselor's agency appear accessible to all and that there are no restrictions that could impede the care of one client just because the client is different in some way.

The impact of welfare reform may augment concern about access issues. This is compounded by the increasing focus on managed care and the decreasing availability of health insurance for the poor. Adding restrictions to a population that is already disenfranchised will require more creativity, patience, and determination on the part of the clinician who is trying to advocate for a client.

In addition, it is important for clinicians to remember that when taking the ethically or morally correct action in a duty-to-treat situation they do not inadvertently create situations where the clinician and agency are legally culpable. Take the example of a counselor who has a substance abuse client who is a minor and engages in prostitution in exchange for drugs. This client is at a high risk of contracting HIV. The counselor feels ethically obligated to treat the client and intervenes to help the client receive clinical treatment or receive information about HIV in a medical setting. Later the client's parents say that they did not approve the medical treatment for their child, and a legal situation is created.

Duty To Warn

In working with HIV-infected substance abusers, there are unique concerns that are raised regarding the duty to warn. Besides the more obvious issues relating to reporting abuse and suicidal or homicidal threats, providers are concerned about clients who are transmitting HIV by not taking necessary precautions. For example, there have been several high profile news reports about individuals with HIV who knowingly infected multiple partners through sexual contact (Richardson, 1998). What does a clinician do if she knows that a client is aware of his HIV-positive status but is still not taking precautions?

Again, counselors must be aware of creating legal culpabilities when taking the ethically or morally correct action in a duty-to-warn situation. For example, if a client has HIV but has not informed his partner about his HIV status, the counselor could be held liable in a civil law suit for knowing and not telling the client's partner. Counselors should consult with their supervisors about agency policy regarding duty-to-warn situations and may report the client to the public health department. Each situation should be examined on a case-by-case basis.

For some counselors, the knowing transmission of HIV is as serious as hearing their client threaten to kill someone. There are some differences, however, between knowingly transmitting HIV and murder. For one, the campaign to stop the transmission of HIV has encouraged people to protect themselves. Therefore, every individual is responsible for safer sex practices, so it is not entirely the responsibility of the person with HIV. Additionally, how can a counselor realistically prevent a client from sharing contaminated syringes or having sex? Finally, there is a greater chance that by using education and counseling, a clinician may be more successful in convincing a client to use protective measures than if the clinician immediately threatened punitive action.

This situation also highlights the conflicts between principles such as beneficence, fidelity, and nonmaleficence. Is the provider "doing good" by reporting a client and trying to help the greater society? Or is the provider doing harm by not working with the client to stop the behavior on a long-term basis? To what extent is the provider breaking the contract with the client by disclosing the client's actions? The ethical nature of these kinds of dilemmas does

not lend itself to an easy decision but requires a case-by-case analysis while looking at the long-term and immediate consequences of action (Reamer, 1991). See Chapter 9 for more information about the legal implications of duty-to-warn issues.

End-of-Life Issues

Treatments for HIV are dramatically lowering the death rate from AIDS, but people are still dying from this disease. When an individual's HIV status is compounded by chronic drug use, her survival is less likely. Thus, a clinician may be faced with dying clients and the ethical dilemmas that relate to dying. Persons with HIV generally have been vocal about their right to self-determination. They have campaigned for access to drugs that are still in the trial stage, they have fought for organizations that advocate for dying individuals, such as the Hemlock Society and Compassion in Dying, and they have been highly effective in organizing a compassionate continuum of care services within certain communities, especially the gay and lesbian communities. Given this activist culture, a client with HIV may decide at a certain point to stop medical interventions and will not expect to be dissuaded in this decision.

In some cases, a client may decide that he wishes to end his life because treatment is not working. Clearly, this has implications for the clinician, who should make it clear that he cannot hold a client's suicide threat confidential. The worker should also tell the client again, at the time the threat is made, that he plans to report it. It is important that the clinician discuss the limitations of his role clearly with the client and that this discussion take place before the client reveals, for example, that she is going to take an overdose of medication. The clinician should explain the professional and agency limitations, and what he would have to do if the client provided certain information. This provides the client with the information needed to make a later decision not to tell the clinician about any such intentions (or, if the client wants intervention, she may decide to tell the clinician, knowing where such information would lead). It is imperative that providers recognize the laws in their own jurisdictions regarding these issues.

For providers who are concerned about liability, it is helpful to note that if a case were to go to court, the provider would be judged on the community standard for that profession. Thus, if the clinician were following the code of ethics for the profession and it was well documented, or if the clinician was adhering to the accepted standards of the institution in which he worked, the chances of being found liable in a lawsuit are greatly reduced. Although there is much concern about liability in the profession of social services, it is extremely rare for a judgment to be made against a clinician who was following appropriate procedures and standards.

Dual Relationships

Dual relationships pose another dilemma that clinicians may find themselves in. Dual relationships, where a provider may have had contact with a client in a social context as well as in a professional role, bring up the ethical issue of boundaries. The line between social and professional roles can become blurred, especially in rural areas or in certain cultural communities. In the treatment provider network, a clinician may be seeing someone with whom she used to socialize or shoot up, or a gay male counselor may be case managing a peer from his community.

Dual relationships should be avoided if possible. A clinician who knows a client via a past social or sexual encounter should not assume a professional role with that client. Some clients may avoid accessing services because they are afraid of seeing someone they know, and the ethical issues regarding disclosure and trust are many. If there is no

other provider available to the client, it is imperative that the clinician clarify what the professional role means, and how the information shared will remain confidential. It may also be necessary throughout the treatment process to frequently check the client's comfort level and to continually emphasize the role and boundaries of the clinician.

Scarce Resources

Given the limited resources available, treatment providers may find it difficult to treat all the clients who seek treatment. Providers will need to plan for the complex decisions that need to be made in such cases. They should consider the following questions:

- How can providers, and society in general, ensure that resources are distributed fairly?
- How can such allocations be free of bias and assumptions about certain individuals, cultures, and populations?

The provider can work to make certain that the method of allocation is objective and applied consistently. This means using objective criteria for access to services or treatment and perhaps instituting a review process to ensure that decisions are not made only on the basis of one provider's recommendation. In some facilities or agencies, for example, there is a team that determines who qualifies for services once certain objective eligibility criteria have been met.

Resources available to many substance abuse treatment providers, particularly for clients with HIV/AIDS, are limited. As interest in HIV has "peaked," organizations serving this population have seen revenues drop. As a result, an agency needing to limit services to a specific number of people may turn down an individual who has failed in treatment a number of times. The justification may be that the resources could be better spent on someone who has a greater likelihood of recovery.

Issues such as these also are affecting the allocation of combination therapies. The provider may block a client's access to the expensive treatments if the client is not up to managing the medication regimen. The case manager or treatment specialist who sees the client on a consistent basis can support or deny the validity of such a decision.

Confidentiality

The issue of confidentiality is the "connecting issue" among the general principles outlined above (NASW, 1997). Ensuring confidentiality is perhaps the strongest element in the foundation of a therapeutic relationship. Clients must feel that what they say to a clinician is protected information. Unfortunately, the nature of managed care requires more extensive justification for treatment, and the number of individuals that need information about a person's treatment is increasing. Additionally, the influx of computerized data can further jeopardize the concept of protected information.

It is the ethical responsibility of the provider to be honest with the client about what data need to be reported to funding sources such as insurance companies, and what information needs to be shared with other agencies or individuals. It is the legal responsibility of the provider to obtain consent for any information shared outside of the client–provider relationship (see Chapter 9). A provider must ensure that clients understand the agreement they are entering into by accepting treatment from the agency or provider. Clients should have all the information they need to make decisions about the services being provided, including to what specific amount and types of disclosure they are willing to consent.

This does not mean that the provider has no control over what is disclosed to others about the client. It is imperative that the provider use discretion in conversations with individuals outside of the therapeutic relationship and only report what is relevant to the situation. The provider also should use discretion in documentation of work with the client. Some providers document everything in detail in case they are sued. The provider should only document what is essential. For example, if a client comes into treatment for substance abuse, the provider should document the client's substance abuse history, motivation for entering treatment, any medical or emotional issues that relate to the treatment, and the plan for service. But there is a significant difference between an entry that states, "Client is upset regarding recent divorce," and an entry that reads, "Client claims his ongoing promiscuity has caused his wife to leave him." The latter may be of interest, and perhaps even relevant to treatment, but it should not be documented until it is necessary treatment information.

A Step-by-Step Model for Making Ethical Decisions

All programs should have a consistent process for dealing with ethical concerns. Although ethical issues are usually complex enough to require a case-by-case evaluation, agency practices should provide for a routine process for approaching an ethical issue. For example, an agency might have, as a policy and procedure, a practice where the employee consults with a supervisor or an ethics consultation team within the agency, within a specified timeframe, and guidelines are provided for how to document such discussions. There could also be agency protocols for situations that have arisen in the past, such as a client's admission that she is suicidal or homicidal, clients who come to the facility intoxicated and insist on driving home, or clients who admit to illegal activity. Given the ambiguous nature of ethical dilemmas, it is helpful to clarify the process for resolving dilemmas, even if the resolution may differ from case to case.

NASW's *Ethical Issues, HIV/AIDS, and Social Work Practice* training manual (NASW, 1997) outlines a process for working through ethical issues. By practicing the following steps, suggested by the NASW, the clinician can move to a more rational level of decisionmaking.

- **Identify the clinical issues.** When an ethical issue arises, the provider should review the larger picture in her work with the client or system. Identifying the clinical issues is the first step. What are the clinical needs of the client? How does the ethical dilemma relate to what the client presented with initially? It is important to assess the clinical issues so that pertinent information is not missed. For example, if a client with advanced AIDS is asking for help in ending his life, the provider would review the client's previous mental health history and current emotional issues, look for any significant changes in the client's support system, and determine if the client is experiencing social or psychological issues that might influence his decision. Until this is done, it is impossible for the clinician to address the ethical issue regarding end of life.

- **Identify the legal issues.** There can be significant legal issues to consider. Has the clinician reviewed the State and local laws regarding the issue? If necessary, has the clinician checked with an attorney for consultation or informed his supervisor of possible liability questions?

- **Identify the system issues.** What are the policies and procedures of the clinician's agency regarding the ethical question? In some agencies, the answers may be hard to find, but they can shed light on any restrictions the clinician may face or make the choices clear. For example, if it is against policy to accept a gift from a client, the clinician can avoid a personal rejection by

referring to the policy. Agency policy also can help a clinician in a legal challenge. For example, if the clinician followed agency policy, it is less likely that the clinician can be challenged legally for actions pertaining to that policy (although the agency can still be challenged).

- **Identify the cultural issues.** Cultural issues often are glossed over in the midst of a dilemma or crisis. Yet cultural issues are significant for understanding the client's motivation and whether or not the client will act according to the proposed treatment plan. For example, a gay, African American client may have difficulty dealing with his homosexuality and as a result may be having anonymous unprotected sex impulsively. In the African American culture it can be especially difficult for men to acknowledge their homosexuality. If the client is HIV positive, there is an ethical need to educate him about protecting others. If the clinician does not acknowledge the client's discomfort on a cultural level, the education process will be limited and the clinician will miss the "larger picture."

- **Identify the ethical issues.** What is the clinician's reaction to the situation? Ethical issues often are revealed when there is a "gut instinct" that something is not right. Confusion, anxiety, or uncertainty about what to do next with the client are indicators that an ethical issue is at stake. If basic principles seem to be compromised, the clinician should stop and evaluate further. A significant step is for the clinician to examine her own feelings about the situation. The clinician needs to identify any countertransference issues regarding the situation to ensure that the issue can be viewed objectively.

- **Review what principles are at stake.** What is the true dilemma? Is there a dilemma at all? So much can be occurring with a client that it is difficult to see the real issue, or whether the issue is significant. Is harm being done either by the client or to the client? Can the client make her own decisions, and is she not being allowed to do so? Is the client being treated fairly regardless of race, culture, or lifestyle? Is there a threat to the client's confidentiality? These are the questions relating to basic ethical principles.

- **What are the possible options?** By this point, the clinician's next step may be clear already. Or, there may be choices of possible options. It is useful to simply list all of the possible options and then examine them.
- **Review the pros and cons of each option.** List the pros and cons of each possible option, noting the impact of the options on the welfare of the client, the clinician, the agency, and others involved in the situation, such as the client's support system.
- **Act.** At this point, the clinician should be ready to make a decision. Sometimes the decision may not be one that everyone is comfortable with, but it may be the least objectionable plan. The client should understand the rationale for the clinician's decision, and there should be evidence of the clinician's thought process in the documentation of consultations, discussions with the client, and supervisory meetings.
- **Follow up and evaluate.** An ethical decision should be evaluated and the impact to the client monitored. For example, if the clinician decided to breach confidentiality for the protection of the client, how has this affected the clinical work with the client? These issues should be considered once an initial crisis has passed.

Additional Resources for Ethical Problemsolving

This section identifies several resources that can provide professional guidance on ethical issues.

Consultation

Consultation can be formal or informal. A supervisor is an obvious choice but may not always be available in some resource-strapped agencies or facilities. In lieu of formal supervision, there can be consultation with peers, lead workers, or other providers within the community who understand what the clinician does. For cultural questions, it is vital to use the community that represents that culture; however, the clinician should be cautious about consulting individuals who claim to represent the community but in actuality do not. The clinician also needs to ensure confidentiality with any consultation. If there is a chance that the information cannot be shared without divulging confidentiality, the provider may have to contact resources from another city, county, or State to ensure that the client's confidentiality is not threatened. Without the client's consent, however, the provider should never share identifying information.

Professional Standards or Codes of Ethics

Professional standards, and the documents that reflect them, are another resource. Social work, medicine, nursing, and psychology are examples of professions that have professional standards and codes of ethics. These documents do not provide answers to every ethical dilemma, but they do provide parameters for what is allowed or disallowed by the profession. They may also provide substantive questions to guide a provider toward making a decision. To find such documents, contact the association office for the particular professional group.

Legal Consultation

For many providers, obtaining legal advice may seem unrealistic given limited resources, but there are low-cost strategies for obtaining advice in some situations. Most bar associations have a pro bono legal component that may provide consultation at no charge or at a reduced rate. Legal service agencies that operate as a social service to the community may have expertise regarding certain ethical dilemmas. Another often untapped resource is the board of the organization that employs the clinician. The

board is legally responsible for any impact to the agency, so it would have a vested interest in assisting with a decision that could have legal repercussions. Many boards have attorneys as members.

It is worthwhile to examine the agency board, discover the specialty areas of the individuals who make up the board, and talk with the agency administration about building a relationship with those board members in advance of a legal issue. In addition, there is a Single State Authority charged with funding and regulating the field of substance abuse treatment. Such an entity may have an attorney available who can assist with legal issues relating to treatment.

9 Legal Issues

A number of legal issues can affect HIV-infected clients and the operations of substance abuse treatment programs. With multiple sets of rules governing HIV/AIDS as well as substance abuse treatment, compliance can be tricky. This chapter examines legal issues (many of them with ethical implications) in two main areas:

1. Access to services and programs, as well as employment opportunities for recovering substance abusers and persons living with HIV/AIDS
2. Confidentiality, or the protection of clients' right to privacy

Both of these areas are covered by Federal and State laws, which are often attempts to address the ethical concerns involved.

Access to Treatment— Issues of Discrimination

Substance abuse treatment providers may encounter discrimination against their clients as they try to connect them with services. Although people have come a long way from the early days of the AIDS pandemic (when people were afraid to have any contact with someone infected with HIV), there are still many instances in which people living with HIV/AIDS are shunned, excluded from services, or offered services under discriminatory conditions. As recently as 1998, the United States Supreme Court considered a case against a dentist who refused to treat a patient in his office. He stated he would only treat her in a hospital (although her situation did not warrant an admission) and that she would have to incur those costs herself.

People in substance abuse treatment also may encounter outright rejection or discrimination because of their history of drug or alcohol use. A hospital might be unwilling to admit a client who relapses periodically. Or a long-term care facility may be reluctant to accommodate a client who is maintained on methadone.

Individuals living with HIV/AIDS and persons in substance abuse treatment may also encounter discrimination in employment. A school may refuse to hire a teacher who is HIV positive, or a business may fire a secretary when it discovers she once was treated for alcoholism.

This section outlines the protections Federal law currently affords people with substance abuse problems and people living with HIV/AIDS, as well as the limitations of those protections. State laws that outlaw discrimination against individuals with disabilities are also mentioned.

Federal Statutes Protecting People With Disabilities

Two Federal statutes protect people with disabilities: the Federal Rehabilitation Act (29 United States Code [U.S.C.] §791 et seq. [1973]) and the Americans With Disabilities Act (ADA) (42 U.S.C. 12101 et seq. [1992]). (In this section these are referred to collectively as "the acts.") Together, these laws prohibit discrimination based on disability by private and public entities that provide most of the benefits, programs, and services a substance abuser or person living with HIV/AIDS is likely to need or seek. They also outlaw discrimination by a wide range of employers. For a general discussion about these Federal statutes, see TIP 29, *Substance Use Disorder Treatment for People With Physical and Cognitive Disabilities* (CSAT, 1998c).

Protections for substance abusers and persons living with HIV/AIDS

The issue for treatment providers is whether substance abusers and people living with HIV/AIDS are included in the definition of "individual with a disability." The answer is yes in many, but not all, instances.

Alcohol abusers

In general, these acts protect alcohol abusers who are seeking benefits or services from an organization or agency covered by one of the statutes (29 U.S.C. §706(8)(C)(iii) and 42 U.S.C. §12110(c)), if they are "qualified" and do not pose a direct threat to the health or safety of others (28 Code of Federal Regulations [CFR] §36.208(a)). This means that an organization or program cannot refuse to serve an individual unless

- The individual's alcohol use is so severe, or has resulted in other debilitating conditions, that he no longer "meets the essential eligibility requirements for the receipt of services or the participation in programs...with or without reasonable modifications to rules, policies, or practices ...." (42 U.S.C. §12131(2)).
- The individual poses "a significant risk to the health or safety of others that cannot be eliminated by a modification of policies, practices, or procedures, or by the provision of auxiliary aids or services" (36 CFR §36.208(b); Supplemental Information 28 CFR

Part 35, Section-by-Section Analysis, §35.104).

For example, a hospital might take the position that an alcohol-dependent client with dementia was not "qualified" to participate in occupational therapy because he could not follow directions. Or an alcohol abuser whose drinking results in assaultive episodes that endanger elderly residents in a long-term care facility might pose the kind of "direct threat" to the health or safety of others that would permit his exclusion.

The Rehabilitation Act also permits programs and activities providing services of an educational nature to discipline students who use or possess alcohol (29 U.S.C. §706(8)(C)(iv)).

Abusers of illegal drugs

The acts divide abusers of illegal drugs into two groups: former abusers and current abusers.

Former abusers. Individuals who no longer are engaged in illegal use of drugs and have completed or are participating in a drug rehabilitation program are protected from discrimination to the same extent as alcohol abusers (29 U.S.C. §706(8)(C)(ii); 42 U.S.C. §12210(b)). In other words, they are protected so long as they are "qualified" for the program, activity, or service and do not pose a "direct threat" to the health or safety of others. Service providers may administer drug tests to ensure that an individual who once used illegal drugs no longer does so (28 CFR §36.209(c); 28 CFR §35.131(c)).

Current abusers. Individuals currently engaging in illegal use of drugs are offered full protection only in connection with health and drug rehabilitation services (28 CFR §36.209(b) and 28 CFR §35.131(b)). (However, drug treatment programs may deny participation to individuals who continue to use illegal drugs while they are in the program (28 CFR §36.209(b)(2)).) The laws explicitly withdraw protection with regard to other services, programs, or activities (29 U.S.C. §706(8)(C)(i) and 42 U.S.C. §2210(a)). Current illegal use of drugs is defined as "illegal use of drugs that occurred recently enough to justify a reasonable belief that a person's drug use is current or that continuing use is a real and ongoing problem" (28 CFR §35.104 and 28 CFR §35.104).

For example, a hospital that specializes in treating burn victims could not refuse to treat a burn victim because he uses illegal drugs, nor could it impose a surcharge on him because of his addiction. However, the hospital is not required to provide services that it does not ordinarily provide; for example, drug abuse treatment (Appendix B to 28 CFR Part 36, Section-by-Section Analysis, §36.302). On the other hand, a homeless shelter could refuse to admit an abuser of illegal drugs, unless the individual has stopped and is participating in or has completed drug treatment.

The Rehabilitation Act also permits programs and activities providing educational services to discipline students who use or possess illegal drugs (29 U.S.C. §706(8)(C)(iv)).

Individuals living with HIV/AIDS

Although alcohol and drug abuse are mentioned in both of the acts, HIV/AIDS is not. However, on June 25, 1998, the United States Supreme Court held that asymptomatic HIV infection is a "disability" under the ADA (*Bragdon* v. *Abbott*, 524 U.S. 624 [1998]. See also 28 CFR §35.104 and §36.104; 28 CFR Part 35, Section-by-Section Analysis, §35.104 and Appendix B to 28 CFR Part 36, Section-by-Section Analysis, §36.104). In this case, a woman with asymptomatic HIV disease sued a dentist who denied her equal service.

The *Bragdon* v. *Abbott* decision means that individuals living with HIV/AIDS are protected from discrimination under both of the acts, so long as they are "qualified" for the service, program, or benefit and do not pose a "direct threat" to the health or safety of others. (See also 28 CFR §36.208; Supplemental Information

28 CFR Part 35, Section-by-Section Analysis, §35.104.) An individual who is too ill to participate in a program, even with reasonable modifications, might not be "qualified."

The "direct threat" question has received the most public attention. Can a "public accommodation," a restaurant, hospital, school, or funeral home, refuse to provide services to someone living with HIV/AIDS because the person poses a "direct threat" to the health and safety of others? Because HIV is not transmitted by casual contact, and most programs and services provided by "public accommodations" involve only casual contact, the answer in most cases should be "no." Even when contact with bodily fluids is likely to occur, public health authorities advise health care professionals to treat HIV-positive clients in the normal setting and to use universal precautions with all clients. Moreover, in those cases where a public accommodation could argue that an HIV-positive individual poses a direct threat, it would also have to show that the threat could not be eliminated by a modification of policies, practices, or procedures, or by the provision of auxiliary aids or services.

Protections in the area of employment

Alcohol-dependent and alcohol-abusing persons. The acts provide limited protection against employment discrimination to individuals who abuse alcohol but who can perform the requisite job duties and do not pose a direct threat to the health, safety, or property of others in the workplace (29 U.S.C. §706(8)(C)(v); 42 U.S.C. §12113(b); 42 U.S.C. §12111(3)). For example, the acts would protect an alcoholic secretary who binges on weekends but reports to work sober and performs her job safely and efficiently. However, a truck driver who comes to work inebriated and unable to do his job safely would not be protected. The employee whose promptness or attendance is erratic would not be protected either, unless the employer tolerated nonalcoholic-employee lateness and absences from work.

The ADA also permits an employer to

- Prohibit all use of alcohol in the workplace
- Require all employees to be free from the influence of alcohol at the workplace
- Require employees who abuse alcohol to maintain the same qualifications for employment, job performance, and behavior that the employer requires other employees to meet, even if any unsatisfactory performance is related to the employee's alcohol abuse (42 U.S.C. §12114(c))

Abusers of illegal drugs. Those who use or have used illegal drugs stand on a different footing. Former abusers who have completed or are participating in a drug rehabilitation program are offered some protection. The acts protect employees and prospective employees who

- Have successfully completed a supervised drug rehabilitation program or otherwise been rehabilitated and are no longer engaging in the illegal use of drugs
- Are participating in a supervised rehabilitation program and are no longer engaging in illegal drug use
- Are erroneously regarded as engaging in illegal drug use (29 U.S.C. 706(8)(C)(ii); 42 U.S.C. §12210(c))

Employers may administer drug testing to ensure that someone who has a history of illegal drug use is no longer using (29 U.S.C. §706(8)(C)(ii); 42 U.S.C. §12210(b); 28 CFR §36.209(c); 28 CFR §35.131(c)).

The ADA also permits an employer to

- Prohibit all use of illegal drugs in the workplace
- Require all employees to be free from the influence of illegal drugs at the workplace
- Require an employee who engages in the illegal use of drugs to maintain the same

qualifications for employment, job performance, and behavior that the employer requires other employees to meet, even if any unsatisfactory performance is related to the employee's drug abuse (42 U.S.C. §12114(c))

The Drug-Free Workplace Act

Another Federal law, the Drug-Free Workplace Act (41 U.S.C. §701), may also affect clients in recovery. The Act requires employers who receive Federal funding through a grant (including block grant or entitlement grant programs) or who hold Federal contracts to certify they will provide a substance-free workplace. The certification means that affected employers must

- Notify employees that "the unlawful manufacture, distribution, dispensing, possession, or use of a controlled substance is prohibited in the workplace and specify the actions that will be taken against employees [who violate the] prohibition"
- Establish an ongoing substance-free awareness program to inform employees of the dangers of substance abuse in the workplace, the availability of any substance abuse counseling or employee assistance program, and the penalties that may be imposed for violations of the employer's policy
- Take appropriate action against an employee convicted of a substance abuse offense when the offense occurred in the workplace
- Notify the Federal funding agency in writing when such a conviction occurs

Current abusers have no protection against discrimination in employment, even if they are "qualified" and do not pose a "direct threat" to others in the workplace (29 U.S.C. §706(8)(C)(i); 42 U.S.C. §12210(a)).

People living with HIV/AIDS. The Supreme Court's decision in *Abbott*, that "disability" includes symptomatic and asymptomatic HIV disease, should apply in the area of employment. See also 28 CFR §35.104; Appendix to 29 CFR Part 1630C Interpretive Guidance on Title I of the Americans with Disabilities Act, §1630.2(j) ("impairments...such as HIV infection, are inherently substantially limiting"). This means that an individual living with HIV/AIDS is protected from employment discrimination as long as he is "qualified," that is, he can, with or without reasonable accommodation, perform the essential functions of the job and does not pose a "direct threat" to others in the workplace.

Reasonable accommodation can include a modified work schedule or reassignment to a vacant position. The "direct threat" issue has been most controversial and was left undecided by the court in *Abbott*. Can an employer running a restaurant, school, beauty salon, or construction company refuse to hire a person living with HIV/AIDS on the basis that the person poses a "direct threat" to coworkers, customers, or others in the workplace? Not if it bases its judgment solely on the individual's HIV/AIDS status. Because most employment involves only casual contact, an HIV-infected individual does not pose a risk to other employees, diners, students, or customers. Even in cases where an employer could argue that an HIV-infected individual poses a direct threat, it would also have to show that the threat could not be eliminated through a reasonable accommodation.

Therefore, in most cases, an employer could not refuse to hire and retain a person living with HIV/AIDS. However, if a person living with HIV/AIDS suffers from a physical condition such as blurred vision or dizziness that might pose a risk if he operates dangerous equipment, the employer might be justified in refusing to hire the person or curtailing the employee's activities after making the individualized assessment required by regulation (29 CFR §1630.2(r)).

The Civil Rights Division of the U.S. Department of Justice has issued a useful "Q & A" about the ADA's protections for persons living with HIV/AIDS. It poses and answers questions about employment discrimination and discrimination by "public accommodations" and State and local governments and gives many helpful examples. It also contains a listing of places to find help. It can be found on the Internet at http://www.usdoj.gov/crt/ada/pubs/hivqanda.txt.

State Laws

Most States have also enacted laws to protect people with disabilities (or "handicaps"). Some State laws protect alcohol abusers, drug abusers, and persons living with HIV/AIDS. Each State's laws are different, and a treatment provider seeking help under State law should make contact with the State or local agency charged with enforcing State civil rights laws. Such agencies often have the words "civil rights," "human rights," or "equal opportunity" in their titles.

Enforcement

Discrimination against substance abusers and individuals living with HIV/AIDS continues despite the existence of the acts. However, these laws offer those who believe they have suffered discrimination a choice of remedies.

For discrimination by program or activity

Filing a complaint with the Federal agency that funds the program, activity, or service (42 U.S.C. §12133; 29 U.S.C. §794(a); 28 CFR Part 35, Subparts F and G). For example, if the program is educational, it may receive funding from the Department of Education; if it involves health care, it may be funded by the U.S. Department of Health and Human Services (DHHS). Once a complaint is filed, one or more of the following actions will be taken:

- The agency will investigate and attempt an informal resolution.
- If a resolution is reached, the agency drafts a compliance agreement enforceable by the U.S. Attorney General.
- If no resolution is achieved, the agency issues a "Letter of Findings." The Letter of Findings contains findings of fact, conclusions of law, a description of the suggested remedy, and a notice of the complainant's right to sue. A copy is sent to the U.S. Attorney General.
- The agency must then approach the offending program about negotiating. If the program refuses to negotiate or negotiations are fruitless, the agency refers the matter to the U.S. Attorney General with a recommendation for action.

Advantages: A complaint to the Federal funding agency may get the offending program's attention (and change its decision) because the funding agency has the power to deny future funding to those who violate the law. It is also inexpensive (no lawyer is necessary); however, if the complainant opts to be represented by an attorney, he may be awarded attorneys' fees if he prevails.

Disadvantage: Depending on the kind of complaint and which Federal agency has jurisdiction, this may not be the most expeditious route.

Filing a complaint with the State administrative agency charged with enforcement of the antidiscrimination laws (42 U.S.C. §12201(b)). Such agencies often have the words "civil rights," "human rights," or "equal opportunity" in their titles.

Advantage: This recourse is inexpensive.

Disadvantages: Some of these agencies have large backlogs that generally preclude speedy resolution of complaints. Depending on the State, remedies may be limited.

Filing a case in State or Federal court. One can file a court case requesting injunctive relief (temporary or permanent) and/or monetary damages. The court has the discretion to appoint a lawyer to represent the plaintiff (42 U.S.C. §§12188 and 2000a-3(a); 28 CFR §36.501).

Advantages: The complainant can ask for injunctive relief (a court order requiring the program to change its policy) and/or monetary damages. It may give the complainant a better sense of control over the process. A lawyer may produce results relatively quickly. A lawyer's approach to an offending program can have prompt and salutary effects. No one likes to be sued; it is costly, unpleasant, and often very public. It is often easier to re-examine one's position and settle the case quickly out of court.

Disadvantages: Unless one can find a not-for-profit organization that is interested in the case, a lawyer willing to represent the aggrieved party pro bono, or a lawyer willing to take the case on contingency or for the attorneys' fees the court can award the side that prevails, this may be an expensive alternative. It also may take a long time.

The advantages and disadvantages of filing a case in State court depend on State law, State procedural rules, and the speed with which cases are resolved.

Requesting enforcement action by the U.S. Attorney General. The Attorney General can file a lawsuit asking for injunctive relief, monetary damages, and civil penalties (42 U.S.C. §12188 and 2000a-3(a); 28 CFR §36.503).

For employment discrimination

Filing a complaint with the Federal Equal Employment Opportunity Commission (EEOC) (42 U.S.C. §12117) or the State administrative agency charged with enforcement of antidiscrimination laws (42 U.S.C. §12201(b)).

- If the EEOC finds reasonable cause to believe that the charge of discrimination is true, and it cannot get agreement from the party charged, it can bring a lawsuit against any private entity. If the offending entity is governmental, the EEOC must refer the case to the U.S. Attorney General, who may file a lawsuit. The complainant can intervene in any court case brought by either the EEOC or the U.S. Attorney General.

- The EEOC or the U.S. Attorney General can also seek immediate relief by filing a motion for a preliminary injunction in a Federal court.
- The court can order injunctive relief, including reinstatement or hiring, back pay, and attorneys' fees (42 U.S.C. §2000e-5).

Advantage: A complaint to the EEOC, the U.S. Department of Justice, a State or local antidiscrimination agency, or State Attorney General is relatively inexpensive because it does not require a lawyer.

Disadvantage: Some of these agencies have large backlogs that generally preclude speedy resolution of complaints.

Filing a lawsuit in State or Federal court. After an aggrieved party has filed a complaint with the State administrative agency and/or the EEOC, he can file a lawsuit (42 U.S.C. §2000e-5(f)).

Advantages: It may give the complainant better control over the process. The complainant can ask for injunctive relief (a court order requiring the employer to change its policy) and/or monetary damages. It can get relatively fast results. A lawyer's approach to an offending employer can have salutary effects. No one likes to be sued—it is costly, unpleasant, and often very public. It is often easier to re-examine one's position and settle the case quickly out of court.

Disadvantages: Unless one can find a not-for-profit organization that is interested in the case, a lawyer willing to represent the aggrieved party pro bono, or a lawyer willing to take the case on contingency or for the attorneys' fees the court can award the side that prevails, this may

be an expensive alternative. It may also take a long time.

The alternatives listed here must be pursued within certain time limits established by State and Federal laws. An individual who is considering filing a complaint with any one of the agencies mentioned above should consult an attorney at an early date to determine when a complaint must be filed.

Summary of Protections

Federal law provides broad protection against discrimination by programs, services, and employers for individuals in substance abuse treatment who are also living with HIV/AIDS. Many States also have laws prohibiting discrimination against "individuals with disabilities" or "handicaps," and some of these statutes also protect recovering substance abusers and individuals living with HIV/AIDS. To learn more about State law, the protections it offers, and the available remedies, providers can call the State or local "human rights," "civil rights," or "equal opportunity" agency. Advocacy groups for individuals with disabilities are also a good source of information. (An AIDS advocacy group would be particularly well informed.) Finally, local legal services offices, law school faculties, or bar associations may also have information available or may be able to provide an individual lawyer willing to make a presentation to staff.

Confidentiality of Information About Clients

Programs providing substance abuse treatment for clients living with HIV/AIDS frequently must communicate with individuals and organizations as they gather information, refer clients for services the program does not provide, and coordinate care with other service providers. On occasion, they are required to report information to the State. This section outlines the laws protecting client confidentiality and examines how staff can continue to provide appropriate treatment services, comply with State reporting laws, and protect client privacy.

Information about clients in substance abuse treatment who are living with HIV/AIDS is subject to two sets of laws:

- Federal statutes and regulations that guarantee the confidentiality of information about all persons applying for or receiving alcohol and drug abuse prevention, screening, assessment, and treatment services (42 U.S.C. §290dd-2; 42 CFR, Part 2)
- State laws governing the confidentiality of HIV/AIDS-related information. (State laws protecting HIV-related information vary in the protection they offer; some guard clients' privacy closely, others are more lenient. State laws also protect the confidentiality of other medical and mental health information. These laws, however, are likely to be less stringent than statutes dealing specifically with information about HIV/AIDS.)

The remainder of this chapter describes what these laws require and examines their impact on substance abuse treatment programs. The first section contains an overview of the Federal law protecting the right to privacy of any person who seeks or receives substance abuse treatment services. Because the Federal law applies throughout the country and preempts less restrictive State laws, this discussion focuses on how the Federal rules apply in a variety of situations, then addresses related State laws in those contexts. Next is an examination of the rules surrounding the use of consent forms to obtain a client's permission to release information, including ways to handle requests

for disclosure when the client's file contains both substance abuse and HIV/AIDS information.

The third section reviews situations that commonly arise when a client in substance abuse treatment is living with HIV/AIDS, including how communications among agencies providing services to the client can be managed. The fourth section discusses exceptions in the Federal confidentiality rules that, in limited circumstances, permit disclosure of information about clients (e.g., reporting child abuse or neglect). The chapter ends with a few additional points concerning the requirement that clients receive a notice about the confidentiality regulations, clients' right to review their own records, and security of records.

Federal and State Laws Protect the Client's Right to Privacy

A Federal law and a set of regulations guarantee strict confidentiality of information about all persons who seek or receive alcohol and substance abuse assessment and treatment services. The legal citations for the laws and regulations are 42 U.S.C. §290dd-2 and 42 CFR Part 2. (Citations below in the form "§2..." refer to specific sections of 42 CFR Part 2.)

The Federal law and regulations are designed to protect clients' privacy rights in order to attract people into treatment. The regulations restrict communications tightly; unlike either the doctor–patient or the attorney–client privilege, the substance abuse treatment provider is prohibited from disclosing even the client's name. Violating the regulations is punishable by a fine of up to $500 for a first offense or up to $5,000 for each subsequent offense (§2.4).

The Federal rules apply to any program that specializes, *in whole or in part*, in providing treatment, counseling, or assessment and referral services for people with alcohol or drug problems (42 CFR §2.12(e)). Although the

Federal regulations apply only to programs that receive Federal assistance, this includes indirect forms of Federal aid such as tax-exempt status, or State or local government funding coming (in whole or in part) from the Federal Government. Whether the Federal regulations apply to a particular program depends on the kinds of services the program offers, not the label the program chooses. Calling itself a "prevention program" or "outreach program" or "screening program" does not absolve a program from adhering to the confidentiality rules.

In the wake of the HIV/AIDS pandemic, many States have adopted laws protecting HIV/AIDS information. These laws are designed to encourage people at risk for HIV/AIDS to be tested, determine their HIV/AIDS status, begin medical treatment early, and change risky behaviors. Many State laws were passed with the concern that those who are seropositive will suffer discrimination in employment, medical care, insurance, housing, and other areas if their status becomes known. (Other State laws protect information about individuals' health, mental health status, or treatment, as well as information about other infectious diseases.)

The primary aim of confidentiality rules is to allow the client (and not the provider) to determine when and to whom information about medical or mental health, substance abuse, or HIV infection will be disclosed. Most of the nettlesome problems that may crop up under the State and Federal laws and regulations can be avoided through planning ahead. Familiarity with the rules will ease communication. It can also reduce the confidentiality-related conflicts among program, client, and outside agency or person to a few relatively rare situations.

General rules pertaining to confidentiality

Federal protections for substance abuse-related information

The Federal confidentiality law and regulations protect any information about a client who has applied for or received any service related to substance abuse treatment from a program that is covered under the law. Services can include screening, referral, assessment, diagnosis, individual counseling, group counseling, or treatment. The regulations are in effect from the time the client applies for or receives services or the program first conducts an assessment or begins to counsel the client. *The restrictions on disclosure apply to any information that would identify the client as an alcohol or drug abuser, either directly or by implication.* They also apply to former clients or patients. The rules apply whether or not the person making an inquiry about the client already has the information, has other ways of getting it, has some form of official status, is authorized by State law, or comes armed with a subpoena or search warrant. It should be noted, however, that if the person requesting information has a "special authorizing court order," he does have the right to receive confidential information according to 42 CFR, Part 2.[1]

State protections for HIV/AIDS-related information

Whereas the Federal confidentiality rules apply throughout the country, each State has a different set of rules regarding disclosure of HIV/AIDS information. When substance abuse treatment programs hold HIV/AIDS-related information about clients, that information is protected by the Federal confidentiality regulations as well as by State law protecting HIV/AIDS-related information.

State protections for other medical and mental health-related information

State laws also offer general protection to some medical and mental health information. While any HIV/AIDS-specific confidentiality law is likely to be more stringent, providers should be aware of these more general statutes.[2]

When may confidential information be shared with others?

Although Federal and State law protect information about clients, the laws do contain exceptions. The most commonly used exception is the client's written consent. Although the Federal law protecting information about clients in substance abuse treatment and State laws protecting HIV/AIDS-related information both permit a client to consent to a disclosure, the consent requirements are likely to differ. Therefore, whenever providers contemplate making a disclosure of information about a client in substance abuse treatment who is living with HIV/AIDS, they must consider both Federal and State laws.

Federal Rules About Consent

The Federal regulations regarding consent are strict, somewhat unusual, and must be carefully followed. A proper consent form must be in writing and must contain *each* of the items below (§2.31):

1. The name or general description of the program(s) making the disclosure
2. The name or title of the individual or organization that will receive the disclosure
3. The name of the client who is the subject of the disclosure
4. The purpose or need for the disclosure
5. How much and what kind of information will be disclosed
6. A statement that the client may revoke (take back) the consent at any time, except to the

extent that the program has already acted on it
7. The date, event, or condition upon which the consent expires if not previously revoked
8. The signature of the client
9. The date on which the consent is signed

A general medical release form, or any consent form that does not contain all of the elements listed above, *is not acceptable*. (See sample consent form in Figure 9-1.) Most disclosures of information about a client in substance abuse treatment are permissible if the client has signed a valid consent form that has not expired or been revoked. (One exception to this statement may be when a client's file contains HIV/AIDS information, as discussed below.)

Items 4 through 7 in the above list deserve further explanation and are discussed in the sections that follow. Two other issues are also considered: the required notice to the recipient of the information that it may not be disclosed and the effect of a signed consent form.

Purpose of the disclosure and how much and what kind of information will be disclosed

These two items are closely related. All disclosures, and especially those made pursuant to a consent form, must be limited to the information necessary to accomplish the need or purpose for the disclosure (§2.13(a)). It is improper to disclose everything in a client's file if the recipient of the information needs only one specific piece of information.

A key step in completing the consent form is specifying the purpose or need for the communication of information. Once the purpose has been identified, it is easier to determine how much and what kind of information will be disclosed and to tailor it to what is essential to accomplish that particular purpose or need.

Figure 9-1
Sample Consent Form

Consent for the Release of Confidential Information

I, _____, authorize XYZ Clinic to receive from/
        (name of client or participant)

disclose to _____
                    (name of person and organization)

for the purpose of _____

_____
                    (need for disclosure)

the following information _____
                    (nature of the disclosure)

_____

_____

I understand that my records are protected under the Federal and State confidentiality regulations and cannot be disclosed without my written consent unless otherwise provided for in the regulations. I also understand that I may revoke this consent at any time except to the extent that action has been taken in reliance on it and that in any event this consent expires automatically on _____
unless otherwise specified below.   (date, condition, or event)

Other expiration specifications:

_____

_____

_____
Date executed

_____
Signature of client

_____
Signature of parent or guardian, where required

Client's right to revoke consent

Federal regulations permit the client to revoke consent at any time, and the consent form must include a statement to this effect. Revocation need not be in writing. If a program has already made a disclosure prior to the revocation, the program has acted in reliance on the consent and is not required to retrieve the information it has already disclosed.

Expiration of consent form

The Federal rules require that the consent form contain a date, event, or condition on which it will expire if not previously revoked. A consent form must last "no longer than reasonably necessary to serve the purpose for which it is given" (§2.31(a)(9)). If the purpose of the disclosure is expected to be accomplished in 5 or 10 days, it is better to fill in that amount of time rather than a longer period. It is best to determine how long each consent form should run rather than impose a set time period such as 60 or 90 days. When uniform expiration dates are used, agencies can find themselves in a situation requiring disclosure, after the client's consent form has expired. This means at the least that the client must return to the agency to sign a new consent form. At worst, the client has left or is unavailable (e.g., hospitalized), and the agency will not be able to make the disclosure.

The consent form need not contain a specific expiration date, but may instead specify an event or condition. For example, a form could expire after a client has seen a specific referred health care provider, or a consent form permitting disclosures to an employer might expire at the end of the client's probationary period.

The signature when the client is a minor (and the issue of parental consent)[3]

Minors must always sign the consent form in order for a program to release information, even with a parent's or guardian's consent. The program must obtain the parent's signature in addition to the minor's signature only if the program is required by State law to obtain parental permission before providing treatment to minors (§2.14). ("Parent" includes parent, guardian, or other person legally responsible for the minor.)

In other words, if State law does not require the program to obtain parental consent to provide services to a minor, then parental consent is not required to make disclosures (§2.14(b)). If State law requires parental consent to provide services to a minor, then parental consent is required to make any disclosures. *The program must always obtain the minor's consent for disclosures and cannot rely on the parent's signature alone.* Substance abuse treatment programs should consult with their Single State Authority or a local lawyer to determine whether they need parental consent to provide services to minors. For more information about minors, see TIP 31, *Screening and Assessing Adolescents for Substance Use Disorders* (CSAT, 1999a), and TIP 32, *Treatment of Adolescents With Substance Use Disorders* (CSAT, 1999b).

Required notice against redisclosing information

Once the consent form is properly completed, one last requirement remains. Any disclosure made with client consent must be accompanied by a written statement that the information disclosed is protected by Federal law and that the recipient of the information cannot further disclose it unless permitted by the regulations (§2.32). This statement, not the consent form itself, should be delivered and explained to the recipient at the time of disclosure or earlier.

The prohibition on redisclosure is clear and strict. Those who receive the notice are prohibited from re-releasing information except as permitted by the regulations. (Of course, a client may sign a consent form authorizing such a redisclosure.)

Note on the effect of a signed consent form

Programs may not disclose information when a consent form has expired, is deficient, is invalid or has been revoked (§2.31(c)). The other rules about how programs should respond to a signed consent form depend upon whether the disclosure will be to a third party or to the client himself and whether the client is a minor.

Disclosures to third parties

Programs subject to the Federal confidentiality rules are not required to disclose information *to a third party* about a client who has signed a consent form authorizing release of information unless the program has *also* been served with a subpoena or court order that meets the requirements of §2.3(b) and §2.61(a)(b). If the client consenting to disclosure is a minor (an issue governed by State law), the same rule applies. However, whether a consent form signed by a minor is valid depends upon whether State law permits a minor to enter treatment without parental consent. If State law permits a minor to enter treatment without parental consent, the program can rely on the minor client's signature on the consent form to make a disclosure to a third party. If State law requires parental consent for minors to enter treatment, then the program must get the signature of *both* parent and client. The minor must always sign the form.

Whenever a program releases information to a third party, it should disclose only what is necessary, and only as long as necessary, keeping in mind the purpose of the communication.

Disclosures to clients

If a client signs a consent form authorizing the program to disclose records *directly to the client* and *State law requires the program to honor such a request*, then the program must release the records *to the client*. (Note that the Federal law does not require clients to sign a proper consent

form to obtain their own records, but State law may.) If the client signing the consent form authorizing release of information is a minor and the disclosure will be to his parent, guardian or other person or entity legally responsible for him, the program should make the disclosure. State law may mandate the disclosure and once the minor has consented, the program must follow the State rule. Even in States without such a rule mandating disclosure, only extraordinary circumstances could justify withholding information from a parent or guardian once the minor has consented to its release.

Special consent rules for clients mandated into treatment by the justice system

Substance abuse treatment programs treating clients who are involved in the criminal justice system (CJS) must also follow the Federal confidentiality regulations. However, some special rules apply when a client comes for assessment or treatment as an official condition of probation, sentence, dismissal of charges, release from detention, or other disposition of a criminal justice proceeding.

A consent form (or court order) is still required before a program can disclose information about a client who is the subject of CJS referral. For more detailed information about consent for clients within the CJS, see TIP 17, *Planning for Alcohol and Other Drug Abuse Treatment for Adults in the Criminal Justice System* (CSAT, 1995c).

State Rules About Consent

State laws that protect disclosure of HIV/AIDS-related information also contain an exception permitting most disclosures when the client consents. However, some States have strict requirements governing the content of the consent form. It is important, therefore, that programs providing substance abuse treatment to people living with HIV/AIDS become familiar with those requirements.

Which set of rules applies when a substance abuse treatment client with HIV/AIDS consents to a disclosure? This depends on what information is to be released, as illustrated in the following examples.

Example 1. Suppose a client's file contains both substance abuse treatment information and HIV/AIDS information, and the client wants to consent to disclosure of information about substance abuse to an outside agency but not information about HIV/AIDS status. This problem could be handled in several ways:

- The federally required consent form can be drafted narrowly so that the purpose for the disclosure and the kind of information to be disclosed are limited to substance abuse treatment.
- The program can maintain a filing system that isolates substance abuse and HIV/AIDS-related information in two different "treatment" or "medical" files and discloses only information from the "treatment" file. (This solution may not be practical, however, in States that regulate how and where HIV/AIDS-related information must be charted.)
- The program can send the client's file without the HIV/AIDS-related information to the outside agency and include the following notice (with the federally required notice of the prohibition on redisclosure):

  This file does not contain any information protected by section ___ of the [State] law. The fact that this notice accompanies these records is NOT an indication that this client's file contains any information protected by section ___.

Example 2. If the client wants the program to release information about his HIV/AIDS status, the answer will be different. Clearly the State's form must be used. However, if the disclosure

of the client's HIV/AIDS-related information will *by implication or otherwise* reveal that the client is in substance abuse treatment, the Federal form must also be used. For example, if the Satellite City Drug and Alcohol Program is the agency releasing HIV/AIDS-related information with a client's consent, the fact that the information came from a substance abuse treatment program will alert the recipient that the client is not only HIV positive but is also in substance abuse treatment. The program, therefore, must use a consent form that complies with both Federal and State requirements. It should not be necessary for clients to sign two separate forms in this kind of situation; a form that complies with both sets of requirements should be drafted.

Example 3. Finally, what happens when a client signs a proper consent form permitting disclosure of information about her substance abuse treatment, and the information she consents to release would also disclose her HIV/AIDS status? Can the program release the information? Not unless the program has complied with State consent requirements. Even if a client has signed a consent form permitting disclosure of substance abuse information, the program may not release information about HIV/AIDS unless it has also satisfied State requirements.

Strategies for Communication With Others About Clients

Some of the practical questions that affect program operations include the following:

- How can substance abuse treatment providers seek information from collateral sources about clients they are screening, assessing, or treating?
- How can providers comply with State mandatory reporting laws?
- How should providers deal with insurance companies and other third-party payors?

- How can providers respond to requests for information about clients who have died or become incompetent?
- How should programs deal with clients' risk-taking behavior? Do programs have a duty to warn potential victims or law enforcement agencies of clients' threats to plan to infect someone else with HIV/AIDS, and if so, how do they communicate the warning?
- Can staff members of substance abuse treatment programs comply with mandatory State child abuse reporting laws?

Seeking information from collateral sources

Making inquiries of family members, employers, schools, doctors, and other health care entities might seem to pose no risk to a client's right to confidentiality. This is not the case. When program staff seek information from other sources, they are letting these sources know that the client has asked for substance abuse treatment services. The Federal regulations generally prohibit this kind of disclosure unless the client consents.

How should a substance abuse treatment program proceed? The easiest way is to obtain the client's consent to contact the employer, family member, school, health care facility, etc. Or, the program could ask the client to sign a consent form that permits it to make a disclosure for the purpose of seeking information from other sources to any one of a number of organizations or persons listed on the consent form. Note that this combination form must still include "the name or title of the individual or the name of the organization" for each source the program contacts. Whichever method the program chooses, it must use the consent form required by the regulations, not a general medical release form.

If the client is living with HIV/AIDS, the program must check State laws to see whether they impose additional requirements. For example, an alcohol and drug counselor wishing

to talk to a client's primary care physician must first find out whether State law protecting HIV/AIDS-related information requires that additional provisions be added to the consent form the client signs.

Making mandatory reports to public health authorities

All States require that AIDS and tuberculosis (TB) be reported to public health authorities, and some States also require that new cases of HIV infection be reported. The reports are forwarded to the Centers for Disease Control and Prevention (CDC). All States also use the TB report to perform contact tracing, or finding others to whom an infected person may have spread the disease; some States use HIV/AIDS reporting similarly.

In each State, what must be reported for which diseases, who must report, and the purposes for which the information is used vary. Therefore, providers must be familiar with their State laws regarding (1) whether they or any of their staff members are mandated to report, (2) when reporting is required, (3) what information must be reported and whether it includes client-identifying information, and (4) what will be done with the information reported.

Reporting HIV/AIDS and TB cases

If client-identifying information must be reported, how can programs comply with State laws mandating the reporting of TB and HIV/AIDS cases? Several ways are listed below.

Reporting with consent

The easiest way to comply is to obtain the client's consent. Note that if the public health authority plans to redisclose the information to the CDC, the consent form must be drafted to permit such redisclosure. The consent form can also be drafted to authorize the program to communicate on an ongoing basis with the public health department to help them find, counsel, monitor, or treat a client or coordinate a client's TB care.

Reporting without making a client-identifying disclosure

If State law permits the use of a code rather than the client's name, the program can make the report without the client's consent because no client-identifying information is being revealed. If the program is part of another health care facility, general hospital, or a mental health program, the report can include the client's name, if it does so under the name of the parent agency and releases no information that links the client with substance abuse treatment. (See the discussion below in "Communications that do not disclose client-identifying information.")

Reporting through a Qualified Service Organization Agreement

A substance abuse treatment program can enter into a Qualified Service Organization Agreement (QSOA) with the State or local public health department charged with receiving mandatory reports. The QSOA (explained in more detail later in this chapter) permits the program to report names of clients to the health department and, if properly drafted, allows ongoing communication between the program and public health officials.

A program that is required to report TB or AIDS cases to a public health department can also enter into a QSOA with a general medical care facility or a laboratory that conducts testing or provides care to the program's clients. The QSOA would permit the program to report the names of clients to the medical care facility or laboratory, which can then report the information (including the clients' names) to the public heath department, without any information that would link those names with substance abuse treatment. Note that State confidentiality laws might impose additional

requirements. Also, an agreement with a medical care facility or laboratory would not permit public health authorities to follow up on cases with the treatment program.

Reporting under the audit and evaluation exception

One exception to the general rule prohibiting disclosure without a client's consent permits programs under certain conditions to disclose information to auditors and evaluators (§2.53). (For an explanation of the requirements of §2.53, see TIP 14, *Developing State Outcomes Monitoring Systems for Alcohol and Other Drug Abuse Treatment* [CSAT, 1995a].) DHHS has written two opinion letters that approve the use of the audit and evaluation exception to report HIV/AIDS-related information to public health authorities (see Pascal, 1988, and Zagame, 1989). Together, these two letters suggest that substance abuse treatment programs may report client-identifying information even if that information will be used by the public health department to conduct contact tracing, so long as the health department does not disclose the name of the client to "contacts" it approaches. The letters also suggest that public health authorities could use the information to contact the infected substance abuse disorder client directly.

However, some authorities may not agree with these opinion letters. As its title "audit and evaluation" implies, §2.53 is intended to permit an outside entity, such as a peer review organization or an accounting firm, to examine a program's records to determine whether it is operating appropriately. It is not intended to permit an outside entity such as the public health authority to gain information for other social ends, such as tracing the spread of disease. It can be argued that such use distorts the purpose of the audit and evaluation exception.

Getting a court order

A program could apply to a court for an order authorizing it to disclose information to a public health department. The court order provision is discussed further under "Exceptions that permit disclosures," below. Since obtaining a court order requires drawing up legal papers, it is not likely to be a program's first choice.

Using the medical emergency exception

The Federal regulations permit a program to disclose information without client consent to medical personnel "who have a need for information about a client for the purpose of treating a condition which poses an immediate threat to the health" of the client or any other individual. The regulations define "medical emergency" as a situation that poses an immediate threat to health and requires immediate medical intervention (§2.51). (This exception is explained more fully later in this chapter.) Because any disclosure under this exception is limited to true emergencies, a program cannot routinely use the medical emergency exception to make mandatory reports. Because immediate medical intervention is unlikely to prevent or cure HIV infection, it is not an advisable way to make mandatory HIV/AIDS reports to public health departments.

For a more complete exploration of these options see TIP 18, *The Tuberculosis Epidemic: Legal and Ethical Issues for Alcohol and Other Drug Abuse Treatment Providers* (CSAT, 1995d).

Dealing with client risk-taking behavior

Does a program have a "duty to warn" others when it knows that a client is infected with HIV? When would that "duty" arise? Even where no duty exists, should providers warn others at risk about a client's HIV status? Finally, how can others be warned without violating the Federal confidentiality regulations and State confidentiality laws?

These questions raise complex legal issues that are discussed below. But first it must be noted that "warning" someone about a client's HIV status without his consent has potential consequences. Successful substance abuse treatment depends on clients' willingness to expose shameful things about themselves to program staff. The news that the program has "warned" a spouse, lover, or someone else that a client is HIV positive will spread quickly among the client population. Such news could destroy clients' trust in the program and its staff. Any counselor or program considering "warning" someone of a client's HIV status without the client's consent should carefully analyze whether there is, in fact, a "duty to warn" and whether it is possible to persuade the client to discharge this responsibility himself or consent to the program's doing so.

Is there a duty?

The answer is a matter of State law. Courts in some States hold that health care providers have a duty to warn third parties of behavior of persons under their care that poses a potential danger to others. In addition to these court decisions, some States have laws that either permit or require health care providers to warn certain third parties. Usually, these State laws prohibit disclosure of the infected person's identity but allow the provider to tell the person at risk that she may have been exposed. It is important that providers consult with an attorney familiar with State law to learn whether the law imposes a duty to warn, as well as whether State law prescribes the ways a provider can notify the person at risk. The law in this area is still developing and may expand; thus, it is important to keep abreast of changes. One source of information about State codes with regard to the duty to warn is each State's Web site (available at http://janus.state.me.us/states.htm). (If there is no State statute or court decision on this issue, it is best to consult with a

lawyer or someone with expertise in this area
who can help the program determine the best
course to take. Such a consultation is
particularly helpful because of the competing
obligations the program may have to protect a
third party who may be in danger and to
safeguard its client's confidentiality.)

When does the duty arise?

Two behaviors of infected persons can put
others at risk of infection: unprotected sex
involving the exchange of bodily fluids and
syringe sharing. Because HIV is not transmitted
by casual contact, the simple fact that a client is
infected would not give rise to a duty to warn
the client's family or acquaintances who are not
engaged in sex or syringe sharing with the
client.

This still leaves open the question as to when
duty arises. Is it when a client tells a counselor
that he wants to or plans to infect others? Or
when a client tells the counselor that he has
already exposed others to HIV? These are two
different questions.

Threat to expose others

A counselor whose client threatens to infect
others should consider four questions in
determining whether there is a "duty to warn":

1. Is the client making a threat or "blowing off
steam?" Sometimes, wild threats are a way
of expressing anger. However, for example,
if the client has a history of violence or of
sexually abusing others, the threat should be
taken seriously.
2. Is there an identifiable potential victim?
Most States that impose a "duty to warn" do
so only when there is an identifiable victim
or class of victims. However, unless public
health authorities have the power to detain
someone in these circumstances there is
little reason to inform them.

3. Does a State statute or court decision impose
a duty to warn in this particular situation?
4. Even if there is no State legal requirement
that the program warn an intended victim
or the police, does the counselor feel a moral
obligation to do so?

Clearly, there are no definitive answers in
this area. Each case depends on the particular
facts presented and on State law. If a provider
believes she has a "duty to warn" under State
law, or that there is real danger to a particular
individual, she should do so in a way that
complies with both the Federal confidentiality
regulations and any State law or regulation
regarding disclosure of medical or HIV/AIDS-
related information. Because a client is unlikely
to consent to disclosure to the potential victim,
to comply with the Federal regulations a
provider could act as follows:

■ Seek a court order authorizing the disclosure.
The program must take care that the court
abide by the requirements of the Federal
confidentiality regulations, which are
discussed below in detail. It should also
consult State law to determine whether it
imposes additional requirements.
■ Make a disclosure that does not identify the
person as a client in substance abuse
treatment. This can be accomplished either
by making an anonymous report or, for a
program that is part of a larger nonsubstance
abuse treatment facility, by making the
report in the larger facility's name.
Counselors at freestanding alcohol or drug
programs cannot give the name of the
program. (Non–client-identifying
disclosures are discussed more fully under
"Exceptions that permit disclosure," below.)

In these circumstances, the counselor should
also limit the way he makes the warning to

minimize the exposure of the client's identity as HIV positive.

Recounting an exposure

Suppose an HIV-infected client tells his counselor that he has had unprotected sex or shared syringes with someone. If the counselor knows who the person is, does she have a "duty to warn" that person (or law enforcement)? This is not a true duty to warn case because the exposure has already occurred. The purpose of the "warning" is not to prevent a criminal act but to notify an individual so that she can take steps to monitor health status. Thus, it is probably not helpful to call a law enforcement agency. Rather, the counselor might want to let the public health authorities know, particularly in States with mandatory partner notification laws. Public health officials can then find the person at risk and provide appropriate counseling.

How can programs notify the public health department without violating confidentiality regulations? In some areas of the country, programs have signed QSOAs with public health departments that provide services to the program. A QSOA enables providers to report exposures to the department in situations like these. The public health department can then not only help the person the counselor believes was exposed but also trace other contacts the client may have exposed. In doing so, the public health department often does not identify the person who has put his contacts at risk. The public health department would not have to tell the contact that the person is in substance abuse treatment, and the QSOA would prohibit it from doing so. (A treatment program must also make sure that reporting an exposure by a client through a QSOA complies with any State law protecting medical or HIV/AIDS-related information.)

If the provider does not have a QSOA with the public health department, it might try one of the following methods:

- **Consent.** The provider could inform the health department with the client's consent. The consent form must comply with both the Federal confidentiality regulations and any State requirements governing client consent to release of HIV/AIDS information, as well as any other State law governing consent (e.g., whether a parent also must consent).
- **"Anonymous" notification.** If the program notifies the public health department in a way that does not identify the client as a substance abuser, this constitutes complying with the Federal regulations.
- **Court order.** Again, State law must be consulted to determine whether it imposes requirements in addition to those imposed by the Federal regulations.

One of the above methods should enable the provider to alert the public health department, which is the most effective way to notify someone who may have been exposed.

The program should document the factors that impelled the decision to warn an individual of impending danger of exposure or to report an exposure to the public health department. If the decision is later questioned, notes made at the time of the decision could prove invaluable.

As noted earlier, whenever a program proceeds without a client's consent to warn someone of a threat the client made or to report an exposure that has already occurred, the program may be undermining the trust of other clients and thus its effectiveness. This may be particularly true for a program serving HIV-positive clients. This is not to say that a disclosure should not be made, particularly when the law requires it. It is to say that a disclosure should not be made without careful thought.

Circumstances in which a "duty to warn" or "duty to notify" arises may change over time, as scientists learn more about the virus and its transmission and as more effective treatments are developed. There is little doubt that the law also will change, as States adopt new statutes and their courts apply statutes to new situations.

Programs should develop a protocol about "duty to warn" cases, so that staff members are not left to make decisions on their own about when and how to report threats or past occurrences of HIV transmission. Ongoing training and discussions can also assist staff in sorting out what should be done in any particular situation. Figure 9-2 provides a decision tree about the duty to warn.

Disclosures to insurers, HMOs, and other third-party payors

Traditional health insurance companies offering reimbursement to clients for treatment expenses require clients to sign claim forms containing language consenting to the release of information about their care. Can a program release information after a client has signed one of these standard consent forms? It cannot do so unless the form contains all the elements required by §2.31 of the regulations. Also, when the disclosure includes any HIV/AIDS-related information, the consent form must comply with State law.

Health maintenance organizations (HMOs) do not require clients to submit claim forms with language consenting to the release of information. Instead, clients in systems run by managed care organizations (MCOs) generally agree when they enter the "system" that the HMO or MCO can review records or request information about treatment at any time.

A substance abuse treatment program cannot rely on the fact that the client agreed when he signed on with the HMO that it could review his records and talk to doctors and other care providers whose fees it is covering. Federal regulations prohibit any communication unless the client has signed a proper consent form or the communication fits within another of the regulatory exceptions. State laws protecting HIV/AIDS-related information may also prohibit release of information in such circumstances.

As managed care becomes more prevalent, substance abuse treatment providers (and other professionals in the field of counseling and mental health) are finding that in order to monitor care and contain costs, third-party payors are demanding more information about clients and about the treatment provided them. The demand for information or records often comes when a provider requests authorization to continue or extend treatment. Providers are becoming all too familiar with the kinds of information they need to supply to HMOs and MCOs to obtain authorization to treat (or continue to treat) a client.

In many instances, simply getting the client's signature on a consent form that complies with the Federal rules and any State law governing the release of HIV/AIDS-related information will not resolve the ethical dilemma raised by the demand for greater and more detailed information. Providers faced with the question, "To disclose or not to disclose?" can be torn between their client's real need for continued treatment and the client's right to privacy. Should the provider disclose all information the HMO requests, perhaps shading it to ensure authorization, or should the provider protect the client's privacy, thereby jeopardizing the client's opportunity to obtain needed treatment services?

The better practice is to discuss the dilemma frankly with the client and to allow the client to decide whether and how much to disclose. To make an informed decision, the client will have to know what information the provider is being asked to disclose to obtain authorization to treat or continue treatment. The client and provider should discuss the likely consequences of the alternatives open to the client—disclosure and refusal to disclose. The client should understand that disclosure of the information

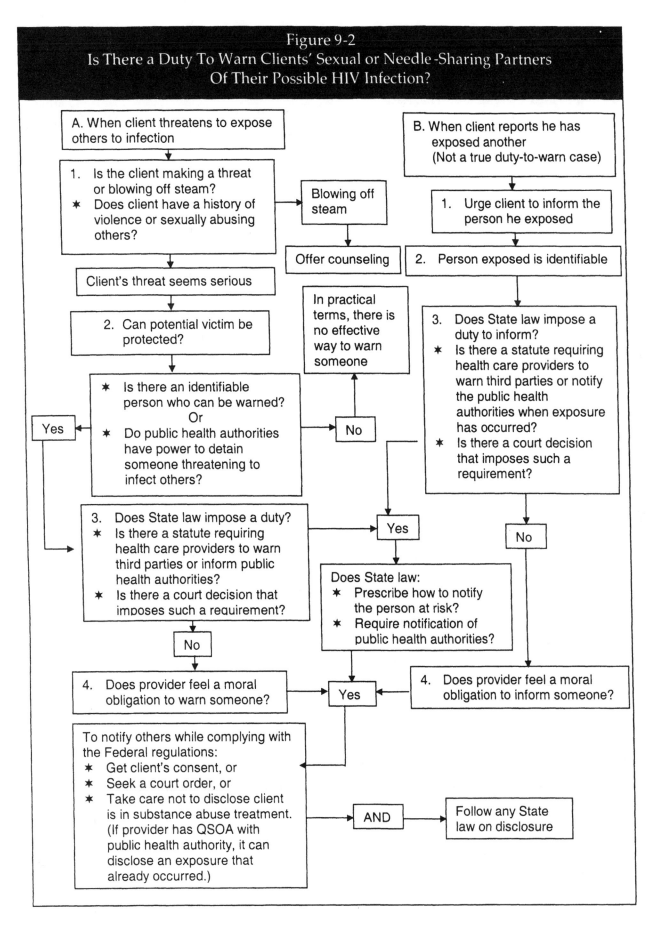

Figure 9-2
Is There a Duty To Warn Clients' Sexual or Needle-Sharing Partners
Of Their Possible HIV Infection?

the HMO seeks may be the only way to get the HMO to cover his treatment. Refusal to comply with the request for information will likely result in the HMO's refusal to cover at least some of the services the client needs.

On the other hand, the client may be more concerned that once his insurer learns she has a substance abuse problem or is HIV positive, she will lose her insurance coverage and be unable to obtain other coverage. For example, if in response to a demand from an HMO the provider releases information that the client's substance abuse has included use of both alcohol and illegal drugs, the HMO may deny benefits, arguing that since its policy does not cover treatment for abuse of drugs other than alcohol, it will not reimburse treatment when abuse of both alcohol and drugs is involved. A client whose employer is self-insured may fear being fired, demoted, or disciplined if the employer suspects he has abused substances or is HIV positive.

The process of helping the client weigh the available choices allows the client to make a decision based on his understanding of his own best interests.

Even a decision as simple as whether to submit a claim for HIV testing should be preceded by a discussion about the pros and cons of requesting coverage from an insurance company or HMO. The insurance company or HMO may infer from the fact that the client has had a test that he has engaged in risky behavior.

A client who fears the loss of employment or insurance may decide to pay for HIV testing or substance abuse treatment out of pocket. Or she may agree to a limited disclosure and ask the provider to inform her if more information is requested. If a client does not want the insurance carrier or HMO to be notified and is unable to pay for treatment, the program may refer her to a publicly funded program, if one is available. Programs should consult State law to learn whether they may refuse to admit a client

who is unable to pay and who will not consent to the necessary disclosures to her insurance carrier.

Disclosing information about clients who have died or become incompetent

The Federal regulations apply to any disclosure of information that would identify a deceased client as a substance abuser, and programs may not release information unless an executor, administrator, or other personal representative appointed under State law has signed a consent form authorizing the release of information. If no such appointment has been made, the client's spouse, or if there is no spouse, any responsible member of the client's family can sign a consent form (§2.15(b)(2)). An exception is that the regulations do permit a program to disclose client-identifying information that relates to a client's cause of death pursuant to laws requiring the collection of death or other vital statistics or permitting an inquiry into the cause of death (§2.15(b)(1)).

How can programs handle disclosures about incompetent clients? If the client has been adjudicated as lacking the capacity to manage his affairs, a consent form can be signed by his guardian or other individual authorized by State law to act on his behalf. If the client has not been adjudicated incompetent but suffers from "a medical condition that prevents knowing or effective action on his own behalf," the program director can sign a consent form but only for the purpose of getting payment for services from a third-party payor (§2.15(a)).

Exceptions that permit disclosures

The Federal confidentiality regulations' general rule prohibiting disclosure of client-identifying information has a number of exceptions. Reference has already been made to some of these exceptions: consent, disclosures that do not identify someone as a client in substance abuse treatment, disclosures pursuant to a

QSOA, disclosures during a medical emergency, disclosures authorized by special court order, and disclosures of information to auditors. The rules governing these exceptions are described in the pages that follow. Also explained is another exception, not yet mentioned, that permits disclosure of information among program staff.

Communications that do not disclose client-identifying information

The Federal regulations permit programs to disclose information about a client if the program reveals no client-identifying information. "Client-identifying" information identifies someone as an alcohol or drug abuser. Thus, a program may disclose information about a client if that information does not identify her as an alcohol or drug abuser or support anyone else's identification of the client as an alcohol or drug abuser.

A program may make such a disclosure in two basic ways. First, a program can report aggregate data about its population (summary information that gives an overview of the clients served in the program) or some portion of its populations. Thus, for example, a program could tell the newspaper that in the last 6 months it screened 43 clients, 10 female and 33 male.

The second way was mentioned above: A program can communicate information about a client in a way that does not reveal the client's status as a substance abuse disorder client (§2.12(a)(i)). For example, a program that provides services to clients with other problems or illnesses as well as substance abuse may disclose information about a particular client as long as the fact that the client has a substance abuse problem is not revealed. More specifically, a program that is part of a general hospital could ask a counselor to call the police about a violent threat made by a client, as long as the counselor does not disclose that the client

has a substance abuse problem or is a client of the treatment program.

Programs that provide only alcohol or drug services cannot disclose information that identifies a client under this exception—letting someone know a counselor is calling from the "Capital City Drug Program" automatically identifies the client as someone who received services from the program. However, a free-standing program can sometimes make "anonymous" disclosures, that is, disclosures that do not mention the name of the program or otherwise reveal the client's status as an alcohol or drug abuser.

Programs using this exception to disclose HIV/AIDS-related information about a client must also consult State law to determine if this kind of disclosure is permitted.

Disclosures to an outside agency that provides services to the program: QSOA

If a program routinely needs to share certain information with an outside agency that provides services to the program, it can enter into what is known as a *qualified service organization agreement*, or "QSOA." This is a written agreement between a program and a person providing services to the program, in which that person

- Acknowledges that in receiving, storing, processing, or otherwise dealing with any client records from the program, she is fully bound by the Federal confidentiality regulations
- Promises that, if necessary, she will resist in judicial proceedings any efforts to obtain access to client records except as permitted by these regulations (§2.11, §2.12(c)(4))

A sample QSOA is provided in Figure 9-3. A QSOA should be used only when an agency or official outside of the program provides a service to the program itself. An example is when laboratory analyses or data processing are performed for the program by an outside agency.

Figure 9-3
Qualified Service Organization Agreement

XYZ Service Center ("the center") and the _____
                                                                    (name of the program)
("the program") hereby enter into a qualified service organization agreement, whereby the center agrees to provide

_____
                                        (nature of services to be provided)

_____

_____

   Furthermore, the center:

   (1)   acknowledges that in receiving, storing, processing, or otherwise dealing with any information from the program about the clients in the program, it is fully bound by the provisions of the Federal regulations governing Confidentiality of Alcohol and Drug Abuse Client Records, 42 CFR Part 2; and

   (2)   undertakes to resist in judicial proceedings any effort to obtain access to information pertaining to clients otherwise than as expressly provided for in the Federal Confidentiality Regulations, 42 CFR Part 2.

Executed this ___ day of _____, 20____

_____   _____

President Director   [Name of the Program]
XYZ Service Center

[address]   [address]

A QSOA is not a substitute for individual consent in other situations. Disclosures under a QSOA must be limited to information needed by others so that the program can function effectively. QSOAs may not be used between programs providing alcohol and drug services. Programs that share information with outside agencies by using the QSOA must take care that any information about HIV/AIDS or other infectious diseases is transmitted in accordance with State law.

Medical emergencies

A program may make disclosures to public or private medical personnel "who have a need for information about a client for the purpose of treating a condition which poses an immediate threat to the health" of the client or any other individual. The regulations define "medical emergency" as a situation that poses an immediate threat to health and requires immediate medical intervention (§2.51).

The medical emergency exception permits only disclosure to medical personnel. This means that this exception cannot be used as the basis for a disclosure to family, the police, or other nonmedical personnel.

Whenever a disclosure is made to cope with a medical emergency, the program must document the following information in the client's records:

- The name and affiliation of the recipient of the information
- The name of the individual making the disclosure
- The date and time of the disclosure
- The nature of the emergency

Programs using the medical emergency exception to disclose information about a client's infectious disease or infection with HIV must also consult State law to determine if a disclosure is permitted.

Disclosures authorized by court order

A State or Federal court may issue an order that will permit a program to make a disclosure about a client that would otherwise be forbidden. A court may issue one of these authorizing orders, however, only after it follows certain procedures and makes particular determinations required by the regulations. *A subpoena, search warrant, or arrest warrant, even when signed by a judge, is not sufficient, standing alone, to require or even to permit a program to disclose information* (§2.61).

Before a court can issue a court order authorizing a disclosure about a client, the program and any clients whose records are sought must be given notice of the application for the order and some opportunity to make an oral or written statement to the court. (However, if the information is being sought to investigate or prosecute a client for a crime, only the program need be notified (§2.65). Also, if the information is sought to investigate or prosecute the program, no prior notice at all is

required (§2.66).) Generally, the application and any court order must use fictitious names for any known client, and all court proceedings in connection with the application must remain confidential unless the client requests otherwise (§2.64(a), (b), §2.65, §2.66). Before issuing an authorizing order, the court must find "good cause" for the disclosure. A court can find "good cause" only if it determines that the public interest and the need for disclosure outweigh any negative effect that the disclosure will have on the client, or the doctor–patient or counselor–client relationship, and the effectiveness of the program's treatment services. Before it may issue an order, the court must also find that other ways of obtaining the information are not available or would be ineffective (§2.64(d)). The judge may examine the records before making a decision (§2.64(c)).

There are also limits on the scope of the disclosure a court may authorize, even when it finds good cause. The disclosure must be limited to information essential to fulfill the purpose of the order, and it must be restricted to those persons who need the information for that purpose. The court should also take any other steps that are necessary to protect the client's confidentiality, including sealing court records from public scrutiny (§2.64(e)).

The court may order disclosure of "confidential communications" by a client to the program only if the disclosure

- Is necessary to protect against a threat to life or of serious bodily injury
- Is necessary to investigate or prosecute an extremely serious crime (including child abuse)
- Is in connection with a proceeding at which the client has already presented evidence concerning confidential communications (e.g., "I told my counselor...") (§2.63)

Again, programs using the court order exception to disclose identity or HIV/AIDS information about a client must also consult State law to determine if a disclosure is permitted.

Research, audit, or evaluation

The confidentiality regulations also permit programs to disclose client-identifying information to researchers, auditors, and evaluators without client consent, provided certain safeguards are met (§2.52, §2.53). For a more complete explanation of the requirements of §2.52 and §2.53, see Chapter 6 of TIP 14, *Developing State Outcomes Monitoring Systems for Alcohol and Other Drug Abuse Treatment* (CSAT, 1995a).

Again, State law must be consulted to see that any audit that inspects HIV/AIDS information about a client is conducted in accordance with State law.

Internal program communications

The Federal regulations permit some information to be disclosed to staff members within the same program:

> The restrictions on disclosure in these regulations do not apply to communications of information between or among personnel having a need for the information in connection with their duties that arise out of the provision of diagnosis, treatment, or referral for treatment of alcohol or drug abuse if the communications are (i) within a program or (ii) between a program and an entity that has direct administrative control over that program (§2.12(c)(3)).

In other words, staff who have access to client records because they work for or administratively direct the program, "including full- or part-time employees and unpaid volunteers," may consult among themselves or otherwise share information if their substance abuse treatment work so requires (§2.12(c)(3)). After consent, this is the most commonly invoked exception.

Some States have enacted laws that restrict the staff who are permitted access to HIV/

AIDS-related information. Programs should consult a lawyer familiar with State law and implement a policy that complies with any restrictions on staff access to this information.

Other rules regarding confidentiality

Client notice

The Federal confidentiality regulations require programs to notify clients of their right to confidentiality and to give them a written summary of the regulations' requirements. The notice and summary should be handed to clients when they begin participating in the program or soon thereafter (§2.22(a)). The regulations contain a sample notice.

Client access to records

Programs can decide when to permit clients to view or obtain copies of their records, unless State law grants clients the right of access to records. The Federal regulations do not require programs to obtain written consent from clients before permitting them to see their own records. Programs serving clients living with HIV/AIDS should educate themselves about any State laws or regulations requiring notice to clients and access to records.

Security of records

The Federal regulations require programs to keep written records in a secure room, a locked file cabinet, a safe, or other similar container. The program should establish written procedures that regulate access to and use of client records. Either the program director or a single staff person should be designated to process inquiries and requests for information (§2.16).

Computerization of medical and treatment records complicates the problem of keeping sensitive information private. Currently, protection is afforded by the cumbersome and inefficient paper files that many, if not most, medical, mental health, and social services still store and send from one provider to another.

When records are stored in computers, retrieval can be far more efficient, but computerized records may allow anyone with access to the computer in which the information is stored to copy information without constraint or accountability. Modems that allow communication about clients among different components of a managed care network extend the possibility of unauthorized access. The ease with which computerized information can be accessed can lead to casual gossip about a client, particularly if it is someone of importance in the community, making privacy difficult to preserve. For a brief discussion of some of the issues that computerization raises, see TIP 23, *Treatment Drug Courts: Integrating Substance Abuse Treatment With Legal Case Processing* (CSAT, 1996), pp. 52–53.

Conclusion

For providers of substance abuse treatment to clients living with HIV/AIDS, the rules regarding confidentiality of clients' information are very specific. State laws address disclosure of HIV/AIDS-related information as well as other medical and mental health information. Overlaid on these are the Federal law and regulations regarding confidentiality of substance abuse treatment information.

Generally, no more than two sets of laws apply in any given situation. If only substance abuse treatment information will be disclosed, a program is generally safe in following Federal rules. If HIV/AIDS-related information will be disclosed, and the disclosure will reveal the client is in drug treatment, the program must comply with both sets of laws. When in doubt, the best practice is to follow the more restrictive rules. Whenever possible, providers should try to find resources familiar with State laws to help sort out their responsibilities. The State Department of Health, the Single State Authority, the State Attorney General,

professional associations, a member of the agency's board who is an attorney, advocacy groups for people living with HIV/AIDS, or a local law school or bar association might provide the necessary information.

End Notes

1. If the purpose of seeking the court order is to obtain authorization to disclose information in order to investigate or prosecute a client for a crime, the court must also find that (1) the crime involved is extremely serious, such as an act causing or threatening to cause death or serious injury; (2) the records sought are likely to contain information of significance to the investigation or prosecution; (3) there is no other practical way to obtain the information; and (4) the public interest in disclosure outweighs any actual or potential harm to the client.

2. For a discussion of these kinds of State confidentiality laws, see TIP 24, *A Guide to Substance Abuse Services for Primary Care Clinicians* (CSAT, 1997), Appendix B.

3. There is an exception that allows the director of a substance abuse treatment program to communicate with a minor's parents without the minor's consent, when (1) the minor is applying for services; (2) the program director believes that the minor, because of extreme substance abuse or medical condition, does not have the capacity to decide rationally whether to consent to the notification of her parents or guardian; and (3) the program director believes that the disclosure is necessary to cope with a substantial threat to the life or well-being of the minor or someone else.

   Thus, if a minor applies for services in a State where parental consent is required to provide services, but the minor refuses to consent to the program's notifying his parents or guardian, the regulations permit the program to contact a parent without the minor's consent, if these conditions are met. Otherwise, the program must explain to the minor that although he has the right to refuse to consent to any communication with a parent, the program can provide no services without such communication and parental consent (§2.14(d)). The regulations add a warning, however, that such action might violate a State or local law (§2.14(b)).

10 Funding and Policy Considerations

This chapter provides information on how to find appropriate sources of funding for services and programs related to HIV/AIDS and substance abuse. It will not address sources of funding for individual medical care (see Chapter 6 for a discussion of individual funding). There are several key steps that will increase the likelihood of successfully obtaining funds, regardless of the type of program or service for which support is being sought.

Keys to Successful Grantseeking

Before seeking funding, the substance abuse treatment professional should determine the basic information about the proposed project. The following questions will help focus this information:

- What are the organization's current capabilities, strengths, and areas for improvement?
- What is the organization's target population, and what are their unique or unmet needs?
- What is the proposed action to meet the identified unmet needs? How would the proposed project or service impact those needs? What will be accomplished and in what time period? Have similar projects been done locally or nationally; that is, are

there model or demonstration projects? If so, can these projects be adapted to suit the organization's needs?

- Does the project support and supplement existing activities in the community or target area?
- Can this project actually be carried out? Is the plan realistic and achievable? How much funding is required and for how long? What staff, facility, and service changes or partnerships would be required to carry out the proposed plan?
- What is currently available in the community and who would support—or oppose—the proposed plan? Who is a potential partner and who is a potential competitor for funding?
- How will the success of the project be evaluated?

How To Identify Potential Funding Sources

It can seem a daunting task to identify potential funding sources. There are more than 40,000 private foundations in the United States, and about 37 percent of them have assets of at least $1 million or award $100,000 or more in grants each year. There are many Federal, State, and local government funding sources as well.

On top of that, each funding source has its own funding priorities, eligible services and providers, funding and geographic restrictions, and application deadlines.

There are three types of funding streams: Federal, State and local, and private initiatives. Federal funding sources for substance abuse treatment and HIV/AIDS resources include Ryan White Comprehensive AIDS Resources Emergency (CARE) Act programs, Substance Abuse and Mental Health Services Administration (SAMHSA), the Centers for Disease Control and Prevention (CDC), and U.S. Department of Housing and Urban Development (HUD). Individual State and local health and human services agencies allocate both Federal and State dollars for substance abuse treatment and HIV/AIDS. Private foundations and many corporations also provide grant awards. A discussion of each of three types of funding streams follows.

There are a number of resources to help identify potential funding sources. Many Federal, State and private grantmakers and clearinghouses provide information via the Internet. A list of potentially useful Web sites is provided in Appendix F of this TIP. Other resources include computerized databases, directories, books, periodicals, and newsletters that may offer information on funding sources, proposal writing, program planning, and related topics.

Examples include:

- *The Local/State Funding Report*, a newsletter published weekly by Government Information Services of Thompson Publishing Group. Provides subscribers with updates on Federal and State funding opportunities, *Washington Notes*, and local/State grant and regulation alerts—a listing of funding notes and regulations issued by Federal agencies. For subscription information, call 202-872-4000.

- *Federal Grants & Contracts Weekly*, published by Aspen Publishers, Inc. Subscription information can be obtained by calling 800-638-8437 or online at www.grantscape.com/catalog/Default.html.
- *The Federal Register*, which announces funding initiatives and can be reached online at www.federalregisterdigest.com.
- *The Catalog of Federal Domestic Assistance* provides information on all Federal government programs that award grants, including basic information on the granting agency, applications and award processes, eligibility criteria, addresses, and key contacts.

Check with your public library or local college or university libraries to see if their collections include these or similar grant resources.

A key private initiative resource is the Foundation Center, a nonprofit organization that maintains a comprehensive and up-to-date database on foundations and corporate giving programs. The Center offers free information to the public at five Foundation Center libraries and approximately 200 Cooperating Collections across the country. The two national library collections are located at

- 79 Fifth Avenue/16th Street New York, NY 10003-3076 (212) 620-4230

- 1001 Connecticut Avenue, NW Suite 938 Washington, DC 20036-5588 (202) 331-1400

Regional collections are available in Atlanta, Cleveland, and San Francisco at the following locations:

- 50 Hurt Plaza Suite 150 Atlanta, GA 30303-2914

- 1422 Euclid Avenue
  Suite 1356
  Cleveland, OH 44115-2001

- 312 Sutter Street
  Room 312
  San Francisco, CA 94108-4314

The 200 Cooperating Collections contain a core collection of the Foundation Center's reference works and provide trained staff to direct grantseekers to appropriate funding information resources. Many of the collections maintain information on local funders. A complete list of Cooperating Collections can be obtained by calling (800) 424-9836 or visiting the Center's Web site (http://fdncenter.org).

Foundation Center resources include Internal Revenue Service Information Returns, which are filed annually by all private foundations and contain fiscal data, addresses, and lists of grantees and trustees; directories, books, and periodicals; computer resources including the Center's database on CD-ROM, its Web site, and other software computer programs; grantmaker files; current awareness files on materials of interest to grantseekers organized by subject heading; and a bibliographic database of approximately 13,000 listings.

The five Center libraries offer regular workshops, seminars, and funding panels of interest to both grantseekers and grantmakers.

Many foundations have their own Web sites. These are especially helpful to visit because they often contain the foundation's guidelines and its annual report. The annual report gives the fundseeker a better notion of what kinds of programs the foundation funds. For example, a funding category may be "education," but until the grantseeker looks at the annual report it will not be clear whether or not the foundation is interested in postsecondary education.

Another excellent source of funding ideas is the annual reports of organizations similar to the fundseeker's. For example, if the fundseeker works at a program for people with HIV disease and ex-offenders, he should receive the annual report of any agencies with similar missions. These agencies could be halfway houses for ex-offenders or housing programs for HIV-positive individuals. The annual reports will have a list of funders. This in turn will lead the fundseeker back to the names of foundations he can research at the Foundation Center or on the Internet.

State and Federal Policy Shifts

Dramatic changes in clinical management of HIV/AIDS have resulted in a shift from regarding AIDS as a fatal disease to a chronic one, and as a result funding urgency and need has diminished in the eyes of both policymakers and some segments of the public. Questions have been raised about why AIDS support has been so great given that other disease conditions such as cancer and heart disease kill many more people. Organizations advocating for these conditions have begun to lobby intensively for increased funding, thereby increasing competition for dollars that were allocated to HIV/AIDS.

Welfare reform eliminated Social Security benefits for individuals with a diagnosis of substance abuse or dependence, which has decreased the availability of public benefits and increased the stigma associated with these diagnoses. In 1997, CSAT received 2 years of supplemental funding to help such individuals make the transition to the elimination of benefits. At the end of the 2-year period, individuals with a diagnosis of substance abuse or dependence will no longer be eligible for SSI benefits.

Arrest and incarceration of individuals with substance abuse disorders is increasing at local, State, and Federal levels. People with substance abuse disorders end up in jails and prisons where they may or may not receive appropriate treatment for their substance abuse problems. In addition, prisoners are at increased risk for HIV infection.

The Ryan White CARE Act (P.L. 101-381) was originally passed in 1990 and amended in 1996 (P.L. 104-146). The act, which is reauthorized in 5-year increments, is up for reauthorization in 2000. Public Law 102-321 in 1992 restructured the Alcohol, Drug, and Mental Health Administration (ADAMHA) into SAMSHSA within the U.S. Department of Health and Human Services (DHHS). This law established separate block grants to enhance the delivery of services regarding substance abuse and mental health. The law is periodically reauthorized. For current information regarding HIV/AIDS set-asides, contact the Single State Authority (SSA).

AIDS-related comprehensive treatment planning groups are increasingly recommending the mainstreaming of some services to help address fragmentation of services and funding. In some instances, this takes the form of awarding services under competitive bid processes to private or public organizations that historically have not been identified as HIV/AIDS service organizations. Examples of mainstreaming include

- Awarding Housing Opportunities for Persons With AIDS (HOPWA) contracts to private housing brokers who maintain lists and links of available housing units, manage vendor payments, and provide home management skills training to residents
- Awarding home-based meal services to meal delivery organizations such as Meals on Wheels
- Providing transportation by private bus companies and taxi-jitney services
- Providing contracts to private providers for mental health services and spiritual counseling

- Awarding dollars for return-to-work initiatives to work placement companies such as Goodwill Industries and Manpower Development Services

There are several advantages to mainstreaming:

- Increased familiarity with scopes of work for specific services
- Less time and effort spent in program startup
- Industry-wide standards of care, service, and quality are often already in place

Those considering mainstreaming services may have to address the following challenges:

- Refragmentation of services
- Increase in the size and complexity of multidisciplinary teams
- Reluctance of private sector providers to attend multidisciplinary team meetings without identifying meeting attendance as billable services
- Difficulties in establishing linked entries in Uniform Reporting System from private providers
- Possible exposure of people with HIV/AIDS to providers not trained in cultural competency, HIV/AIDS, or substance abuse treatment

Funders Concerned About AIDS (FCAA) was organized in 1987 to advance the private philanthropic response to HIV/AIDS. This organization seeks not only to sustain but also to increase the philanthropic resources available to fight HIV/AIDS and assists funders in enhancing the strategic nature of their HIV/AIDS-related grantmaking. FCAA works to help funders in the following ways:

- Viewing HIV/AIDS within the larger social context and integrating HIV/AIDS funding into the broader grantmaking agendas of funders

- Broadening the support and understanding of HIV/AIDS at the international, national, and local levels
- Supporting high-quality, effective, collaborative, and nonduplicative programs and services
- Targeting populations that are currently underserved by HIV/AIDS services and related health, welfare, and education services
- Demonstrating explicit support for effective new approaches in the fight against HIV/AIDS

FCAA carries out primary and secondary research into HIV/AIDS funding trends and issues and provides the philanthropic sector with technical assistance. They can be contacted by phone at: (212) 573-5533; or by writing to 50 East 42nd Street, 19th floor, New York, NY 10017.

Obtaining Funds

It is important to be aware that there are three kinds of support: capital (buildings, equipment), general (general program support), and project support. Most funders prefer project support, since they can easily see the results of their funding. Yet even general support can sometimes be cast as "project" support. For example, the fundseeker could add a component to the program or add 10 slots to the program. These can be marketed to the foundation as projects.

To obtain some of the funds discussed in this section, following is a list of suggestions for administrators.

1. Keep up with trend data to give to policymakers.
2. Know the local, State, and Federal politics regarding the pertinent issue and/or the proposal.
3. Be aware of political and philosophical realities for the community.

4. Become active in community task forces and on advisory or planning councils (e.g., Ryan White Planning Council, HIV/AIDS State Task Force). Join subcommittees, bring up substance abuse treatment issues whenever possible, and bring clean and sober clients to meetings to put a face on the disease of addiction.
5. Form coalitions, especially in rural areas.
6. Work with other agencies in the area to eliminate or decrease duplication of services and maximize resources.
7. Form partnerships with local research entities (e.g., universities, private agencies) and community-based organizations.
8. Invite political representatives to tour the agency or discuss ideas before applying for funding. Build support for your application at the grassroots level.
9. Find new partners to apply collaboratively for funding.
10. Add business representatives and other community leaders to the agency's board so that more effective partnerships can be built.
11. Build the board infrastructure so that the organization has a strong foundation before it receives funding. Involve board members in developing funding proposals and in marketing proposals to foundations and other funding sources.
12. On a regular basis, do an exhaustive review of potential funding resources, including nontraditional funding sources.
13. Invite researchers to the program and build relationships before submitting a proposal. Make them true partners in the development of the proposed project's design and evaluation. Researchers can also be helpful in conducting needs assessment. Include funding for evaluation in the proposal.
14. Contact the major pharmaceutical companies that produce HIV/AIDS drugs to determine if they have funding available for

local or State initiatives. Check with the local pharmaceutical representative to discover the appropriate way to contact a specific pharmaceutical company.

15. If a name is available, call the project officer for the grant and clarify any questions. Attend any pre-application workshops offered by the granting organization.

16. Present the proposed project as a model program with potential for replication. Emphasize the innovative and effective aspects of the project. Clearly address the diversity of the program's target population and staff.

17. Along with the application, include a feasible, realistic timeline and budget that provides the granting agency with target dates for achieving key project milestones. Involve the substance abuse treatment agency's financial experts or outside experts in developing a budget to implement the proposed project. Avoid projects that are too costly, but make sure that the budget is sufficient to carry out the project. Include any supply, copying, telephone, and postage charges, meeting costs, and other types of "hidden" costs. Budgets also should include any in-kind contributions.

18. Clearly present the substance abuse treatment organization's experience and expertise. If the funding agency permits supporting documentation, include letters of endorsement and memorandums of agreement from clients, community leaders, and collaborating organizations.

19. Seek funding from more than one resource so that you do not become dependent on one particular funding source.

20. Ask outside reviewers in the community to review the grant application prior to submission. If they do not understand the proposal or have questions, chances are the funding agency will, too. Clarify any issues raised by outside reviewers. Request letters of support from organizations that refer clients to the program or that will work with the project.

21. Make sure that the proposed project meets the needs of the target population and that provided services are culturally competent.

22. Attend grantmaking and proposal-writing workshops.

23. Meet grant application submission deadlines and follow the granting agency's guidelines exactly (e.g., page margins, line spacing, inclusion or exclusion of supporting documentation, page limits).

24. Stay in touch with the funder, even when a report is not due, and notify the funder when a milestone is reached or when the program gets publicity. Call the funder and ask whether the funder wants to visit the program. There may be a special event, like a graduation, that the funder should see.

25. Think "outside the box" when researching potential funders. For example, a program may be for HIV-positive women with children. There may be a funding source that would support a therapy group worker for the children. However, this funder may be primarily interested in mental health, not HIV/AIDS or substance abuse treatment.

Federal Initiatives

Substance Abuse Prevention and Treatment Block Grant Funding

Within DHHS, SAMHSA administers the Substance Abuse Prevention and Treatment (SAPT) Block Grant. SAPT Block Grant funding is allocated by formula to the 50 States, the District of Columbia, and 10 Territories. States and Territories administer the SAPT Block Grant funds through a principal agency, defined as the SSA. The SSA is responsible for planning, carrying out, and evaluating activities to prevent and treat substance abuse and related activities.

Each Principal Agency designates an SSA director as the point of contact for that State or Territory's SAPT Block Grant. SAPT Block Grant funds are subject to certain set-asides and requirements for States, Territories, administrators, and providers of services. States and Territories must expend the Block Grant in accordance with the percentage to be allocated to treatment, prevention, and other activities as prescribed by law.

Funding requirements

States and Territories must spend at least 35 percent of the Block Grant funds for prevention and treatment activities regarding alcohol, 35 percent for prevention and treatment activities regarding other substances, and 20 percent on primary prevention programs. In addition, a certain amount of the Block Grant must be spent on gender-specific women's substance abuse treatment services, including HIV/AIDS services.

Women's services

The amount set aside for women's services is to be spent on individuals who have no financial means of obtaining such services. All programs providing such services will treat the family as a unit and therefore will admit both women and their children into treatment services, if appropriate.

At a minimum, treatment programs receiving funding for women's services must also provide or arrange for the following services for pregnant women and women with dependent children, including women who are trying to regain custody of their children:

- Primary medical care, including referral for prenatal care and child care while the women are receiving such services
- Primary pediatric care for children, including immunizations

- Gender-specific substance abuse treatment and other therapeutic interventions for women that may address issues of relationships, sexual and physical abuse, and parenting, and child care while the women are receiving these services
- Therapeutic interventions for children in custody of women in treatment that may, among other things, address their developmental needs, their issues of sexual and physical abuse, and neglect
- Sufficient case management and transportation to ensure that women and their children have access to services provided

Procedures for the implementation of women's services will be developed in consultation with the State medical director for substance abuse services.

Services for individuals with HIV/AIDS and/or injection drug users

States with a certain rate of AIDS cases must spend at least 5 percent of the total Block Grant funds on HIV/AIDS Early Intervention Services for persons in substance abuse treatment. States so designated have an AIDS rate of 10 or more cases per 100,000 individuals, as indicated by the number of cases reported to and confirmed by the Director of the CDC for the most recent calendar year for which the data are available.

HIV/AIDS Early Intervention Services are defined as

- Appropriate pretest counseling for HIV and AIDS
- Testing services, including tests to confirm the presence of the disease, tests to diagnose the extent of the deficiency in the immune system, and tests to provide information on appropriate therapeutic measures to prevent

and treat the deterioration of the immune system and conditions arising from the disease

■ Appropriate posttest counseling

Designated States must

■ Carry out one or more projects to make early intervention services for HIV/AIDS available at the substance abuse treatment site to individuals undergoing substance abuse treatment

■ Make available from the grant the prescribed money for these activities

■ Carry out such projects only in geographic areas of the State that have the greatest need for the projects

■ Require programs participating in the project to establish linkages with a comprehensive community resource network of related health and social services organizations to ensure a wide-based knowledge of the availability of these services

■ Require any entity receiving money from the Block Grant for operating a substance abuse treatment program to follow procedures developed by the SSA, in consultation with the State medical director for substance abuse services, and in cooperation with the public health agency

If the State plans to carry out two or more HIV/AIDS early intervention projects, the State must carry out one such project in a rural area of the State, unless the requirement is waived.

All entities providing early intervention services for HIV disease to an individual must comply with payment provisions and restrictions on expenditure of grant. The individual will enter services voluntarily (i.e., with informed consent) and will not be required to undergo such services as a condition for receiving substance abuse treatment or any other services.

Capacity of treatment for injecting substance abusers

All programs that receive funding under the grant and that treat individuals for injection drug use (IDU) must notify the State within 7 days upon reaching 90 percent of admission capacity. Each individual who requests and is in need of treatment for IDU must be admitted to a program no later than

■ Fourteen days after requesting admission to such a program, or

■ One hundred and twenty days after the date of the request if no such program has the capacity to admit the individual on the date of the request, or if interim services are made available to the individual no later than 48 hours after the request (including referral for prenatal care)

Outreach requirements

Any organization that receives funding for treatment services for injection drug users must actively encourage individuals in need of such treatment to undergo treatment. The States require organizations to use outreach models that are scientifically sound, or if no such models are available that apply to the local situation, to use an approach that reasonably can be expected to be an effective outreach method. By this definition, all outreach efforts must include the following tasks:

■ Selecting, training, and supervising outreach workers

■ Contacting, communicating, and following up with high-risk substance abusers, their associates, and neighborhood residents, while observing Federal and State confidentiality laws, including 42 CFR (see Chapter 9)

■ Promoting awareness among injection drug users about the relationship between IDU and diseases such as HIV

- Recommending steps to ensure that HIV transmission does not occur
- Encouraging entry into treatment

In turn, the State must

- Establish a capacity management program to enable a program to report quickly to the State when it reaches 90 percent of its capacity—to ensure maintenance of a continually updated record of all reports and make excess capacity information available to such programs
- Establish a waiting list management program that provides systematic reporting of treatment demand
- Require that any program receiving funding from the grant for treatment for injection drug users establish a waiting list that includes a unique client identifier for each injection drug user seeking treatment, including those receiving interim services while waiting for admission to the treatment program
- Ensure that individuals who cannot be placed in treatment within 14 days are enrolled in defined interim services, that mechanisms are developed for maintaining contact with individuals awaiting admission, and that those who remain active on a waiting list are admitted to a treatment program within 120 days
- Ensure that programs consult the capacity management system so that patients on a waiting list are admitted as soon as possible to a program providing such treatment within a reasonable geographic area
- Develop effective strategies for monitoring programs' compliance with SAPT Block Grant requirements
- Report the specific strategies to be used to identify compliance problems and corrective actions to be taken to address those problems

Eligibility and restrictions for funding with SAPT Block Grants

Only public or private nonprofit entities are eligible to receive SAPT Block Grant funding. States cannot spend Block Grant funds to provide inpatient hospital services; make cash payments to intended recipients of services; purchase or improve land; purchase, construct, or improve facilities; purchase major medical equipment; or provide individuals with hypodermic needles or syringes for use of illegal drugs.

References

CFR, Title 45, Volume 1, parts 120 to 137, pages 490–09, revised as of October 1, 1997 contains the regulations regarding the SAPT Block Grant. Subpart L—Substance Abuse Prevention and Treatment Block Grant Authority: 42 U.S.C. 300x-21 to 300x-35 and 300x-51 to 300x-64. Source: 58 Federal Register 17070, March 31, 1993, unless otherwise noted.

Information contact

CSAT, Division of State and Community Assistance. Phone: (301) 443-3820; Fax: (301) 443-8345.

The Ryan White CARE Act

The Ryan White CARE Act of 1990 was created to improve the quality and availability of care for individuals and families affected by HIV/AIDS. The act was amended and reauthorized in 1996.

In 1997, the Health Resources and Services Administration (HRSA) in DHHS consolidated into its new HIV/AIDS Bureau all of the lead programs in the United States that deliver HIV/AIDS health care and support services for low income and uninsured individuals. The Bureau houses all of the programs authorized under the Ryan White CARE Act. Grant applications for all Ryan White CARE Act programs can be obtained from the HRSA Grants Application Center. The center may be contacted by phone at (888) 300-4772 or by e-mail at: HRSA.GAC@ix.netcom.com. The street address is 40 West Gude Drive, Suite 100, Rockville, MD 20850.

Ryan White CARE Act Programs include

- Title I, II, III, and IV grants
- Special Projects of National Significance (SPNS)
- AIDS Education and Training Centers (AETCs)
- Dental Reimbursement Program

Within the HIV/AIDS Bureau, the Division of Service Systems administers Title I, II, and AIDS Drug Assistance Programs; the Division of Community Based Programs administers Title III, IV and the HIV/AIDS Dental Reimbursement Program; and the Division of Training and Technical Assistance administers the AIDS Education and Training Center Program. The SPNS Program is administered by the HIV/AIDS Bureau's Office of Science and Epidemiology.

A description of each Ryan White program follows.

Ryan White Title I

Title I funding provides formula and supplemental grants to eligible metropolitan areas (EMAs) that are disproportionately affected by HIV/AIDS (there were 49 of them in 1997).

Title I eligibility

Metropolitan areas are eligible for funding if they have reported more than 2,000 AIDS cases in the past 5 years and if they have a population of at least 500,000. (This provision does not apply to EMAs funded prior to fiscal year 1997.)

Grantees

Grants are awarded to the chief elected official (CEO) of the city or county administering the health agency that provides services to the greatest number of people with HIV in the EMA. The CEO usually designates an administrative agent, often the local health department, to select service providers and administer contracts. The CEO must establish an HIV/AIDS Health Services Planning Council that is representative of the local epidemic, including health care agencies and community-based providers. At least 25 percent of the council's voting membership must be composed of people with HIV disease.

Funding

The Planning Council sets priorities for the allocation of funds within the EMA, develops a comprehensive plan, and assesses the grantee's administrative mechanism in allocating funds. The councils are not allowed to become involved in the selection of providers to receive Title I funding or in the administration of contracts with selected providers. These are grantee responsibilities.

Eligible services

Title I funding may be used to provide a wide range of community-based services, including

- **Outpatient health care**, including medical and dental care, developmental and rehabilitation services, and mental health and substance abuse treatment services
- **Support services**, such as case management, home health and hospice care, housing and transportation assistance, nutrition services, and day and respite care
- **Inpatient case management services** that expedite discharge and prevent unnecessary hospitalization

Eligible providers

Eligible providers include public or nonprofit entities. Private for-profit entities are eligible only if they are the only available provider of quality HIV/AIDS care in the EMA.

Title I funding has two components: formula and supplemental grants. Formula grants are awarded based on the estimated number of people living with HIV disease in the EMA. Supplemental grants are competitive and based on demonstration of severe need and other criteria, including the ability to use the funds responsibly and cost-effectively; plans to allocate funds in accordance with the local demographics of AIDS; and inclusive planning council membership. Effective fiscal year 1999, Title I will have a single grant application for formula and supplemental funds. Applications will be reviewed internally only and will be considered as noncompeting continuations.

Information contact

Division of Service Systems, HIV/AIDS Bureau, HRSA, 5600 Fishers Lane, Room 7A-55, Rockville, MD 20857. Phone: (301) 443-6745; Fax: (301) 443-8143.

Ryan White Title II

The Title II AIDS Drug Assistance Program (ADAP) provides funds to States to make protease inhibitors and other therapies available to uninsured and underinsured individuals.

Funding

Title II base and supplemental grants are awarded to States, the District of Columbia, Puerto Rico, and eligible U.S. Territories on a formula basis according to the rate of infection. Grants are awarded to the State agency designated by the Governor to administer Title II funding, usually the State health agency.

States receiving Title II funding are required to have a process that periodically convenes individuals with HIV disease, providers, public health agencies, and representatives of other Ryan White CARE Act grantees to develop a Statewide Coordinated Statement of Need (SCSN).

Funding restrictions

States have limited discretion in using formula funds, but must direct some portion of the grant to the provision of therapeutics or to support ADAPs. In addition, States are awarded earmarked Title II ADAP funds, which must all be used for ADAP.

States with more than 1 percent of the total AIDS cases reported nationally during the past 2 years must contribute matching funds, based on a yearly formula. Title II awards include earmarked funds to support the ADAP, which provides medications to low-income individuals with HIV disease who are uninsured or have limited coverage from private insurance or Medicaid. States must document their progress in making HIV/AIDS medications (including drugs for the prevention and treatment of opportunistic diseases) available to eligible people.

Eligible services

States may use Title II funding to support a wide range of support services, including

- Home and community-based health care and support services
- Continuation of health insurance coverage, through a health insurance continuation program (HICP)
- Pharmaceutical therapies, through the ADAP program
- Local consortia that assess needs, organize and deliver HIV/AIDS services in consultation with service providers, and contract for services
- Direct health and support services

Eligibility

Public or nonprofit providers are eligible. Private for-profit providers are eligible only if they are the only available provider of quality HIV/AIDS care in the service area.

The majority of States provide some Title II services directly and others through subcontracts with local Title II HIV/AIDS consortia. Title II defines a consortium as an association of public and nonprofit health care and support service providers and community-based organizations that plans, develops, and delivers services to people living with HIV disease.

Information contact

Division of Service Systems, HIV/AIDS Bureau, HRSA, 5600 Fishers Lane, Room 7A-55, Rockville, MD 20857. Phone: (301) 443-6745; Fax: (301) 443-8143.

Ryan White Title III

Title III grants provide competitive funding to public and private nonprofit entities for outpatient early intervention/primary care services. In 1997, 166 Title III programs were funded to provide early intervention services, and 4 communities were funded as early intervention planning grants. Forty percent are Community Health Centers and Migrant Health Centers, 20 percent are hospital or university-based medical centers, 19 percent are city and county health services, and 18 percent are community-based health centers that are not federally funded. Three percent provide health care for the homeless, family planning clinics, and comprehensive hemophilia diagnostic and treatment centers.

Eligible services

A wide array of services are eligible for funding, including

- Risk-reduction counseling and partner involvement in risk education
- Education to prevent early transmission
- Antibody testing, medical evaluation, and clinical care

- Antiretroviral therapies
- Ongoing medical, oral health, nutritional, psychosocial, and other care for individuals with HIV
- Case management to ensure access to services and continuity of care
- Addressing coepidemics that occur frequently in association with HIV infection, including substance abuse and tuberculosis

Information contact

Division of Community-Based Programs, HIV/AIDS Bureau, HRSA, 4350 East-West Highway, Bethesda, MD 20814. Phone: (301) 594-4444; Fax: (301) 594-2470.

Ryan White Title IV

Title IV grants offer competitive funding to public and private nonprofit entities to coordinate services and enhance access to research for children, youth, women, and families who are infected or affected by HIV and AIDS. Grantees are expected to interface with established service delivery systems to plan and provide a range of services including HIV prevention efforts, counseling and testing, primary medical care, and opportunities for clinical research. In accomplishing this, grantees must identify and address barriers to care for the targeted populations. Applicants who do not propose to serve one or more of the target populations must provide sufficient justification.

Projects funded under Ryan White Title IV are expected to serve not only individual persons, but also family members affected by HIV disease. The family structures range from the traditional, biological family unit to nontraditional family units with partners, significant others, and unrelated caregivers.

Title IV has three priority areas: access to clinical research, activities to reduce perinatal HIV transmission, and consumer involvement.

Funding eligibility

Public and nonprofit entities that provide primary health care directly or through contracts are eligible to apply for funding. Eligible entities include, but are not limited to, State or local health departments, university medical centers, public or nonprofit private hospitals, community health centers receiving support under section 330 of the Public Health Service Act, hemophilia treatment centers, drug abuse treatment agencies, tribal health programs, school-based clinics, and institutions of higher education.

To be eligible, the applicant must either be located in a geographic area not currently funded for comprehensive services by Title IV, or in an area where the existing grantee's project period is ending. Applicants in areas with an existing Title IV project are not eligible for funding. The Comprehensive Family Services Branch should be contacted at (301) 443-9051 regarding questions about geographic areas eligible for Title IV funding.

Availability of funding

Each approved project will have a maximum project period of 3 years and a 12-month budget period, starting August 1. Preference for funding in new areas is given to applicants that help achieve an equitable geographical distribution of programs, especially programs that provide services in rural or underserved communities where the number of HIV-infected and affected women, children, and families is increasing and in areas that receive limited or no Ryan White CARE Act monies.

Information contact

Title IV Program, HRSA, 5600 Fishers Lane, Room 18A-19, Rockville, MD 20857. Phone: (301) 443-9051; Fax: (301) 443-1728.

Special Projects of National Significance (SPNS) Program

SPNS programs explore new care models for national replication. The purpose of SPNS programs is to support demonstrations and evaluations of innovative and replicable models for delivering health care and support services to people living with HIV/AIDS.

Eligibility

Awards are made to nonprofit organizations wishing to evaluate a model of care. A competitive grant award process is used to assure fair and equitable distribution of funds.

Information contact

SPNS Program, Office of Science and Epidemiology, HIV/AIDS Bureau, HRSA, 5600 Fishers Lane, Room 7A-08, Rockville, MD 20857. Phone: (301) 443-9976; Fax: (301) 443-4965.

AIDS Education and Training Centers (AETCs)

The AETC Program is a network of 15 regional centers and 75 associated sites that conduct targeted, multidisciplinary education and training programs for health care providers. The AETCs serve all 50 States, the District of Columbia, the Virgin Islands, and Puerto Rico.

Priority

The AETCs are aimed at training primary health care providers, including physicians, nurses, and dentists. Training is also provided for mental health and allied health professionals.

Funding

The majority of AETC resources have been focused in areas of high HIV prevalence and incidence, with remaining resources allocated to suburban and rural needs. Each AETC involves at least one CARE Act Title I EMA (areas that have high incidence of HIV disease).

AETCs collaborate with other CARE Act–funded organizations, area health education centers community-based HIV/AIDS organizations, medical and health professional organizations, medical and health professional schools, local hospitals, health departments, community and migrant health centers, medical societies, and other professional organizations.

Information contact

AETC Program, HIV/AIDS Bureau, HRSA, 5600 Fishers Lane, Room 9A-39, Rockville, MD 20857. Phone: (301) 443-6364; Fax: (301) 443-9887.

HIV/AIDS Dental Reimbursement Program

The HIV/AIDS Dental Reimbursement Program reimburses accredited schools of dentistry and graduate dental programs for providing dental care to people with HIV. Eligible applicants must have documented uncompensated costs of oral health care for HIV-positive persons, and must be accredited by the Commission on Dental Accreditation.

Funding

This program takes into account the number of patients served by each individual applicant and unreimbursed oral health costs, as compared to the total number of patients served and total costs incurred by all eligible applicants.

Information contact

Division of Community-Based Programs, HIV/AIDS Bureau, HRSA, 4350 East-West Highway, Bethesda, MD 20814. Phone: (301) 594-4444; Fax: (301) 594-2470.

HUD

As part of its Super Notice of Funding Availability (SuperNOFA), HUD makes funding available for housing assistance and supportive services under the HOPWA program. The HOPWA program is intended to provide low-income housing for persons with HIV/AIDS and their families. There are two types of funding assistance: grants for SPNSs and grants for projects that are part of Long-Term Comprehensive Strategies. SPNS grants are intended for projects that may serve as national models in addressing the housing and related special needs of eligible individuals. Long-Term Comprehensive Strategies grants are for eligible persons who need specially tailored support rather than formula allocations.

Eligibility

States, local governments, and nonprofit organizations are eligible for SPNS grants. Certain States and units of local government may be eligible for Long-Term Comprehensive Strategies grants. HOPWA provides both formula and competitive grants. Qualified States and urban areas with the highest number of AIDS cases receive annual formula grants, which comprise 90 percent of total HOPWA funds. The competitive grant program awards the remaining 10 percent of HOPWA funds to projects with a national impact and to projects in areas that do not receive formula funds.

Eligible grantees

Cities with a population of more than 500,000 and at least 1,500 cumulative AIDS cases may apply for the formula grants. States with more than 1,500 cumulative AIDS cases (in areas outside cities eligible to receive HOPWA) may also apply. For competitive grants, States and local governments that do not qualify for formula grants and nonprofit organizations may apply.

Funding

Grants of up to $1 million are available. An additional 10 percent may be allocated for administrative costs, and another $50,000 may be allocated to an applicant to collect project outcome data.

Services

Grants may be used to fund the following:

- Housing information services, including fair housing counseling and project-based or tenant-based assistance
- New construction of a community residence or similar dwelling
- Acquisition, rehabilitation, conversion, lease, or repair of facilities to provide housing and services
- Operating costs for housing
- Short-term rent, mortgage, and utility payments to prevent homelessness
- Supportive services
- Administrative expenses
- Resource identification and technical assistance

Funding may also be used to help communities improve their needs assessment capacity, initiate long-range HIV/AIDS housing planning, and enhance facility operations.

Information contact

For an application kit, supplemental information, or technical assistance, call HUD's SuperNOFA Information Center at (800) 483-8929 or (800) 483-8209 (TDD) for the hearing impaired. Applicants requesting a HOPWA grant application must refer to it specifically. For general information on HUD policies, programs, and initiatives for the homeless, call HUD's toll-free National Homeless Assistance Hotline (800-HUD-1010), which provides callers from across the country with the names and phone numbers of local homeless assistance providers, as well as tips on what individuals can do to help the homeless.

For general information on housing and AIDS, contact the AIDS Housing of Washington National Technical Assistance Project at: (206) 448-5242; or by e-mail at: info@aidshousing.org.

The Centers for Disease Control and Prevention

The CDC, the nation's prevention agency, monitors health, detects and investigates health problems, conducts research to enhance prevention, develops and advocates public health policies, implements prevention strategies, promotes healthy behaviors, and fosters safe and healthful environments.

The CDC's National Center for HIV, STD (sexually transmitted diseases), and TB Prevention (NCHSTP) is responsible for public health surveillance, prevention research, and programs to prevent and control HIV infection and AIDS, other STDs, and TB. Center staff work in collaboration with government and nongovernment partners at community, State, national, and international levels, applying well-integrated multidisciplinary programs of research, surveillance, technical assistance, and evaluation.

Two key CDC services are the CDC National AIDS Clearinghouse (NAC) and the CDC National Prevention Information Network (NPIN). NAC provides information about HIV/AIDS, STDs, and TB to people and organizations working in prevention, health care, research, and support services. All of the clearinghouse's services are designed to facilitate the sharing of information about education, prevention, published materials, and research findings, and news about HIV/AIDS, STD, and TB-related trends. Health information specialists at the clearinghouse answer questions, provide referrals, and offer technical assistance. By using the CDC NAC databases and other CDC resources, staff members help callers find up-to-date information about organizations that provide HIV/AIDS-, STD-, and TB-related services, educational materials, and funding resources. To contact a health information specialist, call (800) 458-5231 (English and Spanish), or (800) 243-7012 (TDD) for the hearing impaired, Monday through Friday, 9 a.m. to 6 p.m. EST.

State and Local Initiatives

Each State has an SSA, such as a department of human resources, which is responsible for allocating State and Federal funds for substance abuse treatment and prevention and for HIV/AIDS services (often located with STD services). Grantseekers should contact their SSA for information regarding the availability of State and local funding initiatives.

At the community level, Join Together, a project of the Boston University School of Public Health, is a national resource for communities working to reduce substance abuse and gun violence. The project assists in locating resource materials, colleagues, or training opportunities. Information is provided about Federal Register announcements, foundation profiles, materials, and online documents available from other organizations, as well as tips for finding grants. A technical assistance team can assist in locating information and provide a directory of more than 75,000 people working in substance abuse treatment throughout the nation. A categorized database provides more than 3,000 Web links to relevant substance abuse treatment information.

Contact Information

Join Together, 441 Stuart Street, Boston, MA 02116. Phone: (617) 437-1500; Fax: (617) 437-9394; e-mail: info@jointogether.org or webmaster@jointogether.org.

Special Populations

Over the past 5 years minorities, women, adolescents, homeless and low-income individuals, and incarcerated persons have become increasingly affected by the HIV/AIDS pandemic. Many funding sources target specific special populations. Directories, such as those published by the Foundation Center and Aspen Publishers, allow grantseekers to search for private foundations and corporate giving by specific subject area, such as substance abuse, women, children and adolescents, and HIV/AIDS. Federal, State, and local funding sources should be contacted directly to determine target population eligibility.

Grantwriting Information

Grantwriters can be helpful in developing an effective grant application. In deciding whether or not to use the services of a grantwriter, it is important to consider cost as well as existing agency staff writing capacity and available funding. If the agency has never used a grantwriter before, it may be helpful to contact other organizations in the area to assist in determining the range of costs associated with grantwriters as well as the names of local grantwriters. Often, grantwriters specialize in a particular field, such as health or education. A grantwriter's prior experience in writing HIV/AIDS or substance abuse treatment grant applications can be very helpful, not only in the writing of an application, but also in the development of the proposed service or project for which funding is sought.

Building agency grantwriting capacity can be an effective alternative to the use of a grantwriter. Check with a local college or university's evening education program to see if classes are offered on grantwriting. A number of grantwriting resources (i.e., workshops, "how-to" books, directories of consultants) are available through the Internet using the key word "grantwriting."

Strategies To Ensure Ongoing Funding

Some funding sources offer one-time funding only; others provide the opportunity for continuation of funding after the initial grant award period. With the latter, especially, it is important that grant recipients have a mutually productive relationship with the funding source during the grant award period, including

- Timely reporting
- Good working relationship with project officer(s)
- Meeting established timelines
- Meeting goals and objectives
- Financial accountability

When applying for continuation funds, the grantee must be able to demonstrate that the program has "made a difference" with prior funding (i.e., project outcomes) and that need still exists for funding and services. The program also needs to adapt to changes in the environment since the initial funding application and to changes within the funding agency itself.

With one-time funding, the grantee should look for new funding sources well before the end of the initial grant award (i.e., at least a year in advance). Grantseekers should keep in mind that potential funding sources may not have the same interests or requirements as the current funder.

Appendix A
Bibliography

AIDS Weekly Plus. Knowledge, attitudes, and behavior: Conspiracy theories about HIV put individuals at risk. November 13, 1995.

Allen, D.M.; Lehman, J.S.; Green, T.A.; Lindegren, M.L.; Onorato, I.M.; and Forrester, W. HIV infection among homeless adults and runaway youth, United States, 1989–1992. *AIDS* 8(11):1593–1598, 1994.

Alliegro, M.B.; Dorrucci, M.; Phillips, A.N.; Pezzotti, P.; Boros, S.; Zaccarelli, M.; Pristera, R.; and Rezza, G. Incidence and consequences of pregnancy in women with known duration of HIV infection. *Archives of Internal Medicine* 157(22):2585–2590, 1997.

Amass, L.; Bickel, W.K.; Higgins, S.T.; and Hughes, J.R. A preliminary investigation of outcome following gradual or rapid buprenorphine detoxification. *Journal of Addictive Diseases* 13(3):33–45, 1994.

American Academy of Neurology, AIDS Task Force. Criteria for diagnosis of HIV-1 associated dementia complex: Nomenclature and research case definitions for neurologic manifestations of HIV-1 infection. *Neurology* 41:778–784, 1991.

American Psychiatric Association (APA). *Diagnostic and Statistical Manual of Mental Disorders*, 4th ed. Washington, DC: APA, 1994.

American Psychiatric Association (APA). *Practice Guidelines for Treatment of Patients With Substance Use Disorders; Alcohol, Cocaine, Opioids.* Washington, DC: APA, 1995.

American Society of Addiction Medicine (ASAM). *Guidelines for HIV Infection and AIDS in Addiction Treatment.* Chevy Chase, MD: ASAM, 1998.

American Thoracic Society. Treatment of tuberculosis in alcoholic patients. *American Review of Respiratory Disease* 116:559–560, 1977.

Americans With Disabilities Act. 42 U.S.C. §12101 et seq. (1992).

Anand, A.; Carmosino, L.; and Glatt, A.E. Evaluation of recalcitrant pain in HIV-infected hospitalized patients. *Journal of Acquired Immune Deficiency Syndromes* 7(1):52–56, 1994.

Angelone, S.M.; Bellini, L.; Di Bella, D.; and Catalano, M. Effects of fluvoxamine and citalopram in maintaining abstinence in a sample of Italian detoxified alcoholics. *Alcohol and Alcoholism* 33(2):151–156, 1998.

Ashery, R.S. Issues in AIDS training for substance abuse workers. *Journal of Substance Abuse Treatment* 9(1):15–19, 1992.

Asim, J. "Black paranoia far-fetched? Maybe, but understandable." *The Phoenix Gazette* Op-Ed:A13, February 23, 1993.

Avins, A.L.; Woods, W.J.; Lindan, C.P.; Hudes, E.S.; Clark, W.; and Hulley, S.B. HIV infection and risk behaviors among heterosexuals in alcohol treatment programs. *JAMA* 271(7):515–518, 1994.

Baker, A.; Kochan, N.; Dixon, J.; Wodak, A.; and Heather, N. HIV risk-taking behaviour among injecting drug users currently, previously, and never enrolled in methadone treatment. *Addiction* 90(4):545–554, 1995.

Ball, J.C.; Lange, W.R.; Myers, C.P.; and Friedman, S.R. Reducing the risk of AIDS through methadone maintenance treatment. *Journal of Health and Social Behavior* 29(3):214–226, 1988.

Ball, J.C., and Ross, A. *The Effectiveness of Methadone Maintenance Treatment*. New York: Springer-Verlag, 1991.

Bandura, A. Self-efficacy: Toward a unifying theory of behavioral change. *Psychological Review* 84(2):191–215, 1977.

Banks, A., and Gartrell, N.K. Lesbians in the medical setting. In: Cabaj, R.P., and Stein, T.S., eds. *Homosexuality and Mental Health: A Comprehensive Review*. Washington, DC: American Psychiatric Press, 1996. pp. 659–671.

Barre-Sinoussi, F.; Chermann, J.C.; Rey, F.; Nugeyre, M.T.; Chamaret, S.; Gruest, J.; Dauguet, C.; Axler-Blin, C.; Vezinet-Brun, F.; Rouzioux, C.; Rozenbaum, W.; and Montagnier, L. Isolation of T-lymphotropic retrovirus from a patient at risk for acquired immunodeficiency syndrome (AIDS). *Science* 220(4599):868–871, 1983.

Bartlett, J.G. *Medical Management of HIV Infection*. Baltimore, MD: Johns Hopkins AIDS Service, 1999. http://www.hopkins-aids.edu/publications/index_pub.html [Accessed August 4, 1999].

Batki, S.L. Treatment of intravenous drug abusers with AIDS: The role of methadone maintenance. *Journal of Psychoactive Drugs* 20(2):213–216, 1988.

Batki, S.L.; Blake, M.; Gruber, V.; Milovitch, E.; Ouye, G.; Nathan, K.; and Warren, R. *Standards of Care: Client Assessment and Treatment Protocol*. Unpublished tool used by the Opiate Treatment Outpatient Program, San Francisco General Hospital, University of California at San Francisco, 1999.

Batki, S.L.; Ferrando, S.J.; Manfredi, L.; London, J.; Pattillo, J.; and Delucchi, K. Psychiatric disorders, drug use, and medical status in injection drug users with HIV disease. *American Journal on Addictions* 5(3):249–258, 1996.

Batki, S.L., and London, J. Drug abuse treatment for HIV-infected patients. In: Sorensen, J.L.; Wermuth, L.A.; Gibson, D.R.; Choi, K.-H., Guydish, J.R.; and Batki, S.L., eds. *Preventing AIDS in Drug Abusers and Their Sexual Partners*. New York: Guilford Press, 1991. pp. 77–98.

Beatty, R.L. "Alcoholism and the adult gay male population of Pennsylvania." Master's thesis. Harrisburg, PA: Pennsylvania State University, 1983.

Beck, A.T., and Steer, R.A. *Beck Depression Inventory*. San Antonio, TX: Psychological Corporation, 1993.

Bell, A.P., and Weinberg, M.S. *Homosexualities: A Study of Diversities Among Men and Women.* New York: Simon & Schuster, 1978.

Bell, A.P.; Weinberg, M.S.; and Hammersmith, S.K. *Sexual Preference; Its Development in Men and Women.* Bloomington, IN: Indiana University Press, 1981.

Berglund, M., and Ojehagen, A. The influence of alcohol drinking and alcohol use disorders on psychiatric disorders and suicidal behavior. *Alcoholism, Clinical and Experimental Research* 22(7 Suppl):333S–345S, 1998.

Berlin, E.A., and Fowkes, Jr., N.C. A teaching framework for cross-cultural health care. *Western Journal of Medicine* 139(6):934–938, 1983.

Bickel, W.K., and Amass, L. The relationship of mean daily blood alcohol levels to admission MAST, clinic absenteeism, and depression in alcoholic methadone patients. *Drug and Alcohol Dependence* 32:113–118, 1993.

Bickel, W.K.; Amass, L.; Higgins, S.T.; Badger, G.J.; and Esch, R.A. Effects of adding behavioral treatment to opioid detoxification with buprenorphine. *Journal of Consulting and Clinical Psychology* 65(5):803–810, 1997.

Bindman, A.B.; Osmond, D.; Hecht, F.M.; Lehman, J.S.; Vranizan, K.; Keane, D.; Reingold, A.; and the Multistate Evaluation of Surveillance of HIV (MESH) Study Group. Multistate evaluation of anonymous HIV testing and access to medical care. *JAMA* 280(16):1416–1420, 1998.

Bloomfield, K. A comparison of alcohol consumption between lesbians and heterosexual women in an urban population. *Drug and Alcohol Dependence* 33(3):257–269, 1993.

Boccellari, A.A.; Chambers, D.B.; Dilley, J.W.; Shore, M.D.; Tauber, M.A.; Moss, A.R.; and Osmond, D.H. Relationship of beta 2 microglobulin and CD4 counts to neuropsychological performance in HIV-1-infected intravenous drug abusers. *Journal of Acquired Immune Deficiency Syndromes* 7(10):1040–1049, 1994.

Boccellari, A.A.; Dilley, J.W.; Chambers, D.B.; Yingling, C.D.; Tauber, M.A.; Moss, A.R.; and Osmond, D.H. Immune function and neuropsychological performance in HIV-1-infected homosexual men. *Journal of Acquired Immune Deficiency Syndromes* 6(6):592–601, 1993a.

Boccellari, A.A.; Dilley, J.W.; Yingling, C.D.; Chambers, D.B.; Tauber, M.A.; Moss, A.R.; and Osmond, D.H. Relationship of CD4 counts to neurophysiological function in HIV-1-infected homosexual men. *Archives of Neurology* 50(5):517–521, 1993b.

Bokos, P.J.; Mejta, C.L.; Mickenberg, J.H.; and Monks, R.L. Case management: An alternative approach to working with intravenous drug abusers. In: Ashery, R.S., ed. *Progress and Issues in Case Management.* NIDA Research Monograph Series, Number 127. DHHS Pub. No. (ADM) 92-1946. Rockville, MD: National Institute on Drug Abuse, 1992. pp. 92–111.

Booth, R.E.; Kwiatkowski, C.; Iguchi, M.Y.; Pinto, F.; and John, D. Facilitating treatment entry among out-of-treatment injection drug users. *Public Health Reports* 113 (Suppl. 1):116–128, 1998.

Booth, R.E., and Wiebel, W.W. Effectiveness of reducing needle-related risks for HIV through indigenous outreach to injection drug users. *American Journal on Addictions* 1(4):277–287, 1992.

Bortolotti, F.; Stivanello, A.; Armi, Dall', A.; Rinaldi, R.; and La Grasto, F. AIDS information campaign has significantly reduced risk factors for HIV infection in Italian drug abusers. *Journal of Acquired Immune Deficiency Syndromes* 1(4):412–413, 1988.

Bozzette, S.A.; Finkelstein, D.M.; Spector, S.A.; Frame, P.; Powderly, W.G.; He, W.; Phillips, L.; Craven, D.; van der Horst, C.; and Feinberg, J. A randomized trial of three antipneumocystis agents in patients with advanced human immunodeficiency virus infection. *New England Journal of Medicine* 332(11):693–699, 1995.

Bradford, J., and Ryan, C. "National Lesbian Health Care Survey: Mental Health Implications." Washington, DC: National Lesbian and Gay Health Foundation, 1987.

Bradley-Springer, L.A. The complex realities of primary prevention for HIV infection in a "just do it" world. *Nursing Clinics of North America* 34(1):49–70, 1999.

Branson, B.M. Home sample collection tests for HIV infection. *JAMA* 280(19):1699–1701, 1998.

Breitbart, W. Suicide risk and pain in cancer and AIDS patients. In: Chapman, C.R., and Foley, K.M., eds. *Current and Emerging Issues in Cancer Pain: Research and Practice.* New York: Raven Press, 1993. pp. 49–65.

Breitbart, W.; Passik, S.; Bronaugh, T.; Zale, C.; Bluestine, S.; Gomez, M.; Galer, B.; and Portney, R. Pain in the ambulatory AIDS patient: Prevalence and psychosocial correlates. *Proceedings of the 38th Annual Meeting, Academy of Psychosomatic Medicine,* Atlanta, GA, October 17–20, 1991.

Brindis, C.; Pfeffer, R.; and Wolfe, A. A case management program for chemically dependent clients with multiple needs. *Journal of Case Management* 4(1):22–28, 1995.

Brindis, C., and Theidon, K.S. The role of case management in substance abuse treatment services for women and their children. *Journal of Psychoactive Drugs* 29(1):79–88, 1997.

Broers, B.; Morabia, A.; and Hirschel, B. A cohort study of drug abusers' compliance with zidovudine treatment. *Archives of Internal Medicine* 154(10):1121–1127, 1994.

Brooner, R.; Kidorf, M.; King, V.; Beilenson, P.; Svikis, D.; and Vlahov, D. Reduced drug use in needle exchange participants. *International Conference on AIDS* 12:671 (Abstract No. 33408), 1998.

Buckingham, S.L., and Van Gorp, W.G. HIV-associated dementia: A clinician's guide to early detection, diagnosis, and intervention. *Families in Society: The Journal of Contemporary Human Services* 75(6):333–345, 1994.

Bux, D.A.; Iguchi, M.Y.; Lidz, V.; Baxter, R.C.; and Platt, J.J. Participation in an outreach-based coupon distribution program for free methadone detoxification. *Hospital and Community Psychiatry* 44(11):1066–1072, 1993.

Cabaj, R.P. Homosexuality and neurosis: Considerations for psychotherapy. *Journal of Homosexuality* 15(1–2):13–23, 1988.

Cabaj, R.P. AIDS and chemical dependency: Special issues and treatment barriers for gay and bisexual men. *Journal of Psychoactive Drugs* 21(4):387–393, 1989.

Cabaj, R.P. Substance abuse in gay men, lesbians, and bisexual individuals. In: Cabaj, R.P., and Stein, T.S., eds. *Textbook of Homosexuality and Mental Health.* Washington, DC: American Psychiatric Press, 1996. pp. 783–799.

Cabaj, R.P. Gays, lesbians, and bisexuals. In: Lowinson, J.H.; Ruiz, P.; Millman, R.B.; and Langrod, J.G., eds. *Substance Abuse: A Comprehensive Textbook*, 3rd ed. Baltimore, MD: Williams & Wilkins, 1997. pp. 725–733.

Cabaj, R.P., and Stein, T.S., eds. *Textbook of Homosexuality and Mental Health.* Washington, DC: American Psychiatric Press, 1996.

California Department of Corrections. What percentage of the California correctional population has a history of substance abuse? *California Correctional Statistics*, CCS 1-98, July 1998. http://www.cdc.state.ca.us/reports/offender.htm [Accessed July 12, 1998].

Calsyn, D.A.; Saxon, A.J.; Freeman, Jr., G.; and Whittaker, S. Ineffectiveness of AIDS education and HIV antibody testing in reducing high-risk behaviors among injection drug users. *American Journal of Public Health* 82:573–575, 1992.

Calzavara, L.M.; Coates, R.A.; Raboud, J.M.; Farewell, V.T.; Read, S.E.; Shephered, F.A.; Fanning, M.M.; and MacFadden, D. Ongoing high-risk sexual behaviors in relation to recreational drug use in sexual encounters. Analysis of 5 years of data from the Toronto Sexual Contact Study. *Annals of Epidemiology* 3(3):272–280, 1993.

Cameron, D.W.; Heath-Chiozzi, M.; Danner, S.; Cohen, C.; Kravcik, S.; Maurath, C.; Sun, E.; Henry, D.; Rode, R.; Potthoff, A.; and Leonard, J. Randomised, placebo-controlled trial of ritonavir in advanced HIV-1 disease. *Lancet* 351(9102):543–549, 1998.

Cameron, D.W.; Pavon, J.; Rodriguez de Castro, F.; Diaz, F.; Julia, G.; Cayla, J.; and Cabrera, P. "Prolongation of life and prevention of AIDS complications in advanced HIV immunodeficiency with ritonavir." Eleventh International Conference on AIDS, Vancouver, Canada, July 7–12, 1996.

Cameron, D.W.; Simonsen, J.N.; D'Costa, L.J.; Ronald, A.R.; Maitha, G.M.; Gakinya, M.N.; Cheang, M.; Ndinya-Achola, J.O.; Piot, P.; and Brunham, R.C. Female to male transmission of human immunodeficiency virus type 1: Risk factors for seroconversion in men. *Lancet* 2(8660):403–407, 1989.

Carpenter, C.C.; Fischl, M.A.; Hammer, S.M.; Hirsch, M.S.; Jacobsen, D.M.; Katzenstein, D.A.; Montaner, J.S.; Richman, D.D.; Saag, M.S.; Schooley, R.T.; Thompson, M.A.; Vella, S.; Yeni, P.G.; and Volberding, P.A. Antiretroviral therapy for HIV infection in 1996. Recommendations of an international panel. *JAMA* 276(2):146–154, 1996.

Carpenter, C.C.; Fischl, M.A.; Hammer, S.G.; Hirsch, M.S.; Jacobsen, D.M.; Katzenstein, D.A.; Montaner, J.S.; Richman, D.D.; Saag, M.S.; Schooley, R.T.; Thompson, M.A.; Vella, S.; Yeni, P.G.; and Volberding, P.A. Antiretroviral therapy for HIV-infection in 1997. Updated recommendations of the International AIDS Society-USA Panel. *JAMA* 277(24):1962–1969, 1997.

Carpenter, C.C.; Fischl, M.A.; Hammer, S.M.; Hirsch, M.S.; Jacobsen, D.M.; Katzenstein, D.A.; Montaner, J.S.; Richman, D.D.; Saag, M.S.; Schooley, R.T.; Thompson, M.A.; Vella, S.; Yeni, P.G.; and Volberding, P.A. Antiretroviral therapy for HIV infection in 1998: Updated recommendations of the International AIDS Society-USA Panel. *JAMA* 280(1):78–86, 1998.

Carroll, J. The negative attitudes of some general nurses towards drug misusers. *Nursing Standard* 9(34):36–38, 1995.

Casadonte, P.P.; Des Jarlais, D.C.; Friedman, S.R.; and Rotrosen, J.P. Psychological and behavioral impact among intravenous drug abusers of learning HIV test results. *International Journal of the Addictions* 25:409–426, 1990.

Castro, K.G.; Ward, J.W.; Slutsker, L.; Buehler, J.W.; Jaffe, H.W.; and Berkelman, R.L. 1993 Revised Classification System for HIV Infection and Expanded Surveillance Case Definition for AIDS Among Adolescents and Adults. *Morbidity and Mortality Weekly Report* 41, December 18, 1992. http://www.cdc.gov/mmwr [Accessed August 20, 1999].

Center for AIDS Prevention Studies. *What Are Women's HIV Prevention Needs?* Fact Sheet #4Er, 1998. http://www.caps.ucsf.edu/womenrev.html [Accessed March 8, 1999].

Center for Substance Abuse Treatment. *Assessment and Treatment of Patients With Coexisting Mental Illness and Alcohol and Other Drug Abuse.* Treatment Improvement Protocol (TIP) Series, Number 9. DHHS Pub. No. (SMA) 94-2078. Washington, DC: U.S. Government Printing Office, 1994a.

Center for Substance Abuse Treatment. *Treatment for Alcohol and Other Drug Abuse: Opportunities for Collaboration.* Technical Assistance Publication (TAP) Series, Number 11. DHHS Pub. No. (SMA) 94-2075. Washington, DC: U.S. Government Printing Office, 1994b.

Center for Substance Abuse Treatment. *Developing State Outcomes Monitoring Systems for Alcohol and Other Drug Abuse Treatment.* Treatment Improvement Protocol (TIP) Series, Number 14. DHHS Pub. No. (SMA) 95-3031. Washington, DC: U.S. Government Printing Office, 1995a.

Center for Substance Abuse Treatment. *Treatment for HIV-Infected Alcohol and Other Drug Abusers.* Treatment Improvement Protocol (TIP) Series, Number 15. DHHS Pub. No. (SMA) 95-3038. Washington, DC: U.S. Government Printing Office, 1995b.

Center for Substance Abuse Treatment. *Planning for Alcohol and Other Drug Abuse Treatment for Adults in the Criminal Justice System.* Treatment Improvement Protocol (TIP) Series, Number 17. DHHS Pub. No. (SMA) 95-3039. Washington, DC: U.S. Government Printing Office, 1995c.

Center for Substance Abuse Treatment. *The Tuberculosis Epidemic: Legal and Ethical Issues for Alcohol and Other Drug Abuse Treatment Providers.* Treatment Improvement Protocol (TIP) Series, Number 18. DHHS Pub. No. (SMA) 95-3047. Washington, DC: U.S. Government Printing Office, 1995d.

Center for Substance Abuse Treatment. *Detoxification From Alcohol and Other Drugs.* Treatment Improvement Protocol (TIP) Series, Number 19. DHHS Pub. No. (SMA) 95-3046. Washington, DC: U.S. Government Printing Office, 1995e.

Center for Substance Abuse Treatment. *Matching Treatment to Patient Needs in Opioid Substitution Therapy.* Treatment Improvement Protocol (TIP) Series, Number 20. DHHS Pub. No. (SMA) 95-3049. Washington, DC: U.S. Government Printing Office, 1995f.

Center for Substance Abuse Treatment. *LAAM in the Treatment of Opiate Addiction.* Treatment Improvement Protocol (TIP) Series, Number 22. DHHS Pub. No. (SMA) 95-3052. Washington, DC: U.S. Government Printing Office, 1995g.

Center for Substance Abuse Treatment. *Treatment Drug Courts: Integrating Substance Abuse Treatment With Legal Case Processing.* Treatment Improvement Protocol (TIP) Series, Number 23. DHHS Pub. No. (SMA) 96-3113. Washington, DC: U.S. Government Printing Office, 1996.

Center for Substance Abuse Treatment. *A Guide to Substance Abuse Services for Primary Care Clinicians.* Treatment Improvement Protocol (TIP) Series, Number 24. DHHS Pub. No. (SMA) 97-3139. Washington, DC: U.S. Government Printing Office, 1997.

Center for Substance Abuse Treatment. *Substance Abuse Among Older Adults.* Treatment Improvement Protocol (TIP) Series, Number 26. DHHS Pub. No. (SMA) 98-3179. Washington, DC: U.S. Government Printing Office, 1998a.

Center for Substance Abuse Treatment. *Comprehensive Case Management for Substance Abuse Treatment.* Treatment Improvement Protocol (TIP) Series, Number 27. DHHS Pub. No. (SMA) 98-3222. Washington, DC: U.S. Government Printing Office, 1998b.

Center for Substance Abuse Treatment. *Substance Use Disorder Treatment for People With Physical and Cognitive Disabilities.* Treatment Improvement Protocol (TIP) Series, Number 29. DHHS Pub. No. (SMA) 98-3249. Washington, DC: U.S. Government Printing Office, 1998c.

Center for Substance Abuse Treatment. *Continuity of Offender Treatment for Substance Use Disorders From Institution to Community.* Treatment Improvement Protocol (TIP) Series, Number 30. DHHS Pub. No. (SMA) 98-3245. Washington, DC: U.S. Government Printing Office, 1998d.

Center for Substance Abuse Treatment. *Screening and Assessing Adolescents for Substance Use Disorders.* Treatment Improvement Protocol (TIP) Series, Number 31. DHHS Pub. No. (SMA) 99-3282. Washington, DC: U.S. Government Printing Office, 1999a.

Center for Substance Abuse Treatment. *Treatment of Adolescents With Substance Use Disorders.* Treatment Improvement Protocol (TIP) Series, Number 32. DHHS Pub. No. (SMA) 99-3283. Washington, DC: U.S. Government Printing Office, 1999b.

Center for Substance Abuse Treatment. *Brief Interventions and Brief Therapies for Substance Abuse.* Treatment Improvement Protocol (TIP) Series, Number 34. DHHS Pub. No. (SMA) 99-3353. Washington, DC: U.S. Government Printing Office, 1999c.

Center for Substance Abuse Treatment. *Enhancing Motivation for Change in Substance Abuse Treatment.* Treatment Improvement Protocol (TIP) Series, Number 35. DHHS Pub. No. (SMA) 99-3354. Washington, DC: U.S. Government Printing Office, 1999d.

Center for Substance Abuse Treatment. *Cultural Issues in Substance Abuse Treatment.* DHHS Pub. No. (SMA) 99-3278. Washington, DC: U.S. Government Printing Office, 1999e.

Center for Substance Abuse Treatment. *Substance Abuse Treatment for Persons With Child Abuse and Neglect Issues.* Treatment Improvement Protocol (TIP) Series, Number 36. DHHS Pub. No. (SMA) 00-3357. Washington, DC: U.S. Government Printing Office, 2000.

Center for Substance Abuse Treatment. *Integrating Substance Abuse Treatment and Vocational Services.* Treatment Improvement Protocol (TIP) Series, Number 38. Washington, DC: U.S. Government Printing Office, in press (a).

Center for Substance Abuse Treatment. *Gay, Lesbian, Bisexual, and Transgender Populations.* Technical Assistance Publication (TAP) Series. Washington, DC: U.S. Government Printing Office, in press (b).

Centers for Disease Control and Prevention. Pneumocystis pneumonia—Los Angeles. *Morbidity and Mortality Weekly Report* 30(21):250–252, 1981.

Centers for Disease Control and Prevention. Unexplained immunodeficiency and opportunistic infections in infants—New York, New Jersey, California. *Morbidity and Mortality Weekly Report* 31(49):665–667, 1982.

Centers for Disease Control and Prevention. Antibody to human immunodeficiency virus in female prostitutes. *Morbidity and Mortality Weekly Report* 36(11):157–161, 1987a.

Centers for Disease Control and Prevention. Recommendations for prevention of HIV transmission in health-care settings. *Morbidity and Mortality Weekly Report* 36(Suppl. 2S):1S–18S, 1987b.

Centers for Disease Control and Prevention. Update: Reducing HIV transmission in intravenous-drug users not in drug treatment in the United States. *Morbidity and Mortality Weekly Report* 39(31):529, 536–538, 1990.

Centers for Disease Control and Prevention. 1993 Revised Classification System for HIV Infection and Expanded Surveillance Case Definition for AIDS Among Adolescents and Adults. *Morbidity and Mortality Weekly Report* 41(51):961–962, 1992.

Centers for Disease Control and Prevention. Technical guidance on HIV counseling. *Morbidity and Mortality Weekly Report* 42(RR-2):11–17, 1993.

Centers for Disease Control and Prevention. Recommendations of the U.S. Public Health Service Task Force on the use of zidovudine to reduce perinatal transmission of human immunodeficiency virus. *Morbidity and Mortality Weekly Report* 43(RR-11):1–20, 1994.

Centers for Disease Control and Prevention. U.S. Public Health Service recommendations for human immunodeficiency virus counseling and voluntary testing for pregnant women. *Morbidity and Mortality Weekly Report* 44(RR-7):1–15, 1995.

Centers for Disease Control and Prevention. HIV/AIDS education and prevention programs for adults in prisons and jails and juveniles in confinement facilities—United States, 1994. *Morbidity and Mortality Weekly Report* 45(13):268–271, 1996a.

Centers for Disease Control and Prevention. *HIV/AIDS Surveillance Report* 8(2), 1996b.

Centers for Disease Control and Prevention. Provisional public health service recommendations for chemoprophylaxis after occupational exposure to HIV. *Morbidity and Mortality Weekly Report* 45(22):468–472, 1996c.

Centers for Disease Control and Prevention. 1997 USPHS/IDSA guidelines for the prevention of opportunistic infections in persons infected with human immunodeficiency virus: A summary. *Morbidity and Mortality Weekly Report* 46(RR-12):1–45, 1997a.

Centers for Disease Control and Prevention. HIV/AIDS and women who have sex with women (WSW) in the United States. *CDC Facts,* July 1997b.

Centers for Disease Control and Prevention. *HIV/AIDS Surveillance Report* 9(2), 1997c.

Centers for Disease Control and Prevention. 1998 guidelines for treatment of sexually transmitted diseases. *Morbidity and Mortality Weekly Report* 47(RR-1):1–118, 1998a.

Centers for Disease Control and Prevention. *Assessing Health Risk Behaviors Among Young People: Youth Risk Behavior Surveillance System,* 1998b. http://www.cdc.gov/nccdphp/dash/yrbs/yrbs98.pdf [Accessed May 10, 1999].

Centers for Disease Control and Prevention. Basic Statistics—Ten States/Territories and Cities Reporting Highest Number of AIDS Cases. 1998c. http://www.cdc.gov/nchstp/hiv_aids/stats/topten.htm [Accessed March 18, 1999].

Centers for Disease Control and Prevention. *HIV/AIDS Surveillance Report: U.S. HIV and AIDS Cases Reported Through June 1998* 10(1), 1998d.

Centers for Disease Control and Prevention. *HIV/AIDS Surveillance Report: U.S. HIV and AIDS Cases Reported Through December 1998* 10(2), 1998e.

Centers for Disease Control and Prevention. Prevention and treatment of sexually transmitted diseases as an HIV prevention strategy. *CDC Update,* June 1998f.

Centers for Disease Control and Prevention. Public health service guidelines for the management of health-care worker exposures to HIV and recommendations for postexposure prophylaxis. *Morbidity and Mortality Weekly Report* 47(RR-7):1–28, 1998g.

Centers for Disease Control and Prevention. Public Health Service Task Force recommendations for the use of antiretroviral drugs in pregnant women infected with HIV-1 for maternal health and for reducing perinatal HIV-1 transmission in the United States. *Morbidity and Mortality Weekly Report* 47(RR-2):1–30, 1998h.

Centers for Disease Control and Prevention. *Rapid HIV Tests: Questions/Answers.* March 1998i.

Centers for Disease Control and Prevention. Report of the NIH panel to define principles of therapy of HIV infection. *Morbidity and Mortality Weekly Report* 47(RR-5):1–41, 1998j.

Centers for Disease Control and Prevention. *The HIV/AIDS Epidemic in the United States, 1997–1998,* 1999a. http://www.cdc.gov/nchstp/hiv_aids/ pubs/facts/hivrepfs.htm [Accessed February 15, 1999].

Centers for Disease Control and Prevention. *HIV/AIDS Surveillance Report: U.S. HIV and AIDS Cases Reported Through June 1999* 11(1), 1999b.

Centers for Disease Control and Prevention. *HIV/AIDS Surveillance Supplemental Report* Atlanta, GA: Centers for Disease Control and Prevention, 1999c.

Centers for Disease Control and Prevention. Preventing occupational HIV transmission to health care workers. 1999d. http://www.cdc.gov/nchstp/hiv_aids/pubs/facts/hcw.htm [Accessed January 10, 2000].

Centers for Disease Control and Prevention. Young people at risk—epidemic shifts further toward young women and minorities. 1999e. http://www.cdc.gov/nchstp/hiv_aids/pubs/facts/youth.htm [Accessed January 10, 2000].

Centers for Disease Control and Prevention, Center for Substance Abuse Treatment, National Institute on Drug Abuse. *HIV/AIDS Prevention Bulletin.* Rockville, MD: April 19, 1993.

Centers for Disease Control and Prevention. National Center for Health Statistics. Births and deaths: Preliminary data for 1998. *National Vital Statistics Reports* 47(25), 1999f. http://www.cdc.gov/nchs/data/nvs47_25.pdf [Accessed April 4, 2000].

Chaisson, R.E.; Stanton, D.L.; Gallant, J.E.; Rucker, S.; Bartlett, J.G.; and Moore, R.D. Impact of the 1993 revision of the AIDS case definition on the prevalence of AIDS in a clinical setting. *AIDS* 7:857–862, 1993.

Chandra, P.S.; Ravi, V.; Desai, A.; and Subbakrishna, D.K. Anxiety and depression among HIV-infected heterosexuals—a report from India. *Journal of Psychosomatic Research* 45(5):401–409, 1998.

Chatham, L.R.; Rowan-Szal, G.A.; Joe, G.W.; Brown, B.S.; and Simpson, D.D. Heavy drinking in a population of methadone-maintained clients. *Journal of Studies on Alcohol* 56:417–422, 1995.

Chen, Z.; Branson, B.; Ballenger, A.; and Peterman, T.A. Risk assessment to improve targeting of HIV counseling and testing services for STD clinic patients. *Sexually Transmitted Diseases* 25(10):539–543, 1998.

Chin, D.P.; Osmond, D.; Page-Shafer, K.; Glassroth, J.; Rosen, M.J.; Reichman, L.B.; Kvale, P.A.; Wallace, J.M.; Poole, W.K.; and Hopewell, P.C. Reliability of anergy skin-testing in persons with HIV infection. *American Journal of Respiratory and Critical Care Medicine* 153(6 pt. 1):1982–1984, 1996.

Clark, S.J.; Saag, M.S.; Decker, W.D.; Campbell-Hill, S.; Roberson, J.L.; Veldkamp, P.J.; Kappes, J.C.; Hahn, B.H.; and Shaw, G.M. High titers of cytopathic virus in plasma of patients with symptomatic primary HIV-1 infection. *New England Journal of Medicine* 324:954–960, 1991.

Clayman, C.B., ed. *The American Medical Association Encyclopedia of Medicine.* New York: Random House, 1989.

Clements, K.; Gleghorn, A.; Garcia, D.; Katz, M.; and Marx, R. A risk profile of street youth in northern California: Implications for gender-specific human immunodeficiency virus prevention. *Journal of Adolescent Health* 20(5):343–353, 1997.

Clements, K.; Marx, B.; Guzman, R.; Ikeda, S.; and Katz, M. Prevalence of HIV infection in transgendered individuals in San Francisco. *The International Conference on AIDS* 12:449 (Abstract No. 23536), 1998.

Cochran, S.D., and Mays, V.M. Relation between psychiatric syndromes and behaviorally defined sexual orientation in a sample of the U.S. population. *American Journal of Epidemiology* 151(5):516–523, 2000.

Cockrell, J.R., and Folstein, M.F. Mini Mental State Examination (MMSE). *Psychopharmacology Bulletin* 24:689–692, 1988.

Coffin, J.A. "HIV and viral dynamics." Plenary address presented at the Eleventh International Conference on AIDS, Vancouver, Canada, July 12, 1996.

Cohen, M.S.; Hoffman, I.F.; Royce, R.A.; Kazembe, P.; Dyer, J.R.; Daly, C.C.; Zimba, D.; Vernazza, P.L.; Maida, M.; Fiscus, S.A.; and Eron, Jr., J.J. Reduction of concentration of HIV-1 in semen after treatment of urethritis: Implications for prevention of sexual transmission of HIV-1. *Lancet* 349:1868–1873, 1997.

Colon, H.M.; Robles, R.R.; Marrero, C.A.; Matos, T.D.; Lopez, C.M.; and Orraca, O. Reduction in sexual risk behaviors among HIV seropositve drug abusers in Puerto Rico. *International Conference on AIDS* 11(2):146 (Abstract No. We.C. 3512) 1996.

Condelli, W.S.; Fairbank, J.A.; Dennis, M.L.; and Rachal, J.V. Cocaine use by clients in methadone programs: Significance, scope, and behavioral interventions. *Journal of Substance Abuse Treatment* 8:203–212, 1991.

Conley, L.J.; Bush, T.J.; Buchbinder, S.P.; Penley, K.A.; Judson, F.N.; and Holmberg, S.D. The association between cigarette smoking and selected HIV-related medical conditions. *AIDS* 10:1121–1126, 1996.

Cooper, J.R. Methadone treatment and acquired immunodeficiency syndrome. *JAMA* 262:1664–1668, 1989.

Cornelius, J.R.; Salloum, I.M.; Ehler, J.G.; Jarrett, P.J.; Cornelius, M.D.; Black, A.; Perel, J.M.; and Thase, M.E. Double-blind fluoxetine in depressed alcoholic smokers. *Psychopharmacology Bulletin* 33:165–170, 1997.

Cornelius, J.R.; Salloum, I.M.; Thase, M.E.; Haskett, R.F.; Daley, D.C.; Jones-Barlock, A.; Upsher, C.; and Perel, J.M. Fluoxetine versus placebo in depressed alcoholic cocaine abusers. *Psychopharmacology Bulletin* 34:117–121, 1998.

Cottler, L.B.; Compton, W.M.; Ben Abdallah, A.; Cunningham-Williams, R.; Abram, F.; Fitchenbaum, C.; and Dotson, W. Peer-delivered interventions reduce HIV risk behaviors among out-of-treatment drug abusers. *Public Health Reports* 113(Suppl. 1):31–41, 1998.

Cox, G.B.; Meijer, L.; Carr, D.I.; and Freng, S.A. Systems alliance and support (SAS): A program of intensive case management for chronic public inebriates. *Alcohol Treatment Quarterly* 10(3/4):125–138, 1993.

Cox, J.M. Justice, compassion needed in treating AIDS patients. *Health Program* 67(4):34–37, 1986.

Crespi, T.D., and Sabatelli, R.M. Adolescent runaways and family strife: A conflict-induced differentiation framework. *Adolescence* 28(112):867–878, 1993.

Croop, R.S.; Faulkner, E.B.; Labriola, D.F.; and the Naltrexone Usage Study Group. The safety profile of naltrexone in the treatment of alcoholism. Results from a multicenter usage study. *Archives of General Psychiatry* 54:1130–1135, 1997.

Cross, T.; Bazron, B.; Dennis, K.; and Isaacs, M. *Towards a Culturally Competent System of Care: A Monograph on Effective Services for Minority Children Who Are Severely Emotionally Disturbed.* Washington, DC: Child and Adolescent Service System Program, Technical Assistance Center, Georgetown University Child Development Center, 1989.

Culnane, M.; Fowler, M.G.; Lee, S.S.; McSherry, G.; Brady, M.; O'Donnell, K.; Mofenson, L.; Gortmaker, S.L.; Shapiro, D.E.; Scott, G.; Jimenez, E.; Moore, E.C.; Diaz, C.; Flynn, P.M.; Cunningham, B.; and Oleske, J. Lack of long-term effects of in utero exposure to zidovudine among uninfected children born to HIV-infected women. *JAMA* 281:151–157, 1999.

Deeks, S.G.; Loftus, R.; Cohen, P.; Chin, S.; and Grant, R. Incidence and predictors of virologic failure of indinavir and/or ritonavir in an urban health clinic. *Program and Abstracts of the 37th Interscience Conference on Antimicrobial Agents and Chemotherapy (ICAAC).* Abstract No. LB-02. Toronto, Canada, September 28–October 1, 1997.

Deeks, S.G.; Smith, M.; Holodniy, M.; and Kahn, J.O. HIV-1 protease inhibitors. A review for clinicians. *JAMA* 277:145–153, 1997.

DeHovitz, J.A.; Kelly, P.; Feldman, J.; Sierra, M.F.; Clarke, L.; Bromberg, J.; Wan, J.Y.; Vermund, S.H.; and Landesman, S. Sexually transmitted diseases, sexual behavior, and cocaine use in inner-city women. *American Journal of Epidemiology* 140(12):1125–1134, 1994.

de Monteflores, C. Notes on the management of difference. In: Stein, T.S., and Cohen, C.C., eds. *Contemporary Perspectives on Psychotherapy With Lesbians and Gay Men.* New York: Plenum Press, 1986.

Dennis, M.L.; Ingram, P.W.; Burks, M.E.; and Rachal, J.V. Effectiveness of streamlined admissions to methadone treatment: A simplified time-series analysis. *Journal of Psychoactive Drugs* 26:207–216, 1994.

Dennison, R. Should I have a baby? It may be the most important decision you'll ever make. *W.O.R.L.D. Newsletter*, April 1998.

Des Jarlais, D.C.; Hagan, H.; Friedman, S.R.; Friedmann, P.; Goldberg, D.; Frischer, M.; Green, S.; Tunving, K.; Ljungberg, B.; and Wodak, A. Maintaining low HIV seroprevalence in populations of injecting drug users. *JAMA* 274:1226–1231, 1995.

Des Jarlais, D.C.; Marmor, M.; Paone, D.; Titus, S.; Shi, Q.; Perlis, T.; Jose, B.; and Friedman, S.R. HIV incidence among injecting drug users in New York City syringe-exchange programs. *Lancet* 348:987–991, 1996.

Des Jarlais, D.C.; Wenston, J.; Friedman, S.R.; Sotheran, J.L.; Maslansky, R.; and Marmor, M. Crack cocaine use in a cohort of methadone maintenance patients. *Journal of Substance Abuse Treatment* 9:319–325, 1992.

Diamond, D.L., and Wilsnack, S.C. Alcohol abuse among lesbians: A descriptive study. *Journal of Homosexuality* 4(2):123–142, 1978.

Diaz, R.M.; Stall, R.D.; Hoff, C.; Daigle, D.; and Coates, T.J. HIV risk among Latino gay men in the southwestern United States. *AIDS Education and Prevention* 8(5):415–429, 1996.

Diaz, T.; Buehler, J.W.; Castro, K.G.; and Ward, J.W. AIDS trends among Latinos in the United States. *American Journal of Public Health* 83:504–509, 1993.

Diaz, T., and Klevens, M. Differences by ancestry in sociodemographics and risk behaviors among Hispanics with AIDS. The Supplement to HIV and AIDS Surveillance Project Group. *Ethnicity and Disease* 7(3):200–206, 1997.

Dieterich, D.T. Advances in the pathophysiology and treatment of HIV-associated wasting. *Improving the Management of HIV Disease* 4(5), 1997. http://hivinsite.ucsf.edu/medical/iasusa/2098.2e2e.html [Accessed March 9, 2000].

Dixon, P.S.; Flanigan, T.P.; DeBuono, B.A.; Laurie, J.J.; De Ciantis, M.L.; Hoy, J.; Stein, M.; Scott, H.D.; and Carpenter, C.C. Infection with the human immunodeficiency virus in prisoners: Meeting the health care challenge. *American Journal of Medicine* 95(6):629–635, 1993.

Dole, V.P.; Nyswander, M.E.; and Kreek, M.J. Narcotic blockade. *Archives of Internal Medicine* 118:304–309, 1966.

Doyle, A.; Jefferys, R.; and Kelly, J. *National ADAP Monitoring Project: Interim Technical Report.* March 1998. http://www.aids infonyc.org/adap/report98.html. [Accessed March 12, 1999].

Drake, R.E., and Noordsy, D.L. Case management for people with coexisting severe mental disorder and substance abuse. *Psychiatric Annals* 24(8):427–431, 1994.

Edlin, B.R.; Irwin, K.L.; Faruque, S.; McCoy, C.B.; Word, C.; Serrano, Y.; Inciardi, J.A.; Bowser, B.P.; Schilling, R.F.; and Holmberg, S.D. Intersecting epidemics—crack cocaine use and HIV infection among inner-city adults. *New England Journal of Medicine* 331:1422–1427, 1994.

Edsall, J.R.; Awe, R.J.; Bunyan, S.B.; Hackney, Jr., R.L.; Iseman, M.D.; and Reagan, W.P. Treatment of tuberculosis in alcoholic patients. *American Review of Respiratory Disease* 116(3):559–561, 1977.

El-Bassel, N.; Gilbert, L.; Krishnan, S.; Schilling, R.; Gaeta, T.; Purpura, S.; and Witte, S.S. Partner violence and sexual HIV-risk behaviors among women in an inner-city emergency department. *Violence and Victims* 13(4):377–393, 1998.

El-Bassel, N., and Schilling, R.F. 15-month followup of women methadone patients taught skills to reduce heterosexual HIV transmission. *Public Health Reports* 107(5):500–504, 1992.

Elifson, K.W.; Boles, J.; and Sweat, M. Risk factors associated with HIV infection among male prostitutes. *American Journal of Public Health* 83:79–83, 1993.

Esteban, J.I.; Esteban, R.; Viladomiu, L.; Lopez-Talavera, J.C.; Gonzalez, A.; Hernandez, J.M.; Roget, M.; Vargas, V.; Genesca, J.; and Buti, M., et al. Hepatitis C virus antibodies among risk groups in Spain. *Lancet* 2(8658):294–297, 1989.

European Mode of Delivery Collaboration. Elective caesarean-section versus vaginal delivery in prevention of vertical HIV-1 transmission: A randomised clinical trial. *Lancet* 353(9158):1035–1039, 1999.

European Study Group on Heterosexual Transmission of HIV. Comparison of female to male and male to female transmission of HIV in 563 stable couples. *British Medical Journal* 304:809–813, 1992.

Fairfield, K.M.; Eisenberg, D.M.; Davis, R.B.; Libman, H.; and Phillips, R.S. Patterns of use, expenditures, and perceived efficacy of complementary and alternative therapies in HIV-infected patients. *Archives of Internal Medicine* 158:2257–2264, 1998.

Federal Rehabilitation Act. 29 U.S.C. §791 et seq., 1973.

Fernandez, F. Psychopharmacological interventions in HIV infections. *New Directions in Mental Health Services* 48:43–53, 1990.

Ferrando, S.J., and Batki, S.L. HIV infection: From dual to triple diagnosis. In: Kranzler, H.R., and Rounsaville, B.J., eds. *Dual Diagnosis and Treatment.* New York: Marcel Dekker, 1998. pp. 503–534.

Ferrando, S.J.; Wall, T.L.; Batki, S.L.; and Sorensen, J.L. Psychiatric morbidity, illicit drug use and adherence to zidovudine (AZT) among injection drug users with HIV disease. *American Journal of Drug and Alcohol Abuse* 22(4): 475–487, 1996.

Festinger, D.S.; Lamb, R.J.; Kirby, K.C.; and Marlowe, D.B. The accelerated intake: A method for increasing initial attendance to outpatient cocaine treatment. *Journal of Applied Behavior Analysis* 29:387–389, 1996.

Fifield, L.; De Crescenzo, T.A.; and Latham, J.D. *Alcoholism and the Gay Community.* Los Angeles: Los Angeles Gay Community Services Center, 1975.

Figley, C.R. *Compassion Fatigue: Coping With Secondary Traumatic Stress Disorder in Those Who Treat the Traumatized.* New York: Brunner/Mazel, 1995.

Finnegan, D.G., and McNally, E.B. *Dual Identities: Counseling Chemically Dependent Gay Men and Lesbians.* Center City, MN: Hazelden, 1987.

Folkers, G. IL-2 plus HAART sharply reduces HIV in hiding places. *UniSci Science and Research News,* November 16, 1998. http://unisci.com/stories/19984/1116983.htm [Accessed April 15, 1999].

Folstein, M.F.; Folstein, S.E.; and McHugh, P.R. "Mini Mental State": A practical method for grading the cognitive state of patients for the clinician. *Journal of Psychiatric Research* 12:196–198, 1975.

Forstein, M. The neuropsychiatric aspects of HIV infection. *Primary Care* 19(1):97–117, 1992.

Freedberg, K.A.; Malabanan, A.; Samet, J.H.; and Libman, H. Initial assessment of patients infected with human immunodeficiency virus: The yield and cost of laboratory testing. *Journal of AIDS* 7:1134–1140, 1994.

Friedman, S.R.; Jose, B.; Deren, S.; Des Jarlais, D.C.; and Neaigus, A. Risk factors for human immunodeficiency virus seroconversion among out-of-treatment drug injectors in high and low seroprevalence cities. *American Journal of Epidemiology* 142:864–874, 1995.

Fudala, P.J.; Jaffe, J.H.; Dax, E.M.; and Johnson, R.E. Use of buprenorphine in the treatment of opioid addiction, II: Physiologic and behavioral effects of daily and alternate day administration and abrupt withdrawal. *Clinical Pharmacology and Therapeutics* 47:525–534, 1990.

Fuentes, A. Naming names: Will the squabble over HIV reporting tear us apart? *POZ* March 1999. http://www.thebody.com/poz/columns/3_99/policy.html [Accessed April 15, 1999].

Fultz, J.M., and Senay, E.C. Guidelines for the management of hospitalized narcotic addicts. *Annals of Internal Medicine* 82(6): 815–818, 1975.

Gallo, R.C.; Sarin, P.S.; Gelmann, E.P.; Robert-Guroff, M.; Richardson, E.; Kalyanaraman, V.S.; Mann, D.; Sidhu, G.D.; Stahl, R.E.; Zolla-Pazner, S.; Leibowitch, J.; and Popovic, M. Isolation of human T-cell leukemia virus in acquired immune deficiency syndrome (AIDS). *Science* 220(4599):865–867, 1983.

Gamble, V.N. Under the shadow of Tuskegee: African Americans and health care. *American Journal of Public Health* 87(11):1773–1778, 1997.

Gao, F.; Bailes, E.; Robertson, D.L.; Chen, Y.; Rodenburg, C.M.; Michael, S.F.; Cummins, L.B.; Arthur, L.O.; Peeters, M.; Shaw, G.M.; Sharp, P.M.; and Hahn, B.H. Origin of HIV-1 in the chimpanzee *Pan troglodytes troglodytes*. *Nature* 397(6718):436–441, 1999.

Gary, L.E. Attitudes toward human service organizations: Perspectives from an urban black community. *Journal of Applied Behavior Science* 21(4):445–458, 1985.

Gerbert, B.; Maguire, B.T.; Bleecker, T.; Coates, T.J.; and McPhee, S.J. Primary care physicians and AIDS: Attitudinal and structural barriers to care. *JAMA* 266:2837–2842, 1991.

Gerstein, D.R., and Harwood, H.J., eds. *Treating Drug Problems*. Washington, DC: National Academy Press, 1990–1992.

Gervasoni, C.; Ridolfo, A.L.; Trifiro, G.; Santambrogio, S.; Norbiato, G.; Musicco, M.; Clerici, M.; Galli, M.; and Moroni, M. Redistribution of body fat in HIV-infected women undergoing combined antiretroviral therapy. *AIDS* 13(4):465–471, 1999.

Glassroth, J.; Jordan, M.; Wallace, J.M.; Kvale, P.A.; Follmann, D.A.; Rosen, M.J.; Reichman, L.B.; Mossar, M.; and Hopewell, P.C. Use of preventive interventions by persons infected with type-1 human immunodeficiency virus (HIV-1). The Pulmonary Complications of HIV Study Group. *American Journal of Preventive Medicine* 10(5):259–266, 1994.

Gold, M.S.; Redmond, Jr., D.E.; and Kleber, H.D. Clonidine blocks acute opioid-withdrawal symptoms. *Lancet* 2(8090):599–602, 1978.

Gómez, C.A., and Marín, B.V. Gender, culture and power: Barriers to HIV prevention strategies for women. *Journal of Sex Research* 33(4):355–362, 1996.

Gonsiorek, J.C., ed. *A Guide to Psychotherapy With Gay and Lesbian Clients*. New York: Harrington Park Press, 1985.

Gorman, E.M. Speed use and HIV transmission. *Focus: A Guide to AIDS Research and Counseling* 11(7):4–6, 1996.

Gorman, E.M.; Morgan, P.; and Lambert, E.Y. Qualitative research considerations and other issues in the study of methamphetamine use among men who have sex with other men. In: Lambert, E.Y.; Ashery, R.S.; and Needle, R.H., eds. *Qualitative Methods in Drug Abuse and HIV Research*. NIDA Research Monograph Series, Number 157. NIDA Pub. No. 95-4025. Rockville, MD: National Institute on Drug Abuse, 1995. pp. 156–181.

Gourevitch, M., and Friedland, G. Methadone and antiretroviral medications, part I. *AIDS Clinical Care* 1(4):30–31, 1999a.

Gourevitch, M., and Friedland, G. Methadone and antiretroviral medications, part II. *AIDS Clinical Care* 11(5):37–45, 1999b.

Graham, K.; Timney, C.B.; Bois, C.; and Wedgerfield, K. Continuity of care in addictions treatment: The role of advocacy and coordination in case management. *American Journal of Drug and Alcohol Abuse* 21(4):433–451, 1995.

Graham, N.M.; Zeger, S.L.; Park, L.P.; Vermund, S.H.; Detels, R.; Rinaldo, C.R.; and Phair, J.P. The effects on survival of early treatment of human immunodeficiency virus infection. *New England Journal of Medicine* 326(16):1037–1042, 1992.

Greenblatt, R.M.; Lukehart, S.A.; Plummer, F.A.; Quinn, T.C.; Critchlow, C.W.; Ashley, R.L.; D'Costa, L.J.; Ndinya-Achola, J.O.; Corey, L.; and Ronald, A.R., et al. Genital ulceration as a risk factor for human immunodeficiency virus infection. *AIDS* 2(1):47–50, 1988.

Grella, C.E.; Anglin, M.D.; and Wugalter, S.E. Cocaine and crack use and HIV risk behaviors among high-risk methadone maintenance clients. *Drug and Alcohol Dependence* 37:15–21, 1995.

Griffin, M.M.; Ryan, J.G.; Briscoe, V.S.; and Shadle, K.M. Effects of incarceration on HIV-infected individuals. *Journal of the National Medical Association* 88(10):639–644, 1996.

Haas, D.W.; Morgan, M.E.; and Harris, V.L. Increased viral load and suicidal ideation in an HIV-infected patient. *Annals of Internal Medicine* 126(1):86–87, 1997.

Hagan, H.; Des Jarlais, D.C.; Purchase, D.; Reid, T.; and Friedman, S.R. The Tacoma syringe exchange. *Journal of Addictive Diseases* 10:81–88, 1991.

Hall, J.M. Lesbians and alcohol: Patterns and paradoxes in medical notions and lesbians' beliefs. *Journal of Psychoactive Drugs* 25(2):109–119, 1993.

Hammer, S.M.; Katzenstein, D.A.; Hughes, M.D.; Gundacker, H.; Schooley, R.T.; Haubrich, R.H.; Henry, W.K.; Lederman, M.M.; Phair, J.P.; Niu, M.; Hirsch, M.S.; and Merigan, T.C. A trial comparing nucleoside monotherapy with combination therapy in HIV-infected adults with CD4 cell counts from 200 to 500 per cubic millimeter. AIDS Clinical Trials Group Study 175 Study Team. *New England Journal of Medicine* 335:1081–1090, 1996.

Hardy, W.D.; Feinberg, J.; Finklestein, D.M.; Power, M.E.; He, W.; Kaczka, C.; Frame, P.T.; Holmes, M.; Waskin, H.; Fass, R.J.; and the AIDS Clinical Trials Group Protocol 021. A controlled trial of trimethoprim-sulfamethoxazole or aerosolized penta-midine for secondary prophylaxis of *Pneumocystis carinii* pneumonia in patients with acquired immunodeficiency syndrome.. *New England Journal of Medicine* 327:1842–1848, 1992.

Hartgers, C.; van den Hoek, A.; Krijnen, P.; and Coutinho, R.A. HIV prevalence and risk behavior among injecting drug abusers who participate in "low threshold" methadone programs in Amsterdam. *American Journal of Public Health* 82:547–551, 1992.

Hayter, M. Burnout and AIDS care-related factors in HIV community clinical nurse specialists in the North of England. *Journal of Advanced Nursing* 29(4):984–993, 1999.

Heather, N. Brief intervention strategies. In: Hester, R.K., and Miller, W.R., eds. *Handbook of Alcoholism Treatment Approaches: Effective Alternatives*, 2nd ed. Allyn & Bacon, 1995. pp. 105–120.

Hecht, F.M.; Colfax, G.; Swanson, M.; and Chesney, M.A. "Adherence and effectiveness of protease inhibitors in clinical practice." Paper presented at the fifth Conference on Retroviruses and Opportunistic Infections, Chicago, IL, 1998a.

Hecht, F.M.; Grant, R.M.; Petropoulos, C.J.; Dillon, B.; Chesney, M.A.; Tian, H.; Hellmann, N.S.; Bandrapalli, N.I.; Digilio, L.; Branson, B.; and Kahn, J.O. Sexual transmission of an HIV-1 variant resistant to multiple reverse-transcriptase and protease inhibitors. *New England Journal of Medicine* 339(5):307–311, 1998b.

Heimer, R. Can syringe exchange serve as a conduit to drug treatment? *Journal of Substance Abuse Treatment* 15:183–191, 1998.

Henry, J.A., and Hill, I.R. Fatal interaction between ritonavir and MDMA. *Lancet* 352(9142):1751–1752, 1998.

Herek, G.M. Heterosexism and homophobia. In: Cabaj, R.P., and Stein, T.S., eds. *Textbook of Homosexuality and Mental Health: A Comprehensive Review*. Washington, DC: American Psychiatric Press, 1996. pp. 101–113.

Herz, A. Endogenous opioid systems and alcohol addiction. *Psychopharmacology (Berl)* 129:99–111, 1997.

Higgins, D.L.; Galavotti, C.; O'Reilly, K.R.; Schnell, D.J.; Moore, M.; Rugg, D.L.; and Johnson, R. Evidence for the effects of HIV antibody counseling and testing on risk behaviors. *JAMA* 266:2419–2429, 1991.

Ho, D.D. Time to hit HIV, early and hard. *New England Journal of Medicine* 333:450–451, 1995.

Hodgson, I. HIV and combination therapy: Meeting the challenge of a new era. *British Journal of Nursing* 8(1):39–43, 1999.

Holmberg, S.D. The estimated prevalence and incidence of HIV in 96 large U.S. metropolitan areas. *American Journal of Public Health* 86:642–654, 1996.

Horn, G. Party favors—Do yourself one: Get the dope on the protease effect. *POZ* June 1998. http://www.thebody.com/poz/survival/6_98/warning.html [Accessed April 15, 1999].

Huba, G.J., and Melchior, L.A. *Evaluation of the Effects of Ryan White Title I Funding on Services for HIV-Infected Drug Abusers: Summary Report & Executive Summary for Year 1: Baseline.* A joint project of the Health Resources and Services Administration, the National Institute on Drug Abuse, and the Consortium on Drug Abuse and HIV Services Access. Pub No. HRSA-RD-SP-94-8. Washington, DC: U.S. Department of Health and Human Services, 1994.

Hubbard, R.L.; Marsden, M.E.; and Rachal, J.V. *Drug Abuse Treatment: A National Study of Effectiveness.* Chapel Hill, NC: University of North Carolina Press, 1989.

Hughes, C.P.; Berg, L.; Danziger, W.L.; Coben, L.A.; and Martin, R.L. A new clinical scale for the staging of dementia. *British Journal of Psychiatry* 140:566–572, 1982.

Hull, H.F.; Bettinger, C.J.; Gallaher, M.M.; Keller, N.M.; Wilson, J.; and Mertz, G.J. Comparison of HIV-antibody prevalence in patients consenting to and declining HIV-antibody testing in an STD clinic. *JAMA* 260(7):935–938, 1988.

Human Rights Campaign. The Ryan White CARE Act . . . Caring for People With HIV/AIDS. http://www.hrcusa.org/issues/aids/ryan/ [Accessed May 19, 1999].

Humphry, D. *Final Exit: The Practicalities of Self-Deliverance and Assisted Suicide for the Dying.* Secaucus, NJ: The Hemlock Society, 1991.

Ickovics, J.R., and Rodin, J. Women and AIDS in the United States: Epidemiology, natural history, and mediating mechanisms. *Health Psychology* 11:1–16, 1992.

Iguchi, M.Y. Drug abuse treatment as HIV prevention: Changes in social drug use patterns might also reduce risk. *Journal of Addictive Diseases* 17(4):9–18, 1998.

Iguchi, M.Y.; Belding, M.A.; Morral, A.R.; Lamb, R.J.; and Husband, S.D. Reinforcing operants other than abstinence: An effective alternative for reducing drug use. *Journal of Consulting and Clinical Psychology* 65:421–428, 1997.

Iguchi, M.Y.; Bux, Jr., D.A.; Lidz, V.; French, J.F.; Baxter, R.C.; and Platt, J.J. Changes in HIV-risk behaviors among injecting drug abusers: Impact of 21 vs. 90 days of methadone detoxification. *AIDS* 10:1719–1728, 1996.

Iguchi, M.Y.; Handelsman, L.; Bickel, W.K.; and Griffiths, R.R. Benzodiazepine and sedative use/abuse by methadone maintenance clients. *Drug and Alcohol Dependence* 32:257–266, 1993.

Iguchi, M.Y.; Platt, J.J.; French, J.; Baxter, R.C.; Kushner, H.; Lidz, V.M.; Bux, D.A.; Rosen, M.; and Musikoff, H. Correlates of HIV seropositivity among injection drug users not in treatment. *Journal of Drug Issues* 22:849–866, 1992.

Iguchi, M.Y., and Stitzer, M.L. Predictors of opiate drug abuse during a 90-day methadone detoxification. *American Journal of Drug and Alcohol Abuse* 17:279–294, 1991.

Institute of Medicine. *Pathways of Addiction: Opportunities in Drug Abuse Research.* Washington, DC: National Academy Press, 1996.

International Association for the Study of Pain. Subcommittee of Taxonomy. Classification of chronic pain. Descriptions of chronic pain syndromes and definitions of pain terms. *Pain Suppl* 3:S1–S226, 1986.

International Perinatal HIV Group. The mode of delivery and the risk of vertical transmission of human immunodeficiency virus type 1—A meta-analysis of 15 prospective cohort studies. *New England Journal of Medicine* 340(13):977–987, 1999.

Jackson, J.F.; Rotkiewicz, L.G.; Quinones, M.A.; and Passannante, M.R. A coupon program—drug treatment and AIDS education. *International Journal of the Addictions* 24(11):1035–1051, 1989.

James, J.S. Protease inhibitors: Drug resistance and cross-resistance overview. *AIDS Treatment News* No. 235, November 17, 1995.

Janikowski, T.P., and Glover, N.M. Incest and substance abuse: Implications for treatment professionals. *Journal of Substance Abuse Treatment* 11(3):177–183, 1994.

Janiri, L.; Gobbi, G.; Mannelli, P.; Pozzi, G.; Serretti, A.; and Tempesta, E. Effects of fluoxetine at antidepressant doses on short-term outcome of detoxified alcoholics. *International Clinical Psychopharmacology* 11:109–117, 1996.

Joe, G.W., and Simpson, D.D. Mortality rates among opioid addicts in a longitudinal study. *American Journal of Public Health* 77:347–348, 1987.

Joe, G.W.; Simpson, D.D.; and Hubbard, R.L. Treatment predictors of tenure in methadone maintenance. *Journal of Substance Abuse* 3:73–84, 1991.

Joint Commission on Accreditation of Healthcare Organizations (JCAHO). *1999–2000 Comprehensive Accreditation Manual for Behavioral Health Care.* Oakbrook Terrace, IL: JCAHO, 1999.

Junge, B.; Vlahov, D.; Riley, E.; Huettner, S.; Brown, M.; and Beilenson, P. Pharmacy access to sterile syringes for injection drug users: Attitudes of participants in a syringe exchange program. *Journal of the American Pharmaceutical Association* 39(1):17–22, 1999.

Kail, B.L.; Watson, D.D.; and Ray, S. Needle-using practices within the sex industry. *American Journal of Drug and Alcohol Abuse* 21:241–255, 1995.

Kalichman, S.C., and Hospers, H.J. Efficacy of behavior-skills enhancement HIV risk-reduction interventions in community settings. *AIDS* 11 Suppl A:S191–S199, 1997.

Kalichman, S.C., and Stevenson, L.Y. Psychological and social factors associated with histories of risk for human immunodeficiency virus infection among African-American inner-city women. *Journal of Womens Health* 6(2):209–217, 1997.

Kanof, P.D.; Aronson, M.J.; and Ness, R. Organic mood syndrome associated with detoxification from methadone maintenance. *American Journal of Psychiatry* 150(3):423–428, 1993.

Karkabi, B. Blacks' health problems addressed. *The Houston Chronicle* Lifestyle:3, April 10, 1994.

Kedes, D.H.; Ganem, D.; Ameli, N.; Bacchetti, P.; and Greenblatt, M. The prevalence of serum antibody to human herpesvirus 8 (Kaposi sarcoma-associated herpesvirus) among HIV-seropositive and high-risk HIV-seronegative women. *JAMA* 277:478–481, 1997.

Kelly, R.; Kiwanuka, N.; Wawer, M.J.; Serwadda, D.; Sewankambo, N.K.; Wabwire-Mangen, F.; Li, C.; Konde-Lule, J.K.; Lutalo, T.; Makumbi, F.; and Gray, R.H. Age of male circumcision and risk of prevalent HIV infection in rural Uganda. *AIDS* 13(3):399–405, 1999.

Kessler, R.C.; Nelson, C.B.; McGonagle, K.A.; Edlund, M.J.; Frank, R.G.; and Leaf, P.J. The epidemiology of co-occurring addictive and mental disorders: Implications for prevention and services utilization. *American Journal of Orthopsychiatry* 66(1):17–31, 1996.

Khabazz, R.F.; Onorato, I.M.; Cannon, R.O.; Hartley, T.M.; Roberts, B.; Hosein, B.; and Kaplan, J.E. Seroprevalence of HTLV-1 and HTLV-2 among intravenous drug abusers and persons in clinics for sexually transmitted diseases. *New England Journal of Medicine* 326:75–80, 1992.

Khantzian, E.J. The self-medication hypothesis of addictive disorders: Focus on heroin and cocaine dependence. *American Journal of Psychiatry* 142:1259–1264, 1985.

Kipke, M.D.; O'Connor, S.; Palmer, R.; and MacKenzie, R.G. Street youth in Los Angeles. Profile of a group at high risk for human immunodeficiency virus infection. *Archives of Pediatrics and Adolescent Medicine* 149(5):513–519, 1995.

Kitchener, K.S. Ethical principles and decisions in student affairs. In: Cannon, H.J., and Brown, R.D., eds. *Applied Ethics in Student Services.* New Directions for Student Services, No. 30. San Francisco: Jossey-Bass, 1985. pp. 17–29.

Kleber, H.D.; Topazian, M.; Gaspari, J.; Riordan, C.E.; and Kosten, T. Clonidine and naltrexone in the outpatient treatment of heroin withdrawal. *American Journal of Drug and Alcohol Abuse* 13:1–17, 1987.

Kosten, T.R.; Gawin, F.H.; Rounsaville, B.J.; and Kleber, H.D. Cocaine abuse among opioid addicts: Demographic and diagnostic factors in treatment. *American Journal of Drug and Alcohol Abuse* 12:1–16, 1986.

Kreek, M.J. Using methadone effectively: Achieving goals by application of laboratory, clinical, and evaluation research and by development of innovative programs. In: Pickens, R.W.; Leukfeld, C.G.; and Schuster, C.R., eds. *Improving Drug Abuse Treatment.* NIDA Research Monograph Series, Number 106. DHHS Pub. No. (ADM) 91-1754. Rockville, MD: National Institute on Drug Abuse, 1991. pp. 245–266.

Kreek, M.J.; Garfield, J.W.; Gutjahr, C.L.; and Giusti, L.M. Rifampin-induced methadone withdrawal. *New England Journal of Medicine* 294:1104–1106, 1976.

Ku, L.; Sonenstein, F.L.; and Pleck, J.H. Patterns of HIV risk and preventive behavior among teenage men. *Public Health Reports* 107(2):131–138, 1992.

Kübler-Ross, E. *On Death and Dying.* New York: MacMillan, 1969.

Kufeldt, K.; Durieux, M.; Nimmo, M.; and McDonald, M. Providing shelter for street youth: Are we reaching those in need? *Child Abuse and Neglect* 16(2):187–199, 1992.

Laumann, E.O.; Masi, C.M.; and Zuckerman, E.W. Circumcision in the United States. Prevalence, prophylactic effects, and sexual practice. *JAMA* 277(13):1052–1057, 1997.

Laurence, J. T-cell subsets in health, infectious disease, and idiopathic CD4+ T lymphocytopenia. *Annals of Internal Medicine* 119(1):55–62, 1993.

Lebovits, A.H.; Lefkowitz, M.; McCarthy, D.; Simon, R.; Wilpon, H.; Jung, R.; and Fried, E. The prevalence and management of pain in patients with AIDS: A review of 134 cases. *Clinical Journal of Pain* 5:245–248, 1989.

Leigh, B.C. The relationship of substance abuse during sex to high-risk sexual behavior. *Journal of Sex Research* 27(2):199–213, 1990.

Leigh, B.C., and Stall, R. Substance use and risky sexual behavior for exposure to HIV. Issues in methodology, interpretation, and prevention. *American Psychologist* 48:1035–1045, 1993.

Leroy, V.; Newell, M.L.; Dabis, F.; Peckham, C.; Van de Perre, P.; Bulterys, M.; Kind, C.; Simonds, R.J.; Wiktor, S.; and Msellati, P. International multicentre pooled analysis of late postnatal mother-to-child transmission of HIV-1 infection. Ghent International Working Group on Mother-to-Child Transmission of HIV. *Lancet* 352(9128):597–600, 1998.

Lesbian and Gay Substance Abuse Planning Group. *San Francisco Lesbian, Gay, and Bisexual Substance Abuse Needs Assessment: A Report.* San Francisco: EMT Associates, August 1991.

Levine, S. *Who Dies? An Investigation of Conscious Living and Conscious Dying.* Garden City, NY: Anchor Press/Doubleday, 1982.

Lewis, C.E.; Saghir, M.T.; and Robins, E. Drinking patterns in homosexual and heterosexual women. *Journal of Clinical Psychiatry* 43:277–279, 1982.

Lidz, V.; Bux, D.; Platt, J.; and Iguchi, M. Transitional case management: A service model for AIDS outreach projects. In: Ashery, R.S., ed. *Progress and Issues in Case Management.* NIDA Research Monograph Series, Number 127. DHHS Pub. No. (ADM) 92-1946. Rockville, MD: National Institute on Drug Abuse, 1992. pp. 112–144.

Ling, W.; Rawson, R.A.; and Compton, M.A. Substitution pharmacotherapies for opioid addiction: From methadone to LAAM and buprenorphine. *Journal of Psychoactive Drugs* 26:119–128, 1994.

Liuzzi, G.; Chirianni, A.; Clementi, M.; Bagnarelli, P.; Valenza, A.; Cataldo, P.T.; and Piazza, M. Analysis of HIV-1 load in blood, semen, and saliva: Evidence for different viral compartments in a cross-sectional and longitudinal study. *AIDS* 10(14):F51–F56, 1996.

Lohrenz, L.J.; Connelly, J.C.; Cony, L.; and Spare, K.E. Alcohol problems in several midwestern homosexual communities. *Journal of Studies on Alcohol* 39(11):1959–1963, 1978.

Longshore, D.; Anglin, M.D.; Annon, K.; and Hsieh, S. Trends in self-reported HIV risk behavior: Injection drug users in Los Angeles. *Journal of Acquired Immune Deficiency Syndromes* 6(1):82–90, 1993.

Longshore, D.; Annon, J.; and Anglin, M.D. HIV prevalence among injection drug users in three Northern California communities. *Journal of Acquired Immune Deficiency Syndromes and Human Retrovirology* 19(2):200, 1998.

Longshore, D.; Hsieh, S.C.; Anglin, M.D.; and Annon, T.A. Ethnic patterns in drug abuse treatment utilization. *Journal of Mental Health Administration* 19(3):268–277, 1992.

Loue, S.; Lurie, P.; and Lloyd, L.S. Ethical issues raised by needle exchange programs. *Journal of Law, Medicine and Ethics* 23:382–388, 1995.

Lowinson, J.H.; Marion, I.J.; Joseph, H.; and Dole, J.P. Methadone maintenance. In: Lowinson, J.H.; Ruiz, P.; and Millman, R.B., eds. *Substance Abuse: A Comprehensive Textbook*, 2nd ed. Baltimore: Williams & Wilkins, 1992. pp. 550–561.

Lurie, P.G.; Drucker, E.; and Knowles, A. Still working after all these years: Increasing evidence of needle exchange program (NEP) effectiveness in studies published since 1993. *International Conference on AIDS* 12:670 (Abstract No. 33403), 1998.

Lurie, P.G.; Sorensen, J.; Lane, S.; Kahn, J.G.; Guydish, J.; Foley, J.; Chen, D.; Bowser, B.; Jones, T.S.; and Reingold, A.L. The public health impact of needle exchange programs (NEPs). (Abstract No. 564C). *International Conference on AIDS* 10(2):72, August 1994.

Lyketsos, C.G.; Hanson, A.L.; Fishman, M.; Rosenblatt, A.; McHugh, P.R.; and Treisman, G.J. Manic syndrome early and late in the course of HIV. *American Journal of Psychiatry* 150(2):326–327, 1993.

Lyketsos, C.G.; Hutton, H.; Fishman, M.; Schwartz, J.; and Treisman, G.J. Psychiatric morbidity on entry to an HIV primary care clinic. *AIDS* 10(9):1033–1039, 1996.

MacDougall, D.S. HIV/AIDS behind bars: Incarceration provides a valuable opportunity to implement HIV/AIDS treatment and prevention strategies in a high-risk population. *Journal of the International Association of Physicians in AIDS Care* 4(4):8–13, 1998.

MacGowan, R.J.; Brackbill, R.M.; Rugg, D.L.; Swanson, N.M.; Weinstein, B.; Couchon, A.; Scibak, J.; Molde, S.; McLaughlin, P.; Barker, T.; and Voigt, R. Sex, drugs and HIV counseling and testing: A prospective study of behavior-change among methadone-maintenance clients in New England. *AIDS* 11(2):229–235, 1997.

Marck, J. Aspects of male circumcision in sub-equatorial African culture history. *Health Transition Review* 7:357–360, 1997.

Margolick, J.B.; Munoz, A.; Vlahov, D.; Solomon, L.; Astemborski, J.; Cohn, S.; and Nelson, K.E. Changes in T-lymphocyte subsets in intravenous drug abusers with HIV-1 infection. *JAMA* 267(12):1631–1636, 1992.

Marin, B.V. *Analysis of AIDS Prevention Among African Americans and Hispanics in the United States.* National Technical Information Service Order No. PB96-10851 INZ. Washington, DC: Office of Technology Assessment, 1995.

Marlatt, G.A.; Somers, J.M.; and Tapert, S.F. Harm reduction: Application to alcohol abuse problems. In: Onken, L.S.; Blaine, J.D.; and Boren, J.J., eds. *Behavioral Treatments for Drug Abuse and Dependence.* NIDA Research Monograph Series, Number 137. DHHS Pub. No. (ADM) 93-3684. Rockville, MD: National Institute on Drug Abuse, 1993. pp. 147–166.

Martinez, T.E.; Gleghorn, A.; Marx, R.; Clements, K.; Boman, M.; and Katz, M.H. Psychosocial histories, social environment, and HIV risk behaviors of injection and noninjection drug using homeless youths. *Journal of Psychoactive Drugs* 30(1):1–9, 1998.

Maruschak, L. *HIV in Prisons and Jails, 1995.* Bureau of Justice Statistics. Pub. No. NCJ-164260. Washington, DC: U.S. Department of Justice, Office of Justice Programs, 1997. http://www.ojp.usdoj.gov/bjs/pub/ascii/hivpj95.txt [Accessed July 20, 1999].

Maslow, A. Hierarchy of needs. In: Maslow, A., ed. *Motivation and Personality.* New York: Harper & Row, 1970. p. 369.

Mason, B.J.; Kocsis, J.H.; Ritvo, E.C.; and Cutler, R.B. A double-blind, placebo-controlled trial of desipramine for primary alcohol dependence stratified on the presence or absence of major depression. *JAMA* 13:761–767, 1996.

Masur, H.; Michelis, M.A.; Greene, J.B.; Onorato, I.; Stouwe, R.A.; Holzman, R.S.; Wormser, G.; Brettman, L.; Lange, M.; Murray, H.W.; and Cunningham-Rundles, S. An outbreak of community acquired *Pneumocystis carinii* pneumonia: Initial manifestation of cellular immune dysfunction. *New England Journal of Medicine* 305(24):1431–1438, 1981.

Masur, H.; Michelis, M.A.; Wormser, G.P.; Lewin, S.; Gold, J.; Tapper, M.L.; Giron, J.; Lerner, C.W.; Armstrong, D.; Setia, U.; Sender, J.A.; Siebkin, R.S.; Nicholas, P.; Arlen, Z.; Maayan, S.; Ernst, J.A.; Siegal, F.P.; and Cunningham-Rundles, S. Opportunistic infection in previously healthy women. Initial manifestations of a community-acquired cellular immunodeficiency. *Annals of Internal Medicine* 97(4):533–539, 1982.

McCaffery, M. *Nursing Management of the Patient With Pain.* Philadelphia: Lippincott, 1979.

McCann, R.M.; Hall, W.J.; and Groth-Juncker, A. Comfort care for terminally ill patients. The appropriate use of nutrition and hydration. *JAMA* 272(16):1263–1266, 1994.

McCarthy, E.P.; Feldman, Z.T.; and Lewis, B.F. Development and implementation of an interorganizational case management model for substance users. In: Ashery, R.S., ed. *Progress and Issues in Case Management.* NIDA Research Monograph Series, Number 127. DHHS Pub. No. (ADM) 92-1946. Rockville, MD: National Institute on Drug Abuse, 1992. pp. 331–349.

McCoy, H.V.; Dodds, S.; Rivers, J.E.; and McCoy, C.B. Case management services for HIV-seropositive IDUs. In: Ashery, R.S., ed. *Progress and Issues in Case Management*. NIDA Research Monograph Series, Number 127. DHHS Pub. No. (ADM) 92-1946. Rockville, MD: National Institute on Drug Abuse, 1992. pp. 181–207.

McCusker, J.; Bigelow, C.; Stoddard, A.M.; and Zorn, M. Human immunodeficiency virus type 1 antibody status and change among drug abusers. *Annals of Epidemiology* 4:466–471, 1994a.

McCusker, J.; Willis, G.; McDonald, M.; Lewis, B.F.; Sereti, S.M.; and Feldman, Z.T. Admission of injection drug users to drug abuse treatment following HIV counseling and testing. *Public Health Reports* 109:212–218, 1994b.

McGrath, P.J.; Nunes, E.V.; Stewart, J.W.; Goldman, D.; Agosti, V.; Ocepek-Welikson, K.; and Quitkin, F.M. Imipramine treatment of alcoholics with primary depression: A placebo-controlled clinical trial. *Archives of General Psychiatry* 53:232–240, 1996.

McKirnan, D., and Peterson, P.L. Alcohol and drug use among homosexual men and women: Epidemiology and population characteristics. *Addictive Behaviors* 14:545–553, 1989.

McLellan, A.T.; Arndt, I.O.; Metzger, D.S.; Woody, G.E.; and O'Brien, C.P. The effects of psychological services in substance abuse treatment. *JAMA* 269(15):1953–1959, 1993.

McNally, E.B., and Finnegan, D.G. Lesbian recovering alcoholics: A qualitative study of identity transformation. A report on research and applications to treatment. *Journal of Chemical Dependency Treatment* 5(1):93–103, 1992.

McRoy, C.P.; Shorkey, C.T.; and Garcia, L. Alcohol use and abuse among Mexican-Americans. In: Freeman, E.M., ed. *Social Work Practice With Clients Who Have Alcohol Problems*. Springfield, IL: Charles C. Thomas, 1985.

McWhirter, D.P.; Sanders, S.A.; and Reinisch, J.M., eds. *Homosexuality/Heterosexuality: Concepts of Sexual Orientation*. New York: Oxford University Press, 1990.

Mejta, C.L.; Bokos, P.J.; Mickenburg, J.H.; Maslar, M.E.; and Senay, E. Improving substance abuse treatment access and retention using a case management approach. *Journal of Drug Issues* 27(2):329–340, 1997.

Mello, N.K., and Mendelson, J.H. Primate studies of the behavioral pharmacology of buprenorphine. In: Blaine, J.D., ed. *Buprenorphine: An Alternative Treatment for Opioid Dependence*. NIDA Research Monograph Series, Number 121. DHHS Pub. No. (ADM) 92-1912. Rockville, MD: National Institute on Drug Abuse, 1992. pp. 61–100.

Mellors, J.W. Closing in on human immunodeficiency virus. *Nature Medicine* 2(3):274–275, 1996.

Mellors, J.W. "Review of Lago Maggiore resistance meeting." Twelfth World AIDS Conference, Geneva, Switzerland, 1998.

Mellors, J.W., and Kuritzkes, D. "Antiretroviral therapy: Resistance." Eighth Clinical Care Options for HIV Symposium, 1998.

Mellors, J.W.; Munoz, A.; Giorgi, J.V.; Margolick, J.B.; Tassoni, C.J.; Gupta, P.; Kingsley, L.A.; Todd, J.A.; Saah, A.J.; Detels, R.; Phair, J.P.; and Rinaldo, Jr., C.R. Plasma viral load and CD4+ lymphocytes as prognostic markers of HIV-1 infection. *Annals of Internal Medicine* 126:946–954, 1997.

Metzger, D.S.; Woody, G.E.; McLellan, A.T.; O'Brien, C.P.; Druley, P.; Navaline, H.; DePhillipis, D.; Stolley, P.; and Abrutyn, E. Human immunodeficiency virus seroconversion among intravenous drug users in- and out-of-treatment: An 18-month prospective follow-up. *Journal of Acquired Immune Deficiency Syndromes* 6:1049–1056, 1993.

Meyer, C. *Surviving Death.* Mystic, CT: Twenty-Third Publications, 1994.

Miller, N. *In Search of Gay America: Women and Men in a Time of Change.* New York: Atlantic Monthly Press, 1989.

Miller, W.R. Behavioral treatments for drug problems: Lessons from the alcohol treatment outcome literature. In: Onken, L.S.; Blaine, J.D.; and Boren, J.J., eds. *Behavioral Treatment for Drug Abuse and Dependence.* NIDA Research Monograph Series, Number 137. DHHS Pub. No. (ADM) 93-3684. Rockville, MD: National Institute on Drug Abuse, 1993. pp. 167–180.

Mills, T.C.; Stall, R.; Catania, J.A.; and Coates, T.J. Interpreting HIV prevalence and incidence among Americans: Bridging data and public policy. *American Journal of Public Health* 87:864–866, 1997.

Millstein, S.G., and Moscicki, A.B. Sexually-transmitted disease in female adolescents: Effects of psychosocial factors and high risk behaviors. *Journal of Adolescent Health* 17(2):83–90, 1995.

Mirin, S.M.; Weiss, R.D.; Michael, J.; and Griffin, M.L. Psychopathology in substance abusers: Diagnosis and treatment. *American Journal of Drug and Alcohol Abuse* 14(2):139–157, 1988.

Montgomery, K., and Lewis, C.E. Fear of HIV contagion as workplace stress: Behavioral consequences and buffers. *Hospital and Health Services Administration* 40(4):439–456, 1995.

Moody, R., Jr. *Life After Life: The Investigation of a Phenomenon, Survival of Bodily Death.* New York: Bantam Books, 1975.

Moore, B.E., and Fine, B.D. *Psychoanalytic Terms and Concepts.* New Haven, CT: The American Psychoanalytic Association and Yale University Press, 1990.

Morales, E., and Graves, M.A. *Substance Abuse: Patterns and Barriers to Treatment for Gay Men and Lesbians in San Francisco.* San Francisco: San Francisco Department of Public Health, 1983.

Morales, T.; Gomez, C.A.; and Marin B.V. "Freedom and HIV prevention: Challenges facing Latino inmates leaving prison." Paper presented at the 103rd American Psychological Association Convention, New York, 1995.

Moreno, S.; Baraia-Etxaburu, J.; Bouza, E.; Parras, F.; Perez-Tascon, M.; Miralles, P.; Vicente, T.; Alberdi, J.C.; Cosin, J.; and Lopez-Gay, D. Risk for developing tuberculosis among anergic patients infected with HIV. *Annals of Internal Medicine* 119:194–198, 1993.

Mosbacher, D. Lesbian alcohol and substance abuse. *Psychiatric Annals* 18(1):47, 49–50, 1988.

Mosbacher, D. Alcohol and other drug use in female medical students: A comparison of lesbians and heterosexuals. *Journal of Gay and Lesbian Psychotherapy* 2(1):37–48, 1993.

Moses, S.; Bailey, R.C.; and Ronald, A.R. Male circumcision: Assessment of health benefits and risks. *Sexually Transmitted Infections* 74(5):368–373, 1998.

Mumola, C.J. *Substance Abuse and Treatment, State and Federal Prisoners, 1997.* Bureau of Justice Statistics. Pub No. NCJ-172871. Washington, DC: U.S. Department of Justice, Office of Justice Programs, 1999.

Musher, D.M.; Hamill, R.J.; and Baughn, R.E. Effect of human immunodeficiency virus (HIV) infection on the course of syphilis and on the response to treatment. *Annals of Internal Medicine* 113:872–881, 1990.

Myers, T.; Orr, K.W.; Locker, D.; and Jackson, E.A. Factors affecting gay and bisexual men's decisions and intentions to seek HIV testing. *American Journal of Public Health* 83(5):701–704, 1993.

Nahass, R.G.; Weinstein, M.P.; Bartels, J.; and Gocke, D.J. Infective endocarditis in intravenous drug users: A comparison of human immunodeficiency virus type 1-negative and -positive patients. *Journal of Infectious Diseases* 162(4):967–970, 1990.

Nakashima, A.K.; Horsley, R.; Frey, R.L.; Sweeney, P.A.; Weber, J.T.; and Fleming, P.L. Effects of HIV reporting by name on use of HIV testing in publicly funded counseling and testing programs. *JAMA* 280:1421–1426, 1998.

National Association of Social Workers. "Ethical Issues, HIV/AIDS, and Social Work Practice." Workshop sponsored by the HIV/AIDS Spectrum: Mental Health Training and Education of Social Workers Project, 1997.

National Commission on AIDS. *The Challenge of HIV/AIDS in Communities of Color.* Washington, DC: National Commission on AIDS, 1992.

National Institute of Allergy and Infectious Diseases. *HIV and Adolescents.* NIAID Fact Sheet. Washington, DC: National Institutes of Health, February 1999. http://www.niaid.nih.gov/factsheets/hivadolescent.htm [Accessed May 18, 1999].

National Institutes of Health. Effective medical treatment of opiate addiction. *NIH Consensus Statement Online* 15(6):1–38, 1997a. http://text.nlm.nih.gov [Accessed January 4, 2000].

National Institutes of Health. Interventions to prevent HIV risk behaviors. *NIH Consensus Statement Online* 15(2):1–41, 1997b. http://text.nlm.nih.gov/ftrs/tocview [Accessed January 4, 2000].

Needle, R.; Coyle, S.L.; Normand, J.; Lambert, E.L.; and Cesari, H. HIV prevention with drug-using populations: Current status and future prospects: Introduction and overview. *Public Health Reports* 113(Suppl.1):4–18, 1998.

Niccolai, L.M.; Dorst, D.; Myers, L.; and Kissinger, P.J. Disclosure of HIV status to sexual partners: Predictors and temporal patterns. *Sexually Transmitted Diseases* 26(5):281–285, 1999.

Normand, J.; Vlahov, D.; and Moses, L.E., eds. *Preventing HIV Transmission: The Role of Sterile Needles and Bleach.* Washington, DC: National Academy Press, 1995.

North, C.S., and Smith, E.M. A systematic study of mental health services utilization by homeless men and women. *Social Psychiatry and Psychiatric Epidemiology* 28:77–83, 1993.

Nuland, S. *How We Die: Reflections on Life's Final Chapter.* New York: A.A. Knopf, 1994.

Nunes, E.V.; McGrath, P.J.; Quitkin, F.M.; Stewart, J.W.; Harrison, W.; Tricamo, E.; and Ocepek-Welikson, K. Imipramine treatment of alcoholism with comorbid depression. *American Journal of Psychiatry* 150:963–965, 1993.

O'Brien, C.; Greenstein, R.; Ternes, J.; and Woody, G. Clinical pharmacology of narcotic antagonists. *Annals of the New York Academy of Sciences* 311:232–240, 1978.

O'Connor, P.G.; Molde, S.; Henry, S.; Shockcor, W.T.; and Schottenfeld, R.S. Human immunodeficiency virus infection in intravenous drug users: A model for primary care. *American Journal of Medicine* 93:382–386, 1992a.

O'Connor, P.G., and Samet, J.H. The substance-using human immunodeficiency virus patient: Approaches to outpatient management. *American Journal of Medicine* 101(4):435–444, 1996.

O'Connor, P.G.; Samet, J.H.; and Stein, M.D. Management of hospitalized intravenous drug users: Role of the internist. *American Journal of Medicine* 96:551–558, 1994a.

O'Connor, P.G.; Selwyn, P.A.; and Schottenfeld, R.S. Medical care for injection-drug users with human immunodeficiency virus infection. *New England Journal of Medicine* 331(7):450–459, 1994b.

O'Connor, P.G.; Waugh, M.E.; Schottenfeld, R.S.; Diakogiannis, I.A.; and Rounsaville, B.J. Ambulatory opiate detoxification and primary care: A role for the primary care physician. *Journal of General Internal Medicine* 7:532–534, 1992b.

Office of National Drug Control Policy (ONDCP). *High Intensity Drug Trafficking Areas.* http://www.whitehousedrugpolicy. gov/enforce/hidta.html [Accessed August 4, 1999].

O'Malley, S.S.; Jaffe, A.; Chang, G.; Schottenfeld, R.S.; Meyer, R.E.; and Rounsaville, B.J. Naltrexone and coping skills therapy for alcohol dependence. A controlled study. *Archives of General Psychiatry* 49: 881–887, 1992.

Packer, K.L. *HIV Infection: The Facts You Need To Know.* New York: Franklin Watts, 1998.

Page, J.B.; Lai, S.H.; Chitwood, D.D.; Klimas, N.G.; Smith, P.C.; and Fletcher, M.A. HTLV-I/II seropositivity and death from AIDS among HIV-1 seropositive intravenous drug users. *Lancet* 335(8703):1439–1441, 1990.

Pascal, C.B. Letter to John Harkness, M.D., Oklahoma State Department of Health, from the Legal Advisor to the U.S. Alcohol, Drug Abuse, and Mental Health Administration, September 2, 1988. In: Center for Substance Abuse Treatment. *Confidentiality of Patient Records for Alcohol and Other Drug Treatment.* Technical Assistance Publication (TAP) Series, Number 13. DHHS Pub. No. (SMA) 95-3018. Washington, DC: U.S. Government Printing Office, 1995.

Paul, J.P. *Clean and Sober and Safe.* 18th Street Services Continuing Recovery Group Client Workbook. San Francisco: 1991a.

Paul, J.P.; Stall, R.D.; and Bloomfield, K. Gay and alcoholics: Epidemiological and clinical issues. *Alcohol Health and Research World* 15:151–160, 1991b.

Paul, J.P.; Stall, R.D.; Crosby, G.M.; Barrett, D.C.; and Midanik, L.T. Correlates of sexual risk-taking among gay male substance abusers. *Addiction* 89:971–983, 1994.

Paul, J.P.; Stall, R.D.; and Davis, F. Sexual risk for HIV transmission among gay/bisexual men in substance-abuse treatment. *Journal of AIDS Education and Prevention* 5:11–24, 1993.

Perlman, D. Quarter of AIDS patients not getting best therapy. *The San Francisco Chronicle*, June 4, 1998. p. A9.

Pena, J., and Koss-Chioino, J. Cultural sensitivity in drug treatment research with African American males. In: Trimble, J.E.; Bolek, C.S.; and Niemrcyk, S.J., eds. *Ethnic and Multicultural Drug Abuse*. Binghampton, NY: The Haworth Press, 1992. pp. 157–179.

Perez-Arce, P.; Carr, K.D.; and Sorensen, J.L. Cultural issues in an outpatient program for stimulant abusers. *Journal of Psychoactive Drugs* 25(1):35–44, 1993.

Perlman, D.C.; Perkins, M.P.; Solomon, N.; Kochems, L.; Des Jarlais, D.C.; and Paone, D. Tuberculosis screening at a syringe exchange program. *American Journal of Public Health* 87(5):862–863, 1997.

Perry, S.; Jacobsberg, L.; and Fishman, B. Suicidal ideation and HIV testing. *JAMA* 263(5):679–682, 1990.

Peterson, J.L.; Coates, T.J.; Catania, J.A.; Middleton, L.; Hilliard, B.; and Hearst, N. High-risk sexual behavior and condom use among gay and bisexual African American men. *American Journal of Public Health* 82:1490–1494, 1992.

Phillips, K.A., and Coates, T.J. HIV counseling and testing: Research and policy issues. *AIDS Care* 7:115–124, 1995.

Pike, E.C. *Human Immunodeficiency Virus (HIV-1) Guidelines for Chemical Dependency Treatment and Care Programs in Minnesota*. St. Paul, MN: Chemical Dependency Program Division, Minnesota Department of Human Services, 1989.

Pillard, R.C. Sexual orientation and mental disorder. *Psychiatric Annals* 18(1):52–56, 1989.

Pirkola, S.P.; Isometsa, E.T.; Henriksson, M.; Heikkinen, M.E.; Marttunen, M.J.; and Lonnqvist, J.K. The treatment received by substance-dependent male and female suicide victims. *Acta Psychiatrica Scandinavica* 99(3):207–213, 1999.

Polonsky, S.; Kerr, S.; Harris, B.; Gaiter, J.; Fichtner, R.R.; and Kennedy, M.G. HIV prevention in prisons and jails: Obstacles and opportunities. *Public Health Reports* 109:615–625, 1994.

Portenoy, R.K., and Payne, R. Acute and chronic pain. In: Lowinson, J.H.; Ruiz, P.; and Millman, R.B., eds. *Substance Abuse: A Comprehensive Textbook*, 2nd ed. Baltimore: Williams & Wilkins, 1992. pp. 691–721.

Power, R.; Hartnoll, R.; and Daviaud, E. Drug injecting, AIDS, and risk behavior: Potential for change and intervention strategies. *British Journal of Addiction* 83:649–654, 1988.

Preston, K.L., and Bigelow, G.E. Subjective and discriminative effects of drugs. *Behavioral Pharmacology* 2:293–313, 1991.

Price, R.W., and Brew, B.J. The AIDS dementia complex. *Journal of Infectious Diseases* 158(5):1079–1083, 1988.

Price, R.W., and Perry, S.W., III, eds. *HIV, AIDS, and the Brain*. New York: Raven Press, 1994.

Rakower, D., and Galvin, T.A. Nourishing the HIV-infected adult. *Holistic Nursing Practice* 3(4):26–37, 1989.

Rall, T.W. Hypnotics and sedatives: Ethanol. In: Gilman, A.G.; Rall, T.W.; Nies, A.S.; and Taylor, P., eds. *Goodman and Gilman's: The Pharmacological Basis of Therapeutics*, 8th ed. New York: Pergamon Press, 1990. pp. 345–382.

Reamer, F. AIDS, social work, and the "duty to protect." *Social Work* 36(1):56–60, 1991.

Regier, D.A.; Farmer, M.E.; Rae, D.S.; Locke, B.Z.; Keith, S.J.; Judd, L.L.; and Goodwin, F.K. Comorbidity of mental disorders with alcohol and other drug abuse. Results from the Epidemiologic Catchment Area (ECA) Study. *JAMA* 264(19):2511–2518, 1990.

Reilly, P.M.; Banys, P.; Tusel, D.J.; Sees, K.L.; Krumenaker, C.L.; and Shopshire, M.S. Methadone transition treatment: A treatment model for 180-day methadone detoxification. *International Journal of the Addictions* 30:387–402, 1995.

Renton, A.; Whitaker, L.; Ison, C.; Wadsworth, J.; and Harris, J.R. Estimating the sexual mixing patterns in the general population from those in people acquiring gonorrhoea infection: Theoretical foundation and empirical findings. *Journal of Epidemiology and Community Health* 49:205–213, 1995.

Resnick, R.; Schuyten-Resnick, E.; and Washton, A.M. Narcotic antagonists in the treatment of opioid dependence: Review and commentary. *Comprehensive Psychiatry* 20:116–125, 1979.

Richardson, L. Man faces felony charge in HIV case. *New York Times*, August 20, 1998.

Richter, R.; Michaels, M.; Carlson, B.; and Coates, T.J. *Motivators and Barriers to Use of Combination Therapies in Patients With HIV Disease*. CAPS Monograph Series, Occasional Paper No. 5. San Francisco: University of California at San Francisco, Center for AIDS Prevention Studies, 1998.

Rosen, A.D., and Rosen, T. Study of condom integrity after brief exposure to over-the-counter vaginal preparations. *Southern Medical Journal* 92(3):305–307, 1999.

Rotheram-Borus, M.J.; Rosario, M.; Reid, H.; and Koopman, C. Predicting patterns of sexual acts among homosexual and bisexual youths. *American Journal of Psychiatry* 152(4):588–595, 1995.

Rowan-Szal, G.; Joe, G.W.; Chatham, L.R.; and Simpson, D.D. A simple reinforcement system for methadone clients in a community-based treatment program. *Journal of Substance Abuse Treatment* 11:217–223, 1994.

Royce, R.A.; Sena, A.; Cates, W.; and Cohen, M.S. Sexual transmission of HIV. *New England Journal of Medicine* 336(15):1072–1078, 1997.

Russell, N.D., and Sepkowitz, K.A. Primary HIV infection: Clinical, immunologic, and virologic predictors of progression. *The AIDS Reader* 8(4):164–172, 1998.

Saag, M.S. The natural history of HIV-1 infection. In: Broder, S.; Merigan, T.C.; and Bolognesi, D., eds. *Textbook of AIDS Medicine*. Baltimore: Williams & Wilkins, 1994. pp. 45–53.

Sadownick, S. Kneeling at the crystal cathedral: The alarming new epidemic of methamphetamine abuse in the gay community. *Genre* December/January 1994: 40–45, 86–90.

Saghir, M.T., and Robins, E. *Male and Female Homosexuality*. Baltimore: Williams & Wilkins, 1973.

Samet, J.H. Models of medical care for HIV-infected drug users. *Substance Abuse* 16(3):131–139, 1995.

Samet, J.H.; Freedberg, K.A.; Stein, M.D.; Lewis, R.; Savetsky, J.; Sullivan, L.; Levenson, S.M.; and Hingson, R. Trillion virion delay: Time from testing positive for HIV to presentation for primary care. *Archives of Internal Medicine* 158:734–740, 1998.

Samet, J.H.; Libman, H.; Labelle, C.; Steger, K.; Lewis, R.; Craven, D.E.; and Freedberg, K.A. A model clinic for the initial evaluation and establishment of primary care for persons infected with human immunodeficiency virus. *Archives of Internal Medicine* 155:1629–1633, 1995.

Samet, J.H.; Libman, H.; Steger, K.A.; Dhawan, R.K.; Chen, J.; Shevitz, A.H.; Dewees-Dunk, R.; Levenson, S.; Kufe, D.; and Craven, D.E. Compliance with zidovudine therapy in patients infected with human immunodeficiency virus, type 1: A cross-sectional study in a municipal hospital clinic. *American Journal of Medicine* 92(5):495–502, 1992.

Samet, J.H.; Mulvey, K.P.; Zaremba, N.; and Plough, A. HIV testing in substance abusers. *American Journal of Drug and Alcohol Abuse* 25:269–280, 1999.

Samet, J.H.; Muz, P.; Cabral, P.; Jhamb, K.; Suwanchinda, A.; and Freedberg, K.A. Dermatologic manifestations in HIV-infected patients: A primary care perspective. *Mayo Clinic Proceedings* 74(7):658–660, 1999.

Samet, J.H.; O'Connor, P.G.; and Stein, M.D. Alcohol and other substance abuse. *Medical Clinics of North America* 81(4):831–1075, 1997.

Samuel, M.C.; Osmond, D.H.; and Osmond, D.E. Annotation: Uncertainties in the estimation of HIV prevalence and incidence in the United States. *American Journal of Public Health* 86:627–628, 1996.

San Francisco AIDS Foundation. HIV Postexposure Prevention (PEP). *Summary Sheets on HIV Treatment Strategies.* Updated December 18, 1997a. http://www.sfaf.org/treatment/factsheets/pep.html [Accessed April 19, 1999].

San Francisco AIDS Foundation. HIV viral load and CD4 T-cell testing, drug resistance, and adherence to HAART. *Summary Sheets on HIV Treatment Strategies.* Updated December 18, 1997b. http://www.sfaf.org/treatment/factsheets/viral_load.html [Accessed April 23, 1999].

San Francisco AIDS Foundation. Protease inhibitor drugs and new HIV treatment strategies. *Summary Sheets on HIV Treatment Strategies.* Updated December 18, 1997c. http://www.sfaf.org/treatment/factsheets/index.html [Accessed April 19, 1999].

Savin-Williams, R.C. Verbal and physical abuse as stressors in the lives of lesbian, gay male, and bisexual youths: Association with school problems, running away, substance abuse, prostitution, and suicide. *Journal of Consulting and Clinical Psychology* 62(2):261–269, 1994.

Saxinger, W.C.; Levine, P.H.; Dean, A.G.; de The, G.; Lange-Wantzin, G.; Moghissi, J.; Laurent, F.; Hoh, M.; Sarngadharan, M.G.; and Gallo, R.C. Evidence for exposure to HTLV-III in Uganda before 1973. *Science* 227(4690):1036–1038, 1985.

Schlenger, W.E.; Kroutil, L.A.; and Roland, E.J. Case management as a mechanism for linking drug abuse treatment and primary care: Preliminary evidence from the ADAMHA/HRSA linkage demonstration. In: Ashery, R.S., ed. *Progress and Issues in Case Management.* NIDA Research Monograph Series, Number 127. DHHS Pub. No. (ADM) 92-1946. Rockville, MD: National Institute on Drug Abuse, 1992. pp. 316–330.

Schneider, M.M.; Hoepelman, A.I.; Eeftinck Schattenkerk, J.K.; Nielsen, T.L.; van der Graaf, Y.; Frissen, J.P.; van der Ende, I.M.; Kolsters, A.F.; and Borleffs, J.C. A controlled trial of aerosolized pentamidine or trimethoprim-sulfamethoxazole as primary prophylaxis against *Pneumocystis carinii* pneumonia in patients with human immunodeficiency virus infection. The Dutch AIDS Treatment Group. *New England Journal of Medicine* 327:1836–1841, 1992.

Schofferman, J., and Brody, R. Pain in far advanced AIDS. In: Foley, K.M.; Bonica, J.J.; and Ventafridda, V., eds. *Advances in Pain Research and Therapy.* Vol. 16. *Proceedings of the Second International Congress on Cancer Pain.* New York: Raven Press, 1990. pp. 379–386.

Schoofs, M. AIDS: The agony of Africa. Part 4: The virus, past and future. *The Village Voice,* November 24, 1999.

Schuster, C.R., and Silverman, K. Advancing the application of behavioral treatment approaches for drug dependence. In: Onken, L.S.; Blaine, J.D.; and Boren, J.J., eds. *Behavioral Treatment for Drug Abuse and Dependence.* NIDA Research Monograph Series, Number 137. DHHS Pub. No. (ADM) 93-3684. Rockville, MD: National Institute on Drug Abuse, 1993. pp. 5–17.

Schwartz, E.L.; Brechbuhl, A.B.; Kahl, P.; Miller, M.H.; Selwyn, P.A.; and Friedland, G.H. Altered pharmacokinetics of zidovudine in former IV drug-using patients receiving methadone. *International Conference on AIDS* 6(3):194, 1990.

Seil, D. Transsexuals: The boundaries of sexual identity and gender. In: Cabaj, R.P., and Stein, T.S., eds. *Textbook of Homosexuality and Mental Health.* Washington, DC: American Psychiatric Press, 1996. pp. 743–762.

Selwyn, P.A. The impact of HIV infection on medical services in drug abuse treatment programs. *Journal of Substance Abuse Treatment* 13:397–410, 1996.

Selwyn, P.A.; Alcabse, P.; Hartel, D.; Buono, D.; Schoenbaum, E.E.; Klein, R.S.; Davenny, K.; and Friedland, G.H. Clinical manifestations and predictors of disease progression in drug users with human immunodeficiency virus infection. *New England Journal of Medicine* 327:1697–1703, 1992.

Selwyn, P.A.; Budner, N.S.; Wasserman, W.C.; and Arno, P.S. Utilization of on-site primary care services by HIV-seropositive and seronegative drug users in a methadone maintenance program. *Public Health Reports* 108:492–500, 1993.

Selwyn, P.A.; Feingold, A.R.; Iezza, A.; Satyadeo, M.; Colley, J.; Torres, R.; and Shaw, J.F. Primary care for patients with human immunodeficiency virus (HIV) infection in a methadone maintenance treatment program. *Annals of Internal Medicine* 111:761–763, 1989.

Selwyn, P.A., and O'Connor, P.G. Diagnosis and treatment of substance users with HIV infection. *Primary Care* 19(1):119–156, 1992.

Shaffer, N.; Bulterys, M.; and Simonds, R.J. Short courses of zidovudine and perinatal transmission of HIV. *New England Journal of Medicine* 340(13):1042–1043, 1999.

Shelton, D. Naming names. *American Medical News* 41(13):11, April 6, 1998.

Sherman, D.W., and Kirton, C.A. Hazardous terrain and over the edge: The survival of HIV-positive heterosexual, minority men. *Journal of the Association of Nurses AIDS Care* 9(4):23–34, 1998.

Sherman, D.W., and Ouellette, S. Moving beyond fear: Lessons learned through a longitudinal review of the literature regarding health care providers and the care of people with HIV/AIDS. *Nursing Clinics of North America* 34(1):1–48, 1999.

Siegel, K., and Meyer, I.H. Hope and resilience in suicide ideation and behavior of gay and bisexual men following notification of HIV infection. *AIDS Education and Prevention* 11(1):53–64, 1999.

Silverman, K.; Higgins, S.T.; Brooner, R.K.; Montoya, I.D.; Cone, E.J.; Schuster, C.R.; and Preston, K.L. Sustained cocaine abstinence in methadone maintenance patients through voucher-based reinforcement therapy. *Archives of General Psychiatry* 53:409–415, 1996.

Simon, F.; Mauclere, P.; Roques, P.; Loussert-Ajaka, I.; Muller-Trutwin, M.C.; Saragosti, S.; Georges-Courbot, M.C.; Barre-Sinoussi, F.; and Brun-Vezinet, F. Identification of a new human immunodeficiency virus type 1 distinct from group M and group O. *Nature Medicine* 4(9):1032–1037, 1998.

Simonsen, J.N.; Cameron, D.W.; Gakinya, M.N.; Ndinya-Achola, J.O.; D'Costa, L.J.; Karasira, P.; Cheang, M.; Ronald, A.R.; Piot, P.; and Plummer, F.A. Human immunodeficiency virus infection among men with sexually transmitted diseases. Experience from a center in Africa. *New England Journal of Medicine* 319(5):274–278, 1988.

Singer, E.J.; Zorilla, C.; Fahy-Chandon, B.; Chi, S.; Syndulko, K.; and Tourtellote, W.W. Painful symptoms reported by ambulatory HIV-infected men in a longitudinal study. *Pain* 54(1):15–19, 1993.

Singh, H.; Squier, C.; Sivek, C.; Wagener, M.; Nguyen, M.H.; and Yu, V.L. Determinants of compliance with antiretroviral therapy in patients with human immunodeficiency virus: Prospective assessment with implcations for enhancing compliance. *AIDS Care* 8:261–269, 1996.

Skinner, W.F. The prevalence and demographic predictors of illicit and licit drug use among lesbians and gay men. *American Journal of Public Health* 84:1307–1310, 1994.

Slaikeu, K., and Lawhead, S. *Up From the Ashes.* Grand Rapids, MI: Zondervan, 1987.

Sonsel, G.E.; Paradise, F.; and Stroup, S. Case management practice in an AIDS service organization. *Social Casework: The Journal of Contemporary Social Work* 69(6):388–392, 1988.

Sorensen, J.L.; Batki, S.L.; Good, P.; and Wilkinson, K. Methadone maintenance program for AIDS-affected opiate addicts. *Journal of Substance Abuse Treatment* 6:87–94, 1989.

Sorensen, J.L.; Costantini, M.F.; Wall, T.L.; and Gibson, D.R. Coupons attract high-risk untreated heroin users into detoxification. *Drug and Alcohol Dependence* 31(3):247–252, 1993.

Soto, B.; Sanchez-Quijano, A.; Rodrigo, L.; del Olmo, J.A.; Garcia-Bengoechea, M.; Hernandez-Quero, J.; Rey, C.; Abad, M.A.; Rodriguez, M.; Sales, G.M.; Gilabert, M.; Gonzalez, F.; Miron, P.; Caruz, A.; Relimpio, F.; Torronteras, R.; Leal, M.; and Lissen, E. Human immunodeficiency virus infection modifies the natural history of chronic parenterally-acquired hepatitis C with an unusually rapid progression to cirrhosis. *Journal of Hepatology* 26(1):1–5, 1997.

St. Lawrence, J.S., and Brasfield, T.L. HIV risk behavior among homeless adults. *AIDS Education and Prevention* 7:22–31, 1995.

Stall, R.D. The prevention of HIV infection associated with drug and alcohol use during sexual activity. *Adv. Alcohol Subst Abuse* 7(2):73–88, 1987.

Stall, R.D.; Hoff, C.; Coates, T.J.; Paul, J.; Phillips, K.A.; Ekstrand, M.; Kegeles, S.; Catania, J.; Daigle, D.; and Diaz, R. Decisions to get HIV tested and to accept antiretroviral therapies among gay/bisexual men: Implications for secondary prevention efforts. *Journal of AIDS and Human Retroviruses* 11:151–160, 1996.

Stall, R.D.; McKusick, L.; Wiley J.; Coates, T.J.; and Ostrow, D.G. Alcohol and drug use during sexual activity and compliance with safe sex guidelines for AIDS: The AIDS Behavior Research Project. *Health Education Quarterly* 13:359–371, 1986.

Stall, R.D.; Paul, J.P.; Barrett, D.C.; Crosby, G.M.; and Bein, E. An outcome evaluation to measure changes in sexual risk-taking among gay men undergoing substance use disorder treatment. *Journal of Studies on Alcohol* 60(6):837–845, 1999.

Stall, R.D., and Wiley, J. A comparison of alcohol and drug use patterns of homosexual and heterosexual men: The San Francisco Men's Health Study. *Drug and Alcohol Dependency* 22:63–73, 1988.

Steer, R.A.; Iguchi, M.Y.; and Platt, J.J. Hopelessness in I.V. drug users not in treatment and seeking HIV testing and counseling. *Drug and Alcohol Dependence* 34(2):99–103, 1994.

Stein, D.S.; Graham, N.M.; Park, L.P.; Hoover, D.R.; Phair, J.P.; Detels, R.; Ho, M.; and Saah, A.J. The effect of the interaction of acyclovir with zidovudine on progression to AIDS and survival. Analysis of data in the Multicenter AIDS Cohort Study. *Annals of Internal Medicine* 121(2):100–108, 1994.

Stein, M.D. Injected drug use: Complications and costs in the care of hospitalized HIV infected patients. *Journal of AIDS* 7:469–473, 1994.

Stein, M.D.; Freedberg, K.A.; Sullivan, L.M.; Savetsky, J.; Levenson, S.M.; Hingson, R.; and Samet, J.H. Sexual ethics. Disclosure of HIV-positive status to partners. *Archives of Internal Medicine* 158:253–257, 1998.

Stein, M.D.; O'Sullivan, P.S.; Ellis, P.; Perrin, H.; and Wartenberg, A. Utilization of medical services by drug abusers in detoxification. *Journal of Substance Abuse* 5:187–193, 1993.

Stein, M.D., and Samet, J.H. Disclosure of HIV status. *AIDS Patient Care and STDs* 13:265–267, 1999.

Stein, M.D.; Urdaneta, M.E.; and Clarke, J. Use of antiretroviral therapies by HIV-infected persons receiving methadone maintenance. *Journal of Addictive Diseases* 19(1):85–94, 2000.

Stimmel, B.; Vernace, S.; and Schaffner, F. Hepatitis B surface antigen and antibody. A prospective study in asymptomatic drug abusers. *JAMA* 234(11):1135–1138, 1975.

Stitzer, M.L.; Iguchi, M.Y.; and Felch, L.J. Contingent take-home incentive: Effects on drug use of methadone maintenance patients. *Journal of Consulting and Clinical Psychology* 60:927–934, 1992.

Storms, D. "Healing the hurt: A conference on homphobia." Paper presented at the Parents, Families, and Friends of Lesbians and Gays (PFLAG) Conference, Houston, TX, 1994.

Stoto, M.A.; Almario, D.A.; and McCormick, M.C. *Reducing the Odds: Preventing Perinatal Transmission of HIV in the United States.* Washington, DC: National Academy Press, 1998. http://www.nap.edu/readingroom/ books/odds [Accessed November 12, 1998].

Strain, E.C.; Stitzer, M.L.; Liebson, I.A.; and Bigelow, G.E. Dose-response effects of methadone in the treatment of opioid dependence. *Annals of Internal Medicine* 119:23–27, 1993.

Stryker, J. Correctional systems. In: Jonsen, A.R., and Stryker, J., eds. *The Social Impact of AIDS in the United States.* Washington, DC: National Academy Press, 1993. pp. 176–200.

Substance Abuse and Mental Health Services Administration. *Summary of Findings from the 1998 National Household Survey on Drug Abuse.* DHHS Pub. No. (SMA) 99-3328. Washington, DC: Government Printing Office, 1999.

Support Center for Nonprofit Management and San Francisco Department of Public Health AIDS Office. *Making the Connection: Standards of Practice for Client-Centered HIV Case Management.* April 1996.

Susser, E.; Valencia, E.; and Conover, S. Prevalence of HIV infection among psychiatric patients in a New York City men's shelter. *American Journal of Public Health* 83:568–570, 1993.

Thomas, S.B., and Quinn, S.C. The Tuskegee Syphilis Study, 1932 to 1972: Implications for HIV education and AIDS risk education programs in the black community. *American Journal of Public Health* 81(11):1498–1505, 1991.

Tiihonen, J.; Ryynanen, O.P.; Kauhanen, J.; Hakola, H.P.; and Salaspuro, M. Citalopram in the treatment of alcoholism: A double-blind placebo-controlled study. *Pharmacopsychiatry* 29:27–29, 1996.

Tondo, L.; Baldessarini, R.J.; Hennen, J.; Minnai, G.P.; Salis, P.; Scamonatti, L.; Masia, M.; Ghiani, C.; and Mannu, P. Suicide attempts in major affective disorder patients with comorbid substance use disorders. *Journal of Clinical Psychiatry* 60 (Suppl) 2:63–69, 1999.

Tong, T.G.; Pond, S.M.; Kreek, M.J.; Jaffery, N.F.; and Benowitz, N.L. Phenytoin-induced methadone withdrawal. *Annals of Internal Medicine* 94:349–351, 1981.

Tuskegee Syphilis Study Legacy Committee. *Report of the Tuskegee Syphilis Study Legacy Committee: Final Report.* May 20, 1996. http://www.med.virginia.edu/hs-library/ historical/apology/report.html. [Accessed December 22, 1999].

Umbricht-Schneiter, A.; Ginn, D.H.; Pabst, K.M.; and Bigelow, G.E. Providing medical care to methadone clinic patients: Referral vs. on-site care. *American Journal of Public Health* 84:207–210, 1994.

Urassa, M.; Todd, J.; Boerma, J.T.; Hayes, R.; and Isingo, R. Male circumcision and susceptibility to HIV infection among men in Tanzania. *AIDS* 11(3):73–80, 1997.

U.S. Bureau of the Census. *Resident Population of the United States: Estimates, by Sex, Race, and Hispanic Origin, With Median Age.* December 28, 1998. http://www.census.gov/population/estimates/nation/intfile3-1.txt [Accessed May 10, 1999].

U.S. Department of Health and Human Services. *Needle Exchange Programs: Part of a Comprehensive HIV Prevention Strategy.* Fact Sheet. April 20, 1998. http://waisgate.hhs.gov/news/press/1998pres/980420a.html [Accessed December 6, 1999].

U.S. Department of Health and Human Services (DHHS) and the Henry J. Kaiser Family Foundation. Panel on Clinical Practices for Treatment of HIV Infection. *Guidelines for the Use of Antiretroviral Agents in HIV-Infected Adults and Adolescents, 1997.* http://hivpositive.com/f-treatment/NIH_Guidelines/NIHguideMenu.html [Accessed December 11, 1998].

U.S. General Accounting Office. *Drug Treatment: Despite New Strategy, Few Federal Inmates Receive Treatment.* Report to the Committee on Government Operations, House of Representatives. GAO/HRD-91-128. Washington, DC: U.S. Government Printing Office, 1991.

U.S. General Accounting Office. *Needle Exchange Programs: Research Suggests Promise as an AIDS Prevention Strategy.* Report to the Chairman, Select Committee on Narcotics Abuse and Control. GAO/HRD-93-60. Washington, DC: U.S. Government Printing Office, 1993.

U.S. General Accounting Office. *Drug Abuse: Research Shows Treatment Is Effective, But Benefits May Be Overstated.* GAO/HEHS-98-72. Washington, DC: U.S. Government Printing Office, 1998.

Van Howe, R.S. Circumcision and HIV infection: Review of the literature and meta-analysis. *International Journal of STD and AIDS* 10(1):8–16, 1999.

Vittinghoff, E.; Scheer, S.; O'Malley, P.; Colfax, G.; Holmberg, S.D.; and Buchbinder, S.P. Combination antiretroviral therapy and recent declines in AIDS incidence and mortality. *Journal of Infectious Diseases* 179(3):717–720, 1999.

Volpicelli, J.R.; Alterman, A.I.; Hayashida, M.; and O'Brien, C.P. Naltrexone in the treatment of alcohol dependence. *Archives of General Psychiatry* 49:876–880, 1992.

Wall, T.L.; Sorensen, J.L.; Batki, S.L.; Delucchi, K.L.; London, J.A.; and Chesney, M.A. Adherence to zidovudine (AZT) among HIV-infected methadone patients: A pilot study of supervised therapy and dispensing compared to usual care. *Journal of Drug and Alcohol Dependence* 37(3):261–269, 1995.

Walsh, S.L.; Preston, K.L.; Stitzer, M.L.; Cone, E.J.; and Bigelow, G.E. Clinical pharmacology of buprenorphine: Ceiling effects at high doses. *Clinical Pharmacology and Therapeutics* 55:569–580, 1994.

Ward, J.W., and Duchin, J.S. The epidemiology of HIV and AIDS in the United States. *AIDS Clinical Review 1997–98*:1–45, 1997–1998.

Wartenberg, A.A. HIV disease in the intravenous drug user: Role of the primary care physician. *Journal of General Internal Medicine* 6:S35–S40, 1991.

Watters, J.K.; Downing, M.; Case, P.; Lorvick, J.; Cheng, Y.; and Fergusson, B. AIDS prevention for intravenous drug users in the community: Street-based education and risk behavior. *American Journal of Community Psychology* 18:587–596, 1990.

Watters, J.K.; Estilo, M.J.; Clark, G.L.; and Lorvick, J. Syringe and needle exchange as HIV/AIDS prevention for injection drug users. *JAMA* 271:115–120, 1994.

Weinberg, M.S., and Williams, C.J. *Male Homosexuals; Their Problems and Adaptations.* New York: Oxford University Press, 1974.

Weissman, G.; Melchior, L.; Huba, G.; Altice, F.; Booth, R.; Cottler, L.; Genser, S.; Jones, A.; McCarthy, S.; Needle, R.; and Smereck, G. Women living with substance abuse and HIV disease: Medical care access issues. *Journal of the American Medical Women's Association* 50(3-4):115–120, 1995.

Weissman, G.; Melchior, L.; Huba, G.; Smereck, G.; Needle, R.; McCarthy, S.; Jones, A.; Genser, S.; Cottler, L.; Booth, R.; and Altice, F. Women living with drug abuse and HIV disease: Drug abuse treatment access and secondary prevention issues. *Journal of Psychoactive Drugs* 27(4):401–411, 1995.

White, J.C. HIV risk assessment and prevention in lesbians and women who have sex with women: Practical information for clinicians. *Health Care for Women International* 18(2):127–138, 1997.

Wiebel, W.W.; Biernacki, P.; Mulia, N.; and Levin, L. Outreach to IDUs not in treatment. In: Brown, B.S., and Beschner, G.M., eds. *Handbook on Risk of AIDS: Injection Drug Users and Sexual Partners.* Westport, CT: Greenwood Press, 1993. pp. 437–444.

Wiegand, M.; Moller, A.A.; Schreiber, W.; Krieg, J.C.; and Holsboer, F. Alterations of nocturnal sleep in patients with HIV infection. *Acta Neurologica Scandinavica* 83(2):141–142, 1991.

Wiley, J., and Samuel, M. Prevalence of HIV infection in the U.S.A. *AIDS* 3 (Suppl) 1:71–78, 1989.

Wilkinson, C.W.; Crabbe, J.C.; Keith, L.D.; Kendall, J.W.; and Dorsa, D.M. Influence of ethanol dependence on regional brain content of beta-endorphin in the mouse. *Brain Research* 378:107–114, 1986.

Wimbush, J.; Amicarelli, A.; and Stein, M. Does HIV test result influence methadone maintenance treatment retention? *Journal of Substance Abuse* 8:263–269, 1996.

Winiarski, M.G. *HIV Mental Health for the 21st Century.* New York: New York University Press, 1997.

Withum, D.J. "High HIV prevalence among female and male entrants to U.S. correctional facilities (1989–1992): Implications for prevention and treatment strategies." Paper presented at the 121st Annual Meeting of the American Public Health Association, San Francisco, CA, October 24–28, 1993.

Wittkowski, K.M.; Susser, E.; and Dietz, K. The protective effect of condoms and nonoxynol-9 against HIV infection. *American Journal of Public Health* 88(4):590–596, 1998.

Wolitski, R.J.; MacGowan, R.J.; Higgins, D.L.; and Jorgensen, C.M. The effects of HIV counseling and testing on risk-related practices and help-seeking behavior. *AIDS Education and Prevention* 9(3 Suppl.): 52–67, 1997.

Woods, W.J.; Avins, A.; Lindan, C.; Hudes, E.; Boscarino, J.; and Clark, W. Predictors of HIV-related risk behaviors among heterosexuals in alcoholism treatment. *Journal of Studies on Alcohol* 57:486–493, 1996.

Woody, G.; O'Hare, K.; Mintz, J.; and O'Brien, C. Rapid intake: A method for increasing retention rate of heroin addicts seeking methadone treatment. *Comprehensive Psychiatry* 16:165–169, 1975.

Word, C.O., and Bowser, B. Background to crack cocaine addiction and HIV high-risk behavior: The next epidemic. *American Journal of Drug and Alcohol Abuse* 23(1):67–77, 1997.

World Health Organization. *HIV and Infant Feeding: A Review of HIV Transmission Through Breastfeeding.* Joint United Nations Programme on HIV/AIDS (UNAIDS), 1998. http://www.unaids.org/publications/documents/mtct/index.html [Accessed August 31, 1999].

Yerly, S.; Schockmel, G.; and Bru, J.P. Frequency of transmission of drug-resistant variants in individuals with primary HIV-1 infection (Abstract No. 32280). 12th World AIDS Conference, Geneva, Switzerland, 1998.

Youle, M.S.; Gazzard, B.G.; Johnson, M.A.; Cooper, D.A.; Hoy, J.F.; Busch, H.; Ruf, B.; Griffiths, P.D.; Stephenson, S.L.; and Dancox, M. Effects of high-dose oral acyclovir on herpesvirus disease and survival in patients with advanced HIV disease: A double-blind, placebo-controlled study. European-Australian Acyclovir Study Group. *AIDS* 8(5):641–649, 1994.

Zagame, S.K. Letter to Peter J. Millock, General Counsel, Department of Health, State of New York, from the Acting General Counsel to the U.S. Department of Health and Human Services, May 17, 1989. In: Center for Substance Abuse Treatment. *Confidentiality of Patient Records for Alcohol and Other Drug Treatment.* Technical Assistance Publication (TAP) Series, Number 13. DHHS Pub. No. (SMA) 95-3018. Washington, DC: U.S. Government Printing Office, 1995.

Zhu, T.; Korber, B.T.; Nahmias, A.J.; Hooper, E.; Sharp, P.M.; and Ho, D.D. An African HIV-1 sequence from 1959 and implications for the origin of the epidemic. *Nature* 391(6667):594–597, 1998.

Ziebold, T.O., and Mongeon, J.E., eds. *Gay and Sober: Directions for Counseling and Therapy.* New York: Harrington Park Press, 1985.

Zolopa, A.R.; Hahn, J.A.; Gorter, R.; Miranda, J.; Wlodarczyk, D.; Peterson, J.; Pilote, L.; and Moss, A.R. HIV and tuberculosis infection in San Francisco's homeless adults. Prevalence and risk factors in a representative sample. *JAMA* 272(6):455–461, 1994.

Appendix B
Glossary

Abstinence: Complete cessation of substance-using behavior.

Acute retroviral syndrome: An array of symptoms that arises after initial infection with HIV that includes fever, sore throat, swollen glands, muscle and joint pain, nausea, and rash.

Adherence: Strict observation of a prescribed treatment regimen, including correct dosage and number of doses per day, as well as taking doses with or without food or other medications.

Agranulocytosis: A sudden, severe drop in white blood cell count that can occur upon the administration of certain HIV medications.

AIDS (acquired immunodeficiency syndrome): AIDS is the end stage of HIV disease and is characterized by a severe reduction in CD4+ T cells. At this point, an infected person has a very weak immune system and is vulnerable to contracting life-threatening infections.

Antiretroviral: A medication that weakens or halts the reproduction of retroviruses such as HIV.

Blood–brain barrier: A physical barrier between the blood vessels and the brain that only allows certain substances to pass through and enter the brain.

CD4+ T cell count: The number of CD4+ T cells in a milliliter of blood. These cells (white blood cells within the immune system) are constantly measured in HIV-infected clients because their number reflects the overall health of the immune system.

Case finding: A component of outreach that identifies individuals at higher risk for HIV infection and that stresses HIV/AIDS prevention, along with the distribution of items to facilitate compliance with risk reduction techniques.

Combination therapy: The treatment of HIV disease with multiple medications. Combinations of three or more different medicines are used to treat a client, with each medicine working in a different way to stop the virus. While this is the most effective treatment to date, once combination therapy is begun, it must not be stopped because the virus could then develop resistance to these medications.

Cross-resistance: Resistance that can develop in the HIV virus once a medication from a certain class is used (e.g., protease inhibitors, nucleosides) to treat it. The virus not only becomes resistant to one particular drug but also becomes resistant to some or all of the other drugs from that class. For this reason, it is widely believed that the best chance for success in HIV treatment is with the first treatment regimen.

Cultural competence: An aspect of treatment that takes into account the cultural heritage of the client. Culturally competent providers recognize the customs, beliefs, and social forms of the racial, religious, or social group to which the client belongs and work within these parameters to interact successfully with the client.

Cytomegalovirus (CMV): Any of the group of herpes viruses that appear as opportunistic infections in patients with HIV disease, generally in the latter stages of AIDS. CMV most commonly causes retinitis, which can lead to blindness if untreated, and may also cause gastrointestinal, adrenal, pulmonary, and other systemic problems.

Drug interaction: The positive or negative effect that one medication has on another when an HIV-infected client is taking both.

Endocarditis: Bacterial endocarditis is a well-recognized complication of unsterile injection drug use that produces inflammation of the endocardium (the lining of the heart). It can also appear as an HIV-related opportunistic infection.

HAART (highly active antiretroviral therapy): Aggressive combination therapy that usually includes a powerful protease inhibitor medication.

Harm reduction: An approach to treatment that emphasizes incremental decreases in substance abuse or HIV risk behaviors as treatment goals. This method attempts to keep clients in treatment even if complete abstinence is not achieved.

Herpes zoster (shingles): A virus that often appears as an initial indication of HIV disease and begins with itching or pain on only one side of the face or body, followed by a rash that looks like chicken pox or poison ivy.

HIV (human immunodeficiency virus): The retrovirus that causes AIDS in humans. HIV is transmitted through direct contact with human bodily fluids; roughly 10 years after infection, AIDS-defining conditions begin to occur. AIDS is characterized by a severe reduction in CD4+ T cells, which greatly weakens the immune system and leaves the patient vulnerable to contracting life-threatening infections. New medicines can control HIV and extend the life of the patient; however, AIDS is inevitably fatal.

Homophobia: An irrational aversion to gay men and lesbians and to their lifestyle.

Hospice: A program or facility that provides care for clients in the last stages of a terminal disease such as AIDS and creates a compassionate environment in which clients can die peacefully.

Leukoplakia: A virus that causes white patches in the mouth and is one of the initial indications of HIV infection.

Lymphadenopathy: Swollen lymph nodes, the most common symptom during the HIV latency period. The lymph nodes can be found around the neck and under the arms and contain cells that fight infections. When an infection is present, lymph nodes usually swell. Inside the lymph nodes HIV is trapped and destroyed, but eventually the HIV breaks down the tissue of the nodes and spills into the rest of the body.

Monotherapy: Treatment of HIV infection with only one medication, usually AZT. This was the standard treatment for HIV before 1995 and is now outdated.

MSMs: Men who have sex with men.

Neutropenia: Bone marrow suppression, which can occur upon the administration of certain HIV medications.

Nonnucleoside reverse transcriptase inhibitor (NNRTI): A type of medication that binds to HIV's reverse transcriptase enzyme and stops the virus from replicating. NNRTI medications include delaviridine, efavirenz, and nevirapine.

Nucleoside analog: A drug that mimics HIV's genetic material and halts it from reproducing. This class of drugs includes AZT, abacavir, didanosine, zalcitabine, stavudine, and lamivudine.

Opportunistic infection: An infection that usually does not harm a healthy person but that can cause a life-threatening illness in someone with a compromised immune system.

Perinatal HIV transmission (vertical transmission): Transmission of HIV from a mother to her child either in the uterus, during birth, or through breast-feeding.

Peripheral neuropathy: A condition in which the peripheral nerves of the hands or feet are afflicted, producing numbness, tingling, pain, or weakness.

Phlebotomy: The act of drawing blood.

Pneumocystis carinii **pneumonia (PCP)**: PCP is the most common AIDS-related infection and is characterized by a dry cough, fever, night sweats, and increasing shortness of breath. Since the late 1980s, the widespread use of PCP prophylaxis has resulted in a dramatic decrease in the incidence of this opportunistic infection. However, despite the availability of effective prophylaxis, PCP is still the most common opportunistic infection; many patients who develop PCP are unaware of their HIV status and hence are not receiving prophylaxis.

Postexposure prophylaxis (PEP): Antiretroviral therapy that is administered within 72 hours after exposure to HIV in an attempt to eradicate the virus from the body.

Protease inhibitor: One of a powerful class of drugs used in combination therapy that acts by interfering with the protease enzyme that cuts HIV proteins into the small pieces required to create new copies of the virus. This slows or halts the replication of HIV. Protease inhibitors include indinavir, nelfinavir, ritonavir, and saquinavir.

Reverse transcriptase inhibitor (RTI): A drug that halts HIV replication by interfering with the reverse transcriptase enzyme used by the HIV virus to transform its genetic material into a form that can be used to produce more viruses. This class of drugs includes nucleoside analogs like AZT and lamivudine.

Risk reduction: An approach to treatment that emphasizes graduated behavior change rather than immediate abstinence. By identifying areas of risk in the client's life, such as sexual risk or needle sharing, the provider can discuss strategies with the client for avoiding or reducing them.

SEPs: Syringe exchange programs.

Seroprevalence: Frequency of presence of antibodies in blood serum as a result of infection.

STDs: Sexually transmitted diseases.

Substance: A drug of abuse, a medication, or a toxin.

Substance abuse: A pattern of substance use that results in harmful consequences for the abuser. This condition is not as severe as substance dependence.

Substance dependence: Repeated self-administration of a substance that usually results in tolerance, withdrawal, and compulsive substance-abusing behavior.

Thrush: Oral candidiasis, or thrush, is a symptom of initial HIV infection and usually appears as white plaques at the back of the mouth. Without treatment, thrush often spreads throughout the mouth and can affect the esophagus in persons with advanced disease, leading to severe pain on swallowing and the need for prolonged systemic treatment.

Toxoplasmosis: An AIDS-defining symptom caused by infection with the protozoan *toxoplasma* and one of the two most common brain infections in HIV. Toxoplasmosis, which produces seizures, usually does not appear until a client's CD4+ T cell count drops below 100.

Triple combination therapy: Treatment involving three medications, which can lower the rate of disease progression and mortality more than can two medicines alone. Triple combination therapy was developed after combination-resistant forms of HIV began to appear.

Viral load: The level of HIV circulating in the bloodstream. This level becomes very high soon after initial infection, then drops until it returns with the onset of AIDS. Drug therapy can keep viral load low or undetectable, but the client can still infect others since the virus still exists—it is simply not visible. Even when testing reveals a low viral load, HIV continues to live inside certain cells in the body and can begin reproducing at any time if the infected person is not on effective treatment. If a person is not in treatment, HIV produces billions of new virions (viral particles) every day.

Appendix C
1993 Revised Classification System For HIV Infection and Expanded AIDS Surveillance Case Definition For Adolescents and Adults

1993 Revised Classification System for HIV Infection and Expanded AIDS Surveillance Case Definition for Adolescents and Adults			
CD4+ T cells	**Clinical Categories**		
	(A) Symptomatic, Acute (Primary) HIV or PGL*	**(B) CD4+ T cells Symptomatic, Not (A) or (C) Conditions**	**(C) AIDS-Indicator Conditions**
(1) ≥500/mL	A1	B1	C1
(2) 200–499/mL	A2	B2	C2
(3) <200/mL AIDS-Indicator T-cell count	A3	B3	C3

(Shaded area indicates that the individual has AIDS.)

PGL-persistent generalized lymphadenopathy. Clinical Category A includes acute (primary) HIV infection.

CD4+ T-Lymphocyte Categories

The three CD4+ T-lymphocyte categories are defined as follows:

- **Category 1:** ≥ 500/mL
- **Category 2:** 200–499/mL
- **Category 3:** <200/mL

These categories correspond to CD4+ T-lymphocyte counts per mL of blood and guide clinical and therapeutic actions in the management of HIV-infected adolescents and adults. The revised HIV classification system also allows for the use of the percentage of CD4+ T cells.

HIV-infected persons should be classified based on existing guidelines for the medical management of HIV-infected persons. Thus, the lowest accurate, but not necessarily the most recent, CD4+ T lymphocyte count should be used for classification purposes.

Clinical Categories

The clinical categories of HIV infection are defined as follows:

Category A

Category A consists of one or more of the conditions listed below in an adolescent or adult ($\geq$ 13 years) with documented HIV infection. Conditions listed in Categories B and C must not have occurred.

- Asymptomatic HIV infection
- Persistent generalized lymphadenopathy
- Acute (primary) HIV infection with accompanying illness or history of acute HIV infection

Category B

Category B consists of symptomatic conditions in an HIV-infected adolescent or adult that are not included among conditions listed in clinical Category C and that meet at least one of the following criteria:

- The conditions are attributed to HIV infection or indicate a defect in cell-mediated immunity
- The conditions are considered by physicians to have a clinical course or to require management that is complicated by HIV infection. Examples of conditions in clinical Category B include, but are not limited to
  - Bacillary angiomatosis
  - Candidiasis, oropharyngeal (thrush)
  - Candidiasis, vulvovaginal: persistent, frequent, or poorly responsive to therapy
  - Cervical dysplasia (moderate or severe)/cervical carcinoma *in situ*
  - Constitutional symptoms, such as fever (38.5° C) or diarrhea lasting >1 month
  - Hairy leukoplakia, oral
  - Herpes zoster (shingles), involving at least two distinct episodes or more than one dermatome
  - Idiopathic thrombocytopenic purpura
  - Listeriosis
  - Pelvic inflammatory disease, particularly if complicated by tubo-ovarian abscess
  - Peripheral neuropathy

For classification purposes, Category B conditions take precedence over those in Category A. For example, someone previously treated for oral or persistent vaginal candidiasis (and who has not developed a Category C disease) but who is now asymptomatic should be classified in clinical Category B.

Category C

Category C includes the clinical conditions listed in the AIDS surveillance case definition (below). For classification purposes, once a Category C condition occurs, the person will remain in Category C.

- Candidiasis of bronchi, trachea, or lungs
- Candidiasis, esophageal
- Cervical cancer, invasive*

- Coccidioidomycosis, disseminated or extrapulmonary
- Cryptococcosis, extrapulmonary
- Cryptosporidiosis, chronic intestinal (>1 month's duration)
- Cytomegalovirus disease (other than liver, spleen, or nodes)
- Cytomegalovirus retinitis (with loss of vision)
- Encephalopathy, HIV-related
- Herpes simplex: chronic ulcer(s) (>1 month's duration); or bronchitis, pneumonitis, or esophagitis
- Histoplasmosis, disseminated or extrapulmonary
- Isosporiasis, chronic intestinal (>1 month's duration)
- Kaposi's sarcoma
- Lymphoma, Burkitt's (or equivalent term)
- Lymphoma, immunoblastic (or equivalent term)
- Lymphoma, primary, of brain
- *Mycobacterium avium complex* or *M. kansasii*, disseminated or extrapulmonary
- *Mycobacterium tuberculosis*, any site (pulmonary or extrapulmonary)
- *Mycobacterium*, other species or unidentified species, disseminated or extrapulmonary
- *Pneumocystis carinii* pneumonia
- Pneumonia, recurrent**
- Progressive multifocal leukoencephalopathy
- Pulmonary pneumonia
- *Salmonella* septicemia, recurrent
- Toxoplasmosis of brain
- Wasting syndrome due to AIDS

*This expanded definition requires laboratory confirmation of HIV infection in persons with a CD4+T lymphocyte count of fewer than 200 cells/mL or with an added clinical condition.

**Added as AIDS-defining illness in the 1993 expansion of the AIDS surveillance case definition, when occurring in persons with HIV infection.

Source: Castro et al., 1992.

Appendix D
Screening Instruments

Symptoms Checklist

Symptoms Checklist	
Symptom	**Question/Action**
■ Fever ■ Loss of appetite ■ Weight loss ■ Night sweats ■ Nausea ■ Diarrhea ■ Lymph node swelling	■ HIV positive? Ask about the possibility of HIV. Get an HIV test. ■ Ask about change in diet. ■ Active drug use? Injection-related bacterial infections, cocaine use, and heroin withdrawal are possible causes. ■ Ask about tuberculosis (suggest the Mantoux Purified Protein Derivative [PPD] test). ■ Ask if the client is taking any new illicit drugs or medications; some symptoms may be side effects. See the medical professional before stopping medicines. ■ Is there another infection? See medical professional for diagnosis and treatment, especially if the CD4+ T cell count is low (< 200).
■ Cough ■ Chest pain ■ Shortness of breath	■ HIV positive? Ask about the possibility of HIV. Get an HIV test. ■ Smoking of tobacco or drugs? ■ Exposure to TB? Cough lasting more than 3 weeks should be checked. ■ Fever and night sweats? Pneumonia usually causes these symptoms along with a fever, with or without chills and night sweats.
■ Forgetfulness ■ Psychosis ■ Seizures	■ HIV positive? Ask about the possibility of HIV. Get an HIV test. ■ Intoxication with drugs or alcohol? Withdrawal? ■ Head injury? Immediate medical attention may be needed. HIV-related infection or cancer in the brain may occur, especially if the CD4+ T cell count is low (< 200). ■ Ask about a history of depressive or dissociative symptoms. ■ Ask about a history of psychotic symptoms.

Symptoms Checklist	
■ Numbness or tingling in the limbs	■ HIV positive? Ask about the possibility of HIV. Get an HIV test. ■ Is didanosine (Videx), zalcitabine (Hivid), or stavudine (D4T) being taken? Contact medical professional immediately. ■ Is there long-term alcohol use or diabetes? See a medical professional. ■ If HIV positive, are antiretroviral medicines working well, are they being taken correctly? Medication resistance or failure to take medicines can make HIV symptoms worse. ■ If there is any numbness or tingling in the limbs, the client should see a medical professional.
■ Rash ■ Itching	■ HIV positive? Ask about the possibility of HIV. Get an HIV test. ■ Hepatitis from drug or alcohol use? See a medical professional. ■ Injection site cellulitis? See a medical professional. ■ Ask if the client is taking any new medications; some symptoms may be side effects. See the medical professional before stopping medicines.

Amsler Grid Test

This instrument is an effective screening tool for early detection of cytomegalovirus. An Amsler grid can help you monitor your central visual field. It can detect early and subtle visual changes resulting from several macular diseases such as age-related macular degeneration and diabetic macular edema. It is also helpful in tracking changes in vision once they have been discovered. The Amsler grid tests each eye separately. This helps you to recognize visual symptoms that are only in one eye.

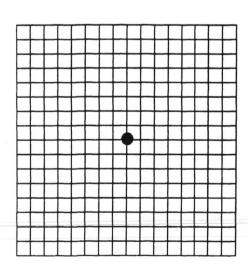 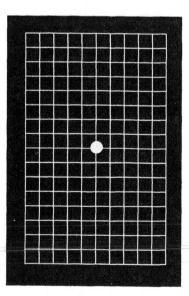

The above are examples of two different Amsler grids. Both are useful for monitoring central vision. The grid on the right is a modified Amsler grid (Yannuzzi card) intended to be carried in the wallet or purse for daily self-assessment.

Instructions

- Test your vision with sufficient lighting.
- Wear your reading glasses or look through the reading portion of your bifocals (if you normally read with spectacles).
- Hold the Amsler grid at normal reading distance (about 14 inches).
- Cover one eye at a time with the palm of your hand.
- Stare at the center dot of the chart at all times.
- Do not let your eye drift from the center dot.

Ask yourself the following questions as you check each eye separately:

- Are any of the lines crooked or bent?
- Are any of the boxes different in size or shape from the others?
- Are any of the lines wavy, missing, blurry, or discolored?

Note: If using a rectangular card like the one on the right above (Yannuzzi card), you should check each eye with the card held both vertically and horizontally.

If the answer to any of these questions is "yes" (and this is a new finding for you), you should contact your doctor immediately for an examination. Sometimes these changes may mean that there is leakage in the back of the eye causing swelling of the retina.

Examples of Abnormal Amsler Grids

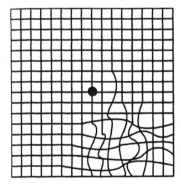

Example of distortion

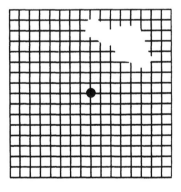

Example of area missing

Appendix E
Sample Codes of Ethics

Code of Ethics for Programs Treating Persons With HIV/AIDS And Substance Abuse Disorders

Nondiscrimination

- In accordance with Federal and State law, this program accords all persons equal access to its facilities and services without regard to race, color, ancestry, or national origin.
- In accordance with Federal and State law, this program accords all persons equal access to its facilities and services without regard to handicap, unless such handicap would render treatment nonbeneficial or hazardous to the patient or others.
- In accordance with Federal and State law, this program accords all persons equal access to its facilities and services without regard to age or gender. (*Or*: In accordance with Federal and State law, this program accords all women, men, and adolescents equal access to its facilities and services without regard to gender or age.)
- This program makes reasonable modifications in policies, practices, and procedures and/or provides assistive services to accommodate clients who are unable to participate in treatment due to language, cultural, or literacy barriers or disabilities, unless doing so would fundamentally alter the nature of the services offered.
- This program offers referral to appropriate service providers for all individuals not admitted to treatment, without regard to race, color, ancestry, national origin, handicap, age, or gender, in accordance with Federal and State law.

Respect for Client Autonomy

- This program respects each client's right to be fully informed about treatment and to make informed treatment decisions. This program provides clients with the information that is reasonably necessary to permit them to make informed decisions regarding treatment, including the information that participation in treatment is voluntary and clients have the right to refuse to participate. If consequences such as termination from other services or benefits or revocation of parole may result from refusal to consent to or continue treatment, the program will so inform the client at the time the client refuses to participate.
- This program respects each client's right to participate in an informed way, alone or with family members or others of his choosing, in planning his participation in treatment and

medical services and reviewing progress toward treatment goals.

Confidentiality and Accuracy Of Records

- This program respects the rights of all clients to confidentiality of all records, correspondence, and information relating to assessment, diagnosis, and treatment in accordance with 42 U.S.C. §290dd-2, 42 CFR Part 2, and State law.
- This program respects the client's right to review and copy his/her records in accordance with State law and regulation and program policy.
- This program respects the rights of all clients to request the correction of inaccurate, irrelevant, outdated, or incomplete information in their records and to submit rebuttal information or memoranda for inclusion in their records.

Competent and Humane Treatment

- This program is dedicated to providing competent and humane services to clients; it recognizes that delivery of competent services requires staff with the knowledge, skill, time, attentiveness, and preparation reasonably necessary to assist clients to achieve their goals for health improvements and recovery from substance abuse.
- This program's employees treat all clients with consideration, respect, and full recognition of their dignity and individuality.
- This program will not permit any client to perform any labor at the program, as a volunteer or in lieu of fees, that is not called for by the client's treatment plan, unless the client agrees in writing and the arrangement complies with regulations of all State agencies sharing oversight of the program.
- This program will not permit any client to participate in any experimental or research project without the full knowledge, understanding, and written consent of that client (and/or legal guardian, when appropriate).
- This program will not participate in any experimental or research project unless it is conducted in full compliance with applicable State and Federal laws, regulations, and guidelines.
- No employee or board member of this program shall
  - Enter into any financial relationship with any client
  - Have a sexual relationship with any client
- No employee of this program shall interfere with any client's
  - Right to seek or have access to legal counsel
  - Exercise of any right accorded by program policy or State law or regulation.
- (For residential programs) No employee of this program shall interfere with any client's right to
  - Visit with family and friends in accordance with the program's written rules
  - Conduct private telephone conversations in accordance with the program's written rules
  - Send and receive uncensored and unopened mail, except that employees may open and inspect a client's mail or package in the client's presence or when the client is not present if the client has consented
  - Wear his or her own clothing in accordance with program rules
  - Bring personal belongings, subject to limitation or supervision by the program
  - Communicate with a personal physician
  - Practice her personal religion or attend religious services, within the program's policies and guidelines

Client Orientation

- All clients entering this program shall be provided with an orientation to the program at or before the time of admission or as soon thereafter as possible.
- The orientation shall include the following information:
  - The program's purpose, a description of the treatment process, and a summary of the medical and other services the program offers
  - Clients' rights as provided by State law and regulations and by 42 CFR Part 2, as outlined in 42 CFR §2.22
  - Clients' responsibilities in the program, including fees, if any
  - The program's hours of operation
  - Relevant program policies, including rules that govern client conduct and the infractions that might result in disciplinary action or discharge
  - The program's grievance procedures
  - Additional areas covered by program policy
  - (For residential programs) information about policies governing visitation, the sending and receiving of mail, and the use of the telephone
- This program will post a copy of the above information in a place accessible to all clients.

Grievance Procedures

- This program has a written procedure for hearing, considering, responding to, and documenting client grievances.
- The written procedure includes
  - Client behavior that constitutes grounds for discharge by the program; and
  - The name, telephone numbers, and address of the State health/substance abuse official in charge of consumer relations.
- The written grievance procedure will be given to each client and/or his

representative upon admission and posted in a place accessible to clients. The grievance procedure shall be available to former clients, upon request.

Discharge Policy

- This program has a written policy that specifies conditions under which clients may be discharged.
- The written discharge policy includes:
  - Client behavior that may constitute grounds for involuntary discharge
  - Procedures consistent with 42 CFR §2.12(c)(5) that staff shall follow when discharging a client involved in the commission of a crime on the premises of the agency or against its staff, including designation of the person who shall make a report to the appropriate law enforcement agency
  - Procedures consistent with 42 CFR Part 2 that staff must follow when a client leaves against medical or staff advice and the client may be dangerous to self or others

Code of Ethics for Therapists and Counselors Who Treat Persons With HIV/AIDS And Substance Abuse Disorders

Nondiscrimination

- Therapists and counselors should accord all persons equal access to program facilities and services without regard to race, color, ancestry, or national origin, in accordance with Federal and State law.
- Therapists and counselors should accord all persons equal access to program facilities and services without regard to handicap,

unless such handicap would render treatment nonbeneficial or hazardous to the patient or others, in accordance with Federal and State law and program policy.

- Therapists and counselors should accord all persons equal access to program facilities and services without regard to age or gender, in accordance with Federal and State law, unless they are employed by a program that holds itself out as specializing in a specific age group or gender.

Respect for Client Autonomy

- Therapists and counselors should respect each client's right to be fully informed about treatment and to make informed treatment decisions.
- Therapists and counselors should provide clients with the information that is reasonably necessary to permit them to make informed decisions regarding treatment, including the information that participation in treatment is voluntary and clients have the right to refuse to participate. Therapists and counselors should inform clients if consequences such as termination from other services or benefits or revocation of parole may result from refusal to consent to or continue treatment.
- Therapists and counselors should respect each client's right to participate in an informed way, alone or with family members or others of her choosing, in planning the receipt of and involvement with treatment and medical services and the review of progress toward treatment goals.

Confidentiality and Accuracy Of Records

- Therapists and counselors should be guided in their dealings with clients and others by the knowledge that confidentiality of information is of the utmost importance to

persons with HIV/AIDS and substance abuse disorders.

- Therapists and counselors should respect the right of all clients to confidentiality of all records, correspondence, and information relating to assessment, diagnosis, and treatment in accordance with 42 U.S.C. §290dd-2, 42 CFR Part 2, and State law.
- Therapists and counselors should respect the client's right to review and copy her records in accordance with State law and regulation and program policy.
- Therapists and counselors should respect the rights of all clients to request the correction of inaccurate, irrelevant, outdated, or incomplete information in their records and to submit rebuttal information or memoranda for inclusion in their records.
- Therapists and counselors should not induce or permit a client to participate in any experimental or research project without the full knowledge, understanding, and written consent of that client (and/or legal guardian, when appropriate).

Competent and Humane Treatment

- Therapists and counselors should provide services only to those clients they can serve in a competent manner and should refrain from counseling any client when they lack the knowledge, skill, time, attentiveness, and preparation reasonably necessary to assist that client to achieve treatment goals.
- Therapists and counselors should be familiar with
  - ♦ Their programs' policies and procedures
  - ♦ State and Federal rules and regulations governing their professions and programs
  - ♦ Any codes of ethics governing their profession
- Therapists and counselors should treat all clients with consideration, respect, and full recognition of their dignity and individuality.

- No therapist or counselor shall
  - ♦ Enter into any financial relationship with any client
  - ♦ Have a sexual relationship with any client
- No therapist or counselor shall interfere with any client's
  - ♦ Right to seek or have access to legal counsel
  - ♦ Exercise of any right accorded by program policy or State law or regulation
- (For those working in residential programs) No therapist or counselor shall interfere with any client's right to
  - ♦ Visit with family and friends in accordance with the program's written rules

- ♦ Conduct private telephone conversations in accordance with the program's written rules
- ♦ Send and receive uncensored and unopened mail, except that staff may open and inspect a client's mail or package in the client's presence or when the client is not present if the client has consented
- ♦ Wear his own clothing in accordance with program rules
- ♦ Bring personal belongings, subject to limitation or supervision by the program
- ♦ Communicate with a personal physician
- ♦ Practice his personal religion or attend religious services, within the program's policies and guidelines

Appendix F
AIDS-Related Web Sites

INFORMATION SOURCES

The National AIDS Treatment Information
Project—
http://www.natip.org/index.html

The Measurement Group—
www.themeasurementgroup.com

JAMA HIV-AIDS information center—
http://www.ama-assn.org/special/
hiv/hivhome.htm

Critical Path AIDS Project—
http://www.critpath.org/critpath.htm

HIV/AIDS Treatment Information Service
(ATIS)—
http://www.hivatis.org

AIDS Clinical Trial Information Service
(ATCTIS)—
http://www.actis.org

Centers for Disease Control and Prevention
(CDC)—
http://www.cdc.gov

SFAF/BETA
San Francisco AIDS Foundation home page—
http://www.sfaf.org

Bulletin of Experimental Treatments for AIDS—
http://www.sfaf.org/beta

Spanish BETA—
http://www.sfaf.org/betaespanol/

Positive News/Noticias Positivas—
http://www.sfaf.org/treatment/positivenews/

Other online sources of BETA:
http://www.critpath.org/newsletters/beta
http://www.aegis.com/search/

LIBRARIES

National Library of Medicine/MEDLINE—
http://www.nlm.nih.gov

Internet Grateful Med—
http://access.nlm.nih.gov -or-
http://igm.nlm.nih.gov

JAMA AIDSLINE search—
http://www.healthgate.com/choice/AMA/
search.html

Medscape HIV/AIDS —
http://HIV.medscape.com/Home/Topics/AIDS
/AIDS.html

Medscape MEDLINE search—
http://www.medscape.com/Clinical/Misc/
FormMedlineInfLive.mhtml

HealthGate MEDLINE search—
http://www.healthgate.com/HealthGate/MEDL
INE/search.shtml

San Francisco Public Library—
http://sfpl.lib.ca.us

UCSF Library (Galen)—
http://www.library.ucsf.edu

University of San Francisco Library—
http://hivinsite.ucsf.edu/

New York Online Access to Health (NOAH)—
http://www.noah.cuny.edu/

AIDS-SPECIFIC SITES

AEGIS: AIDS Education Global Information
System—
http://www.aegis.com/

AIDS Action Committee's subject bibliography to
HIV literature—
http:www.aac.org/hivtreat/index/subj.html

AIDS NYC—
http://www.aidsnyc.org

Asian and Pacific Island Coalition on
HIV/AIDS—
http://www.aidsinfonyc.org/apicha/home.html

The Body HIV/AIDS site—
http://www.thebody.com

Center for AIDS Prevention Studies (UCSF)
CAPSweb—
http://www.epibiostat.ucsf.edu/capsweb

HIV/AIDS Outreach Project (Vanderbilt)—
http://www.mc.vanderbilt.edu/adl/aidsproject

HIVInsite (UCSF)—
http://hivinsite.ucsf.edu

HIVnet, Amsterdam—
http://www.hivnet.org

HIVpositive - comprehensive resource for PWA—
http://www.HIVpositive.com

Immunet, HIV/AIDS information resources for
providers—
http://www.immunet.org

JAMA's HIV/AIDS information center—
http://www.ama-assn.org/special/hiv/
hivhome.htm

News briefings and current articles—
http://www.ama-assn.org/special/hiv/newsline

Johns Hopkins AIDS Service—
http://www.hopkins-aids.edu
http://www.infoweb.org

JRI Health's InfoWeb (Boston)—
http://www.infoweb.org

Marty Howard's AIDS resource page—
http://www.smartlink.net/~martinjh/

Edward King's AIDS pages—
http://www.eking.dircon.co.uk

Queer Resources Directory AIDS links—
http://abacus.oxy.edu/qrd/health/aids

Project Reggie, San Francisco HIV services—
http://www.reggie.org

Search for a Cure—
http:www.searchforacure.org

San Francisco General Hospital AIDS Program—
http://sfghaids.ucsf.edu

AIDS ORGANIZATIONS

ACT UP/Golden Gate—
http://www.actupgg.org

ACT UP/New York—
http://www.actupny.org

AIDS Action Committee, Boston—
http://www.aac.org

AIDS Project Los Angeles—
http://www.apla.org

East Harlem HIV Care Network—
http://www.aidsnyc.org/network

AIDS Research Information Center—
http://www.critpath.org/aric

Critical Path Project, Philadelphia—
http://www.critpath.org

Gay Men's Health Crisis—
http://www.gmhc.org

Harvard AIDS Institute—
http://www.hsph.harvard.edu/Organizations/
hai

The Lambda Center—
http://www.lambdacenter.com/index.htm

National AIDS Treatment Advocacy Project (Jules
Levin)—
http://www.natap.org

Project Inform—
http://www.projinf.org

Stop AIDS Project—
http://www.stopaids.org

Treatment Action Group—
http://www.thebody.com/tag/tagpage.html

UCSF AIDS Health Project—
http://www.ucsf-ahp.org/

AIDS/MEDICAL PUBLICATIONS

AIDS Journal—
http://www.aidsonline.com

AIDS Treatment News—
http://www.aidsnews.org/aidsnews/index.html

AIDS Weekly Plus (CW Henderson) (table of
contents and abstracts)—
http://www.NewsRx.com

British Medical Journal (full text articles)—
http://www.bmj.com/bmj

Clinical Care Options for HIV—
http://www.usc.edu/hsc/nml/e-
resources/info/ClinCarehiv.html

Doctor's Guide to AIDS Information and
resources—
http://www.pslgroup.com/AIDS.htm

International Association of Physicians in AIDS
Care Web site—
http://www.iapac.org

Library of the National Medical Society—
http://www.medical-library.org/

Journal of the American Medical Association
(JAMA) (full text articles available to
registrants)—
http://www.ama-assn.org/public/journals/
jama/jamahome.htm

The Lancet (full text articles available to registrants)—
http://www.thelancet.com

The Merck Manual online—
http://www.merck.com/pubs/

AIDS Knowledge Base—
http://hivinsite.ucsf.edu/

Morbidity & Mortality Weekly Report (full text, requires PDF viewer)—
http://www.cdc.gov/mmwr/

Nature Magazine (summaries and News and Views available)—
http://www.nature.com

Nature Medicine (contents and abstracts available)—
http://medicine.nature.com

New England Journal of Medicine (contents and abstracts available)—
http://www.nejm.org

Science Magazine (contents, abstracts and full text articles available)—
http://sciencemag.org/

Scientific American—
http://www.sciam.com

Treatment Issues (GMHC)—
http://www.gmhc.org/living/treatmnt.html

NEWSPAPERS, MAGAZINES

Multiple newspaper/news service headlines from Aegis—
http://www.aegis.com/newslines.html

CNN Interactive—
http://www.cnn.com

The Gate: San Francisco Chronicle and Examiner—
http://www.sfgate.com
Registration: lizbr/ysw2x

Mercury Center (San Jose Mercury News)—
http://www.sjmercury.com

New York Times On the Web—
http://www.nytimes.com

GOVERNMENT AND NONGOVERNMENT INFO SITES

Centers for Disease Control and Prevention (CDC)—
http://www.cdc.gov

CDC National AIDS Clearinghouse—
http://www.cdcnpin.org/

Wonder, database of CDC reports—
http://wonder.cdc.gov

AIDS Clinical Trials Information Service—
http://www.actis.org or
http://www.hivactis.org

HIV AIDS Treatment Information Service—
http://www.hivatis.org

U.S. Department of Health and Human Services comprehensive health information—
http://www.healthfinder.gov

National Institutes of Health—
http://www.nih.gov

National Institute of Allergies and Infectious Diseases (includes latest news, news archive)—
http://www.niaid.nih.gov

Office of the Federal Register—
http://www.nara.gov/fedreg/

World Health Organization—
http://www.who.org

Joint United Nations Programme on HIV/AIDS—
http://www.unaids.org

HIV/AIDS GLOSSARIES

ATIS Glossary (plain text)—
http://www.cdcnpin.org/

JAMA HIV/AIDS Information Center—
http://www.ama-assn.org/special/hiv

POLICY/ADVOCACY

AIDS Action Council—
http://www.thebody.com/aac/aacpage.html

National Association of People with AIDS (NAPWA)—
http://www.napwa.org/

TREATMENT ACCESS/ADAP

East Harlem HIV Care Network—
http://www.aidsnyc.org/network/

California ADAP—
http://sfghaids.ucsf.edu/research.html

Patient Assistance Programs—
http://sfghaids.ucsf.edu/people.html

Compassionate use, expanded access, and TIND—
http://sfghaids.ucsf.edu/resources.html

CLINICAL TRIALS LISTINGS

AIDS Clinical Trials Information Service—
http://www.actis.org

Centerwatch, international trails listing, information on newly approved drugs—
http://www.centerwatch.com/main.htm

HIV/AIDS trials listing—
http://www.centerwatch.com/CAT2.HTM

Community Programs for Clinical Research on AIDS (CRCRA) home page—
http://www.cpcra.org

Trials Search, California clinical trials—
http://sfghaids.ucsf.edu/research.html

U.S. clinical trials (compiled by Community Consortium)—
http://hivinsite.ucsf.edu/

DRUG/PHARMACEUTICAL SITES

Anti-HIV drug database (HIV Insite)—
http://arvdb.ucsf.edu/

Pharmaceutical Information Network—
http://pharminfo.com/drugdb/db_mnu.html

Drug interactions—
http://www.hivatis.org/fdachart.html

Community Prescription Service—
http://www.prescript.com/

FDA drug information—
http://www.fda.gov/cder/drug/default.htm

Pharminfo (includes drug database)—
http://www.pharminfo.com
http://www.abbott.com
http://www.agouron.com

http://www.fightinfection.com/bms/hiv.htm
http://www.chiron.com
http://www.glaxowellcome.co.uk
http://www.merck.com
http://www.pharmacia.se
http://www.roche.com
http://www.roxane.com/ (Roxane Pain Institute)

GENERAL MEDICAL SITES

Medscape—
http://www.medscape.com

MEDICAL SPECIALTIES

Alternative therapy sites:
http://www.teleport.com/~amrta (AMRTA)
http://www.bastyr.edu/research/buarc/
(Bastyr University)

Cancer information
http://oncolink.upenn.edu/cancernet

Oncolink—
http://www.nci.nih.gov/

NCI's Cancernet—
http://www.graylab.ac.uk/cancernet.html

Hepatitis information site—
http://www.hepnet.com

Pain Management—
http://www.roxane.com

Tuberculosis resources—
http://www.cpmc.columbia.edu/resources/
tbcpp/

Virology information—
http://www.tulane.edu/~dmsander/garryfavwe
bindex.html

New York Times women's health—
http://www.nytimes.com/women

CONFERENCES

Conference on Retroviruses and OI—
http://www.idsociety.org

Conference listings—
http://www.immunet.org/confcalendar

FUNDING

Substance Abuse Prevention and Treatment
Block Grant text (CDC grants and cooperative
agreements on a variety of topics, including
HIV/AIDS)—
www.cdc.gov/funding.htm

National Institutes of Health Funding
Opportunities—
http://grants.nih.gov/grants/

Foundation Center—
www.fdncenter.org

Local/State Funding Report—
www.grantsandfunding.com

HRSA—
www.hrsa.dhhs.gov

HUD—
www.hud.gov

Join Together—
www.jointogether.org

CMHS—
www.samhsa.gov/cmhs

CSAT—
www.samhsa.gov/csat

Substance Abuse Treatment Improvement Exchange—includes a listing of the current SSA Directors—
www.treatment.org

MISCELLANEOUS

AIDS Patent Library—
http://patents.cnidr.org/

The Center Gender Identity Project—
http://www.gaycenter.org/programs/mhss/gip.html

HPP/Prevention Point Needle Exchange—
http://www.sfaf.org/prevention/

Drug Reform Coalition's needle exchange site—
http://www.drcnet.org/gateway/nep.html

North American Syringe Exchange Network—
http://www.nasen.org/NASEN_II/index.html

Safe Works Needle Exchange page—
http://www.safeworks.org

Queer Resources Directory—
http://www.qrd.org/

The Safer Sex Pages—
http://www.safersex.org

Service guide for San Francisco (health clinics, shelters, etc)—
http://thecity.sfsu.edu/~coleman/pguide.html

Appendix G
State and Territorial Health Agencies/Offices of AIDS

*Listed immediately following each State's name is the **State's HIV/AIDS Hotline telephone number**, which provides free and anonymous information and referral to services.*

ALABAMA
Hotline: (800) 228-0469

Alabama Department of Public Health
Division of HIV/AIDS Prevention and Control
RSA Tower
201 Monroe Street
Suite 1400
Montgomery, AL 36104
Phone: (334) 206-5364; Fax: (334) 206-2092
Web site: http://www.alapubhealth.org/inform/hiv/frames7.htm

ALASKA
Hotline: (800) 478-2437

Alaska Department of Health and Social Services
Division of Public Health
350 Main Street, Room 503
Juneau, AK 99801
Phone: (907) 465-3090; Fax: (907) 586-1877
Web site: http://epi.hss.state.ak.us/
(See "Section on Epidemiology" for HIV/AIDS information.)

ARIZONA
Hotline: (800) 352-3792

Arizona Department of Health Services
Bureau of Epidemiology & Disease Control Services
3815 North Black Canyon
Phoenix, AZ 85015
Phone: (602) 230-5808; Fax: (602) 230-5959
Arizona Office of HIV/STD Services
Phone: (602) 230-5819
Web site: http://www.hs.state.az.us/edc/hivpage.html#help

ARKANSAS
Hotline: (800) 482-5400

Arkansas Department of Health
AIDS/STD Section
Arkansas Department of Health
4815 West Markham Street, Mailstop 33
Little Rock, AR 72205-3867
Phone: (501) 661-2111; Fax: (501) 671-1450
Web site: http://health.state.ar.us

CALIFORNIA
Hotline: (800) 367-AIDS
TDD: (888) 225-AIDS

California Department of Health Services
Office of AIDS
611 North 7th Street
P.O. Box 942732
Sacramento, CA 94234-7320
Phone: (916) 445-0553
Web site: http://www.dhs.cahwnet.gov/

COLORADO
Hotline: (800) 252-2437

Colorado Department of Public Health and
   Environment
Disease Control & Environmental Epidemiology
   Division
DCEED-A3
4300 Cherry Creek Drive South
Denver, CO 80246-1530
Phone: (303) 692-2700; Fax: (303) 782-0904
Web site: http://www.cdphe.state.co.us/

CONNECTICUT
Hotline: [not available]

State of Connecticut Department of Public
   Health
Bureau of Community Health
410 Capitol Avenue
P.O. Box 340308, MS #11BCH
Hartford, CT 06134-0308
Phone: (860) 509-7655; Fax: (860) 509-7717
Web site: http://www.state.ct.us/dph/

DELAWARE
Hotline: (800) 422-0429

Delaware Health and Social Services
Division of Public Health, Epidemiology
Federal & Water Streets
P.O. Box 637
Dover, DE 19903
Phone: (302) 739-5617; Fax: (302) 739-6659
Web site: http://www.state.de.us/dhss/irm/
dph/epi1.htm

DISTRICT OF COLUMBIA
Hotline: (800) 322-7432

District of Columbia Department of Health
Administration for HIV/AIDS
717 14th Street NW, 6th Floor
Washington, DC 20036
Phone: (202) 727-2500; Fax: (202) 724-3795
Web site: http://www.dchealth.com/

FEDERATED STATES OF MICRONESIA
Hotline: [not available]

Government of the Federated States of
Micronesia
P.O. Box PS70
Palikir Station
Pohnpei, FSM 96941
Phone: 011 (691) 320-2619; Fax: (690) 320-5263

FLORIDA

Hotline: (800) 352-AIDS
TDD: (888) 503-7118
Spanish: (800) 545-SIDA
Haitian Creole: (800) 243-7101

Department of Health
Bureau of HIV/AIDS
2020 Capital Circle SE, BIN A09
Tallahassee, FL 32399-1715
Phone: (850) 488-9766; Fax: (850) 414-0038
Web site: http://www.doh.state.fl.us/

GEORGIA

Hotline: (800) 551-2728

Georgia Division of Public Health
Epidemiology and Health Information
HIV/STD Surveillance Unit
Two Peachtree Street, NW, Suit 14460
Atlanta, GA 30303-3186
Phone: (404) 657-2624
Web site: http://www.ph.dhr.state.ga.us/epi
epi/aidsunit.shtml

GUAM

Hotline: [not available]

Guam Department of Public Health and Social
    Services
P.O. Box 2816
Agana, GU 96910
Phone: 011 (671) 735-7102; Fax: (671) 734-5910

HAWAII

Hotline: (800) 321-1555

Hawaii Department of Health
Communicable Disease Division
STD/AIDS Information and Prevention
3627 Kileuee Avenue
Suite 305
Honolulu, HI 96816-2399
Phone: (808) 733-9010
Web site: http://www.state.hi.us/health/
resource/comm_dis/std_aids/index.html

IDAHO

Hotline: (800) 677-2437

Idaho Department of Health and Welfare
P.O. Box 83720
450 West State Street, 10th Floor
Boise, ID 83720-0036
Phone: (208) 334-5500
Web site: http://www.state.id.us/
home/health.htm.

ILLINOIS

Hotline: (800) 243-2437
TDD: (800) 782-0423

Illinois Department of Public Health
535 West Jefferson Street
Springfield, IL 62761
Phone: (217) 782-4977; Fax: (217) 782-3987
Web site: http://www.idph.state.il.us/

INDIANA

Hotline: (800) 848-2437
TDD: (800) 972-1846

Indiana State Department of Health
2 North Meridian Street
Indianapolis, IN 46204
Phone: (317) 233-1325
Web site: http://www.state.in.us/isdh/
index.html

IOWA

Hotline: (800) 445-2437

Iowa Department of Public Health
STD/HIV Prevention Program
Lucas State Office Building
321 East 12th Street
Des Moines, IA 50319
Phone: (515) 242-5838; Fax: (515) 281-4570
Web site: http://www.idph.state.ia.us/

KANSAS

Hotline: [not available]

Kansas Department of Health and Environment
Division of Health
Bureau of Epidemiology and Disease
    Prevention, AIDS Section
109 SW 9th Street, Suite 605
Topeka, KS 66612-1271
Phone: (785) 296-6173; Fax: (785) 296-4197
Web site: http://www.kdhe.state.ks.us/aids/

KENTUCKY

Hotline: [not available]

Kentucky Department for Public Health
275 East Main Street
Frankfort, KY 40621
Phone: (502) 564-3970; Fax: (502) 564-6533
Web site: http://cfc-chs.chr.state.ky.us/ph.htm

LOUISIANA

Hotline: (800) 992-4379

TDD: (504) 944-2492

Louisiana Department of Health and
    Hospitals
P.O. Box 3214
Baton Rouge, LA 70821
Phone: (504) 342-8093; Fax: (504) 342-8098
Web site: http://www.dhh.state.la.us/
OPH/index.htm

MAINE

Hotline: (800) 851-2437

Maine Bureau of Health
State House Station 11
157 Capitol Street
Augusta, ME 04333-0011
Phone: (207) 287-8016; Fax: (207) 287-4631
Web site: http://janus.state.me.us/dhs/
boh/index.htm

MARYLAND

Hotline: (800) 638-6252

Metro D.C. and VA: (800) 322-7432

TDD (Baltimore area only): (410) 333-2437

Spanish: (301) 949-0945

State of Maryland Department of Health and
    Mental Hygiene
AIDS Administration
500 North Calvert St.
Fifth Floor
Baltimore, MD 21202
Phone: (410) 767-6505; Fax: (410) 767-6489
Web site: http://www.dhmh.state.md.us/

MASSACHUSETTS

Hotline: (800) 235-2331

TDD: (617) 437-1672

Massachusetts Department of Public Health
250 Washington Street, 2nd Floor
Boston, MA 02108-4619
Phone: (617) 624-5200; Fax: (617) 624-5206
Web site: http://www.magnet.state.ma.us/dph

MICHIGAN

Hotline: (800) 872-2437

TDD: (800) 332-0849

Michigan Department of Community Health
3423 North Martin Luther King, Jr. Boulevard.
P.O. Box 30195
Lansing, MI 48909
Phone: (517) 335-8024; Fax: (517) 335-9476
Web site: http://www.mdch.state.mi.us/

MINNESOTA

Hotline: (800) 248-2437

Minnesota Department of Health
121 East Seventh Place, Suite 450
P.O. Box 9441
St. Paul, MN 55164-0975
Phone: (612) 215-5803; Fax: (612) 215-5801
Web site: http://www.health.state.mn.us/

MISSISSIPPI

Hotline: (800) 826-2961

Mississippi State Department of Health
570 East Woodrow Wilson
P.O. Box 1700
Jackson, MS 39215-1700
Phone: (601) 576-7634; Fax: (601) 960-7931
Web site: http://www.msdh.state.ms.us/
msdhhome.htm

MISSOURI

Hotline: (800) 533-2437

Missouri Department of Health
920 Wildwood
P.O. Box 570
Jefferson City, MO 65102
Phone: (573) 751-6002; Fax: (573) 751-6041
Web site: http://www.health.state.mo.us/

MONTANA

Hotline: (800) 233-6668

Montana Department of Public Health and
    Human Services
P.O. Box 202951
Helena, MT 59620-2951
Phone: (406) 444-5622; Fax: (406) 444-1970
Web site: http://www.dphhs.state.mt.us/

NEBRASKA

Hotline: (800) 782-2437

Nebraska Health and Human Services System
P.O. Box 95007
Lincoln, NE 68509-5007
Phone: (402) 471-3711; Fax: (402) 471-0820
Web site: http://www.hhs.state.ne.us/

NEVADA

Hotline: (800) 842-2437

Nevada State Health Division
505 East King Street, Room 201
Carson City, NV 89701-4797
Phone: (775) 687-3786; Fax: (702) 687-3859
Web site: http://www.state.nv.us/health/

NEW HAMPSHIRE

Hotline: (800) 752-2437

New Hampshire Department of Health and
    Human Services
Six Hazen Drive
Concord, NH 03301-6527
Phone: (603) 271-4372; Fax: (603) 271-4727
Web site: http://www.dhhs.state.nh.us/
Index.nsf?Open

NEW JERSEY

Hotline: (800) 624-2377

TDD: (201) 926-8008

New Jersey Department of Health and Senior
    Services
CN360, Room 805
John Fitch Plaza
Trenton, NJ 08625-0360
Phone: (609) 292-7837; Fax: (609) 292-0053
Web site: http://www.state.nj.us/health/aids/
aidsprv.htm

NEW MEXICO

Hotline: (800) 545-2437

New Mexico Department of Health
P.O. Box 26110
Santa Fe, NM 87502-6110
Phone: (505) 827-2613; Fax: (505) 827-2530
Web site: [not available]

NEW YORK
Hotline: (800) 872-2777, (800) 541-2437;
Spanish: (800) 233-SIDA
TDD: (800) 369-2437

New York State Department of Health
AIDS Institute
Empire State Plaza, 14th Floor
Corning Tower Building
Albany, NY 12237
Phone: (518) 474-2011; Fax: (518) 474-5450
Web site: http://www.health.state.ny.us/
nysdoh/aids/hivtesti.htm

NORTH CAROLINA
Hotline: (800) 342-2437

North Carolina Department of Health and
    Human Services
1601 Mail Service Center
Raleigh, NC 27699-1601
Phone: (919) 733-4984; Fax: (919) 715-3060
Web site: http://www.dhhs.state.nc.us/

NORTH DAKOTA
Hotline: (800) 472-2180

North Dakota Department of Health
600 East Boulevard Avenue
Bismarck, ND 58505-0200
Phone: (701) 328-2372; Fax: (701) 328-4727
Web site: http://www.ehs.health.
state.nd.us/ndhd/

OHIO
Hotline: (800) 332-2437; TDD: (800) 332-3889

Ohio Department of Health
246 North High Street
P.O. Box 118
Columbus, OH 43266-0118
Phone: (614) 466-2253; Fax: (614) 644-0085
Web site: http://www.odh.state.oh.us/

OKLAHOMA
Hotline: (800) 535-2437

Oklahoma State Department of Health
1000 NE 10th Street
Oklahoma City, OK 73117-1299
Phone: (405) 271-4200; Fax: (405) 271-3431
Web site: http://www.health.state.ok.us/
program/hivstd/index.html

OREGON
Hotline: (800) 777-2437 (*For area codes 503, 206
and 208*)
Voice and TDD: (503) 223-2437

Oregon Department of Human Services
800 NE Oregon Street, #21, Suite 925
Portland, OR 97232
Phone: (503) 731-4000; Fax: (503) 731-4078
Web site: http://www.ohd.hr.state.or.us/
hiv/welcome.htm

PENNSYLVANIA
Hotline: (800) 662-6080

Pennsylvania Department of Health
HIV/AIDS Programs
Health and Welfare Building, Room 802
Harrisburg, PA 17120
Phone: (717) 787-6436; Fax: (717) 787-0191
Web site: http://www.health.state.pa.us/
php/HIV/default.htm

PUERTO RICO
Hotline: (800) 981-5721

Puerto Rico Department of Public Health
Commonwealth of Puerto Rico
Building A
Call Box 70184
San Juan, PR 00936
Phone: (809) 274-7600; Fax: (809) 250-6745
Web site: [not available]

RHODE ISLAND
Hotline: (800) 726-3010

Rhode Island Department of Health
Three Capitol Hill, Room 106
Providence, RI 02908-5097
Phone: (401) 222-2577; Fax: (401) 272-3771
Web site: http://www.health.state.ri.us/

SOUTH CAROLINA
Hotline: (800) 322-2437

South Carolina Department of Health and
Environmental Control
2600 Bull Street
Columbia, SC 29201
Phone: (803) 898-3432; Fax: (803) 734-4620
Web site: http://www.state.sc.us/dhec/

SOUTH DAKOTA
Hotline: (800) 592-1861

South Dakota Department of Health
Sigurd Anderson Building
445 East Capitol Avenue
Pierre, SD 57501-3185
Phone: 605-773-3361; Fax: 605-773-5683
Web site: http://www.state.sd.us/doh/
doh.html

TENNESSEE
Hotline: (800) 525-2437

Tennessee Department of Health
Cordell Hull Building, 3rd Floor
425 Fifth Avenue North
Nashville, TN 37247-0101
Phone: (615) 741-3111; Fax: (615) 741-2491
Web site: http://www.state.tn.us/health/

TEXAS
Hotline: (800) 299-2437
TDD: (800) 252-8012

Texas Department of Health
1100 West 49th Street
Austin, TX 78756-7446
Phone: (512) 458-7376; Fax: (512) 458-7477
Web site: http://www.tdh.texas.gov/

UTAH
Hotline: (800) 366-2437

Utah Department of Health
Bureau of HIV/AIDS/TB Control/Refugee
Health
288 North 1460 West
P.O. Box 142105
Salt Lake City, UT 84114-2105
Phone: (801) 538-0696; Fax: (801) 538-6306
Web site: http://hlunix.ex.state.ut.us/els/
hivaids/index.html

VERMONT
Hotline: (800) 464-4343

Vermont Department of Health
108 Cherry Street
Burlington, VT 05402-0070
Phone: (802) 863-7280; Fax: (802) 863-7425
Web site: http://www.state.vt.us/health/
index.htm

U.S. VIRGIN ISLANDS

Hotline: (809) 773-2437

Virgin Islands Department of Social and Health
  Services
48 Sugar Estate
St. Thomas, VI 00802
Phone: (809) 774-0117; Fax: (809) 777-4001
Web site: [not available]

VIRGINIA

Hotline: (800) 533-4148
Spanish: (800) 322-7432

Virginia Department of Health
1500 East Main Street, Suite 214
P.O. Box 2448
Richmond, VA 23219
Phone: (804) 786-3561; Fax: (804) 786-4616
Web site: http://www.vdh.state.va.us/

WASHINGTON

Hotline: (800) 272-2437

Washington State Department of Health
1112 SE Quince Street
P.O. Box 47890
Olympia, WA 98504-7890
Phone: (360) 753-5871; Fax: (360) 586-7424
Web site: http://www.doh.wa.gov/

WEST VIRGINIA

Hotline: (800) 642-8244

West Virginia Department of Health and
  Human Resources
Bureau for Public Health
Surveillance and Disease Control
Room 125
350 Capitol Street
Charleston, WV 25302-3715
Phone: (304) 558-5358; Fax: (394) 558-1035
Web site: http://www.wvdhhr.org/

WISCONSIN

Hotline: (414) 273-2437 or (800) 334-2437

Wisconsin Department of Health and Family
  Services
One West Wilson Street
P.O. Box 309
Madison, WI 53701-0309
Phone: (608) 266-1511; Fax: (608) 267-2832
Web site: http://www.dhfs.state.wi.us/

WYOMING

Hotline: (800) 327-3577

Wyoming Department of Health
117 Hathaway Building
Cheyenne, WY 82002
Phone: (307) 777-7656; Fax: (307) 777-7439
Web site: http://wdhfs.state.wy.us/wdh/

Department of Health	If Phoning Within the State	If Phoning Out of State
Alabama Department of Public Health	(800) 228-0469	(334) 613-5357
Alaska Department of Health and Social Services	(800) 478-AIDS	(907) 276-1400
Arizona Department of Health Services	(602) 234-2752	(602) 234-2752
Arkansas Department of Health	(501) 375-0352	(501) 375-0352
California Department of Health Services	(800) 400-7432	(213) 845-4180
Colorado Department of Public Health and the Environment	(800) 252-AIDS	(303) 692-2720
Connecticut Department of Public Health	(203) 247-AIDS	(203) 624-AIDS
Delaware Department of Health and Social Services	(800) 422-0429	(302) 652-6776
District of Columbia Department of Health	(800) 342-AIDS	(202) 332-AIDS
Florida Department of Health	(800) FLA-AIDS	(904) 681-9131
Georgia Department of Public Health	(800) 551-2728	(404) 876-9944
Hawaii Department of Health	(808) 922-1313	(808) 922-1313
Idaho Department of Health and Welfare	(800) 677-AIDS	(208) 345-2277
Illinois Department of Public Health	(800) 243-AIDS	(773) 929-4357
Indiana Department of Health	(800) 848-AIDS	(317) 383-6743
Iowa Department of Public Health	(800) 445-AIDS	(515) 244-6700
Kentucky Department for Public Health	(800) 840-2865	(606) 278-3935
Louisiana Department of Health and Hospitals	(800) 992-4379	(504) 945-4000
Maine Bureau of Health	(800) 851-AIDS	(207) 774-6877
Maryland Department of Health and Mental Hygiene	(800) 638-6252	(410) 333-AIDS
Massachusetts Department of Public Health	(800) 235-2331	(617) 536-7733
Michigan Department of Community Health	(800) 872-AIDS	(810) 547-3783
Minnesota Department of Health	(800) 248-AIDS	(612) 373-AIDS
Mississippi State Department of Health	(800) 826-2961	(601) 936-6959
Missouri Department of Health	(800) 533-AIDS	(314) 516-2761
Montana Department of Public Health and Human Services	(800) 233-6668	(406) 444-3566
Nebraska Health and Human Services System	(800) 782-AIDS	(402) 342-4233
Nevada State Health Division	(702) 687-4804	(702) 474-AIDS
New Hampshire Department of Health/Human Services	(800) 639-1122	(603) 623-0710
New Jersey Department of Health	(800) 508-7577	(201) 489-2900
New Mexico Department of Health	(800) 545-AIDS	(505) 476-8456
New York State Department of Health	(800) 647-1420	(800) 828-3280
North Carolina Department of Health and Human Services	(800) 346-3731	None
North Dakota Department of Health	(800) 472-2180	None
Ohio Department of Health	(800) 332-AIDS	(513) 421-AIDS
Oklahoma Department of Health	(800) 535-AIDS	(405) 271-4636
Oregon Department of Human Resources	(800) 777-AIDS	(503) 223-AIDS
Pennsylvania Department of Health	(717) 783-0479	None
Rhode Island Department of Health	(800) 726-3010	(401) 831-5522

Department of Health	If Phoning Within the State	If Phoning Out of State
South Carolina Department of Health and Environmental Control	(800) 342-AIDS	(803) 779-7257
South Dakota Department of Health	(800) 738-2301	(605) 773-3364
Tennessee Department of Health	(800) 525-AIDS	(615) 741-7583
Texas Department of Health	(800) 299-AIDS	(512) 490-2535
Utah Department of Health	(800) 366-AIDS	(801) 487-2100
Vermont Department of Health	(800) 882-AIDS	(802) 863-7245
Virginia Department of Health	(800) 533-4148	(804) 371-7455
Washington State Department of Health	(800) 272-AIDS	(360) 586-3887
West Virginia Department of Health and Human Resources	(800) 642-8244	(304) 558-2950
Wisconsin Department of Health and Social Services	(800) 334-AIDS	(414) 273-AIDS
Wyoming Department of Health	(800) 327-3577	(307) 777-5800

Appendix H
Mini Mental State Examination (MMSE)

Date: _____

Patient's Name: _____

Maximum Score	Score	
		ORIENTATION
5	( )	What is the (year) (season) (date) (day) (month)?
5	( )	Where are we: (State) (county) (town or city) (hospital) (floor)?
		REGISTRATION
3	( )	Name 3 common objects (e.g., "apple," "table," "penny"): Take 1 second to say each. Then ask the patient to repeat all 3 after you have said them. Give 1 point for each correct answer. Then repeat them until he/she learns all 3. Count trials and record. Trials:
		ATTENTION AND CALCULATION
5	( )	Spell "world" backwards. The score is the number of letters in correct order. (D__L__R__O__W__).
		RECALL
3	( )	Ask for the 3 objects repeated above. Give 1 point for each correct answer. (Note: Recall cannot be tested if all 3 objects were not remembered during registration.)

LANGUAGE

2	( )	Name a "pencil" and "watch."
1	( )	Repeat the following: "No ifs, ands, or buts."
3	( )	Follow a 3-stage command:

"Take a paper in your right hand,

fold it in half, and

put it on the floor."

1	( )	Read and obey the following:
1	( )	Close your eyes.
1	( )	Write a sentence.
1	( )	Copy the following design:

No construction problem

Total Score: ─────────

Source: Folstein, M.F.; Folstein, S.E.; and McHugh, P.R. "Mini-mental state": A practical method for grading the cognitive state of patients for the clinician. *Journal of Psychiatric Research* 12(3):189–198, 1975.

Appendix I
Standards of Care: Client Assessment/Treatment Protocol

This assessment tool was developed by Steven Batki, M.D.; Marilyn Blake, R.N.; Valerie Gruber, Ph.D.; Ellie Milovitch, R.N.; Gale Ouye, L.C.S.W.; Kalpana Nathan, M.D.; and Richard Warren. It is currently in use at the Opiate Treatment Outpatient Program, San Francisco General Hospital, University of California at San Francisco.

Client name _____   Date _____   Completed by _____

A. CLIENT ASSESSMENT

Physical Health (Measures American Society of Addiction Medicine, Dimension 2: Biomedical Conditions. (Scale is adapted from Karnofsky Scale)
This rating is based on a physician's examination of the client or of the client's file.

5   No signs or symptoms of disease; normal activity

4   Mild signs and/or symptoms of disease; needs only routine medical care; normal activity

3   Moderate signs and/or symptoms of disease; requires medical care more than once per month; requires occasional assistance with activities

2   Disabled, severe signs and symptoms of disease; requires weekly medical and nursing care; requires assistance with activities several times per week

1   Severely disabled, requires daily medical and nursing care; requires daily assistance with activities (e.g., visiting nurses and hospice)

UK   Unknown, cannot be determined at this time

_____

Physical Health Score

Mental Health (ASAM Dimension 3: Emotional/Behavioral Conditions) (Scale is adapted from DSM-IV
   GAF)

This rating is based on a psychiatrist's examination of the client or of the client's file.

5   No psychiatric symptoms, past or present

4   Psychiatric symptoms by history but stable

3   Mild psychiatric symptoms, i.e., change in sleep, appetite, or mood

2   Moderate psychiatric symptoms are present, and behavior may be unpredictable

1   Severe psychiatric symptoms are present; behavior is influenced by serious impairment in
        communication and judgment or inability to function in almost all areas

UK   Unknown, cannot be determined at this time

_____

Mental Health Score

Social Resources (ASAM Dimension 6: Recovery Environment) *Rated by the counselor.*

Social Support

5   Consistently utilizes clean and sober friends/family for support

4   Consistently uses community resources, e.g., support groups, case management, social services

3   Inconsistent utilization of clean and sober friends/family and community resources

2   Rarely utilizes clean and sober friends/family and community resources

1 ´   Never utilizes clean and sober support resources

UK   Unknown, cannot be determined at this time

_____

Social Support Score

Housing

5   Permanent housing (e.g., apartment, home)

4   Long-term SRO hotel (available over 2 years)

3   Temporary housing (91 days to 2 years, e.g., long-term residential facilities)

2   Short-term housing (30-90 days, e.g., shelters, short-term residential facilities)

1   Homeless (e.g., in SRO for less than 30 days, couch surfing, or living outdoors)

UK   Unknown, cannot be determined at this time

_____

Housing Score

Social Resources Score =

    Social Support score: _____

    Housing score: _____

    Average Social Resources score: _____ **divided by 2:** _____

Total = _____

Combined Score =

    Physical Health Score   _____
        +
    Mental Health Score   _____
        +
    Social Resources Score   _____

    Total =   _____

    Average: Divide total by 3:   _____

B. TREATMENT PROTOCOL

General Expectations and Interventions for Methadone/LAAM Maintenance Clients

1. *Attendance*

1a) Target Behavior:
Clients are expected to attend (or cancel with advance notice) 90 percent or more of scheduled clinic visits each month. This includes dosing, counseling, and other visits (e.g., social services, psychiatric services, or medical services).

1b) Initial Interventions:
Clients who attend less than 90 percent of scheduled visits for 1 month will receive counseling and behavior contracts to help them reduce unscheduled absences.

1c) Clinic Response to Continued Nonadherence:
Clients who continue to attend less than 90 percent of scheduled visits despite 6 months of the interventions above will be considered for discharge.

2. *Giving Urine Samples Upon Request*

2a) Target Behavior:
Clients are expected to provide urine samples and Breathalyzer™ tests upon request.

2b) Initial Interventions:
Clients who refuse urine samples or Breathalyzers™ or who no-show on urine collection days once or more per month will receive counseling and behavior contracts to help them reduce refusals and/or no-shows.

2c) Clinic Response to Continued Nonadherence:
Clients who continually refuse urine samples or Breathalyzers™ or who no-show on urine collection days after 6 months of the interventions above will be considered for discharge.

3. *Drug and Alcohol Use*

3a) Target Behavior:
Clients are expected to provide urine samples free of illicit drugs (including opiates and non-opiates) and Breathalyzer™ tests indicating nonsignificant alcohol use no later than after 1 year in the program. Prescribed medications and medicinal marijuana are not counted as illicit drugs.

3b) Initial Interventions:
Clients who provide drug/alcohol positive samples will receive counseling and behavior contracts to help them reduce and stop their drug/alcohol use.

3c) <u>Clinic Response to Continued Nonadherence</u>:
Clients who continue to provide drug/alcohol positive samples for several consecutive months at 2 years in the program, AND show no progress in other areas of their life, will be considered for discharge.

<u>Note</u>:
Clients who are discharged may apply after 1 month to be placed on the waiting list for readmission.

Standards of Care for Clients at Various Levels of Functioning

1. <u>Is Physical Health</u> = 2 or less? (disabled, severe disease, weekly medical care, assistance several times per week)

IF YES → <u>Use Palliative Care Model</u>

These severely medically ill clients are generally expected to meet the expectations above. There are several modifications with these clients:

1a) <u>Modified expectations regarding attendance and urine samples</u>:
On rare occasions, medical problems prevent these clients from attending clinic or providing urine samples.

1b) <u>Modified response to continued use of illicit drugs or alcohol</u>:
Counseling focuses on reducing substance use as well as increasing access to and adherence to medical treatment.

These clients are rarely discharged for continued drug use. This is because methadone/LAAM can prevent the serious health effects of return to heavy heroin use by medically ill clients.

IF NO → <u>Go to 2</u>

2. <u>Is Mental Health</u> = 2 or less? (moderate to severe psychiatric impairment)

IF YES → <u>Use Psychiatric Model</u>

These severely mentally ill clients are generally expected to meet the expectations above. There are several modifications with these clients:

2a) <u>Modified expectations regarding attendance</u>:
The expected clinic attendance is lower for clients with severe psychiatric symptoms such as cognitive impairment, thought disorder, or mood disorder.

2b) <u>Modified response to continued drug or alcohol use</u>:

Counseling focuses on reducing substance use as well as increasing access and adherence to treatment of psychiatric disorder or cognitive deficit.

These clients are rarely discharged for continued drug use. This is because methadone/LAAM can help to maintain functioning and connection to services among clients with severe psychiatric symptoms.

IF NO → Go to 3

3. Are Social Resources = 2 or less? (insufficient or high-risk social support, housing, and/or finances)

IF YES → Use Psychosocial Model

These clients are generally expected to meet the expectations above. There are several modifications with these clients:

3a) Modified expectations regarding attendance:
The expected attendance is lower for clients with severely deficient housing, financial, or transportation resources.

3b) Response to continued drug or alcohol use:
Counseling focuses on reducing substance use as well as accessing housing, finances, and transportation.

Clients who, despite efforts to access housing and other basic resources, continue to be homeless and impoverished are rarely discharged for continued drug use. This is because for these clients, the methadone/LAAM clinic is often one of the last remaining resources, the loss of which may be life threatening.

IF NO → Go to 4

4. If no scale scores are 2 or less, use Standard Treatment Model

These clients are expected to meet the general expectations above.

Appendix J
Resource Panel

Brad Austin
   Public Health Advisor
   Division of State and Community Assistance
   PPG Program Branch
   Center for Substance Abuse Treatment
   Rockville, Maryland

Jose Martin Garcia-Ordoria
   Technical Assistant Manager
   National Latino/a Lesbian and Gay
      Organization
   Washington, D.C.

Patricia Hawkins, Ph.D.
   Associate Executive Director
   Whitman-Walker Clinic
   Washington, D.C.

Adolfo Mata
   Director
   Migrant Health Program
   Community of Migrant Health
   Bureau of Primary Health Care
   Health Resources Services Administration
   Bethesda, Maryland

M. Valerie Mills, M.S.W.
   Associate Administrator for AIDS
   Substance Abuse and Mental Health Services
      Administration
   Rockville, Maryland

Andrea Ronhovde, L.C.S.W.
   Director
   Alexandria Mental Health HIV/AIDS Project
   Alexandria Mental Health Center
   Alexandria, Virginia

Gloria Weissman
   Director
   Program Development Staff
   Division of Community Based Programs
   HIV/AIDS Bureau
   Health Resources and Services
      Administration
   Rockville, Maryland

Appendix K
Field Reviewers

Deborah Wright Bauer, M.P.H., M.L.S.
Health Project Consultant
Georgia Ryan White Title IV Project
Epidemiology and Prevention Branch
Department of Human Resources
Atlanta, Georgia

Margaret K. Brooks, J.D., M.A.
New Perspectives
Montclair, New Jersey

Robert Paul Cabaj, M.D.
Medical Director
San Mateo County Mental Health Services
Mental Health Services Administration
San Mateo, California

Edwin M. Craft, Ph.D.
Program Analyst
Office of Evaluation, Scientific Analysis and
Synthesis, Synthesis Branch
Center for Substance Abuse Treatment
Rockville, Maryland

Michael A. Dawes, M.D.
Assistant Professor of Psychiatry
Child and Adolescent Psychiatry
Western Psychiatric Institute and Clinic
Pittsburgh, Pennsylvania

James Donagher, M.A.
Director
Senior Services
Special Populations of Office of Behavioral
Health
Department of Mental Health and Addiction
Services
Hartford, Connecticut

Michael Fingerhood, M.D.
Associate Professor of Medicine
Center for Chemical Dependence
School of Medicine
Johns Hopkins University
Baltimore, Maryland

Stewart L. Gallas, S.W.A., M.A.
Co-Director, Client Services
AIDS Services of Austin
Austin, Texas

Susan M. Gallego, M.S.S.W., L.M.S.W.-A.C.P.
Trainer, Consultant, and Facilitator
Austin, Texas

Larry M. Gant, Ph.D., C.S.W., M.S.W.
Associate Professor
School of Social Work
University of Michigan
Ann Arbor, Michigan

Brian C. Giddens, M.S.W., A.C.S.W.
Associate Director
Social Work Department
University of Washington Medical Center
Seattle, Washington

Michael Gorman, Ph.D., M.S.W., M.P.H.
Research Scientist/Principal Investigator
Alcohol and Drug Abuse Institute
School of Social Work
University of Washington
Seattle, Washington

Brian L. Greenberg, Ph.D.
Director of Development
Walden House, Incorporated
San Francisco, California

Gregory L. Greenwood, Ph.D., M.P.H.
TAPS Fellow
Center for AIDS Prevention Studies
University of California at San Francisco
San Francisco, California

Susan Haikalis, A.C.S.W., M.S.W., L.C.S.W.
Director
HIV Services and Treatment Support
San Francisco AIDS Foundation
San Francisco, California

William F. Haning, III, M.D.
Department of Psychiatry
School of Medicine
University of Hawaii
Honolulu, Hawaii

Peter Hayden
Director
TURNING POINT
National Chairperson
National Black Alcoholism and Addictions
Council
Minneapolis, Minnesota

Warren W. Hewitt, Jr., M.S.
Planner
Office of Policy Coordination and Planning
Center for Substance Abuse Treatment
Rockville, Maryland

Donna Johnson, L.M.S.W.
Hospice Social Worker
Denson Community Health Services Hospice
League City, Texas

Murali R. Jonnalagadda, M.D., M.P.H., F.A.P.A.
Jacksonville, North Carolina

Karen Kelly-Woodall, M.S., M.A.C., N.C.A.C.II
Criminal Justice Coordinator
Addiction Technology Transfer Center
Morehouse School of Medicine
Atlanta, Georgia

Sherry Knapp, Ph.D.
Associate Director
Division of Substance Abuse
Rhode Island Department of Health
Providence, Rhode Island

Marshall K. Kubota, M.D.
Director
Family Practice Residency Program
Sutter Medical Center of Santa Rosa
Santa Rosa, California

Susan LeLacheur, M.P.H., P.A.-C.
Assistant Professor of Health Care Sciences
and Health Sciences
The George Washington University
Physician Assistant Program
Washington, D.C.

Yvette Lindsey
HIV Community Coalition
Washington, D.C.

Russell P. MacPherson, Ph.D., C.A.P., C.A.P.P.,
   President
   RPM Addiction Prevention Training
   Deland, Florida

John J. McGovern, C.S.W.
   Director
   Clinical Services
   HELP/Project Samaritan, Inc.
   Bronx, New York

Lisa A. Melchior, Ph.D.
   Vice President
   The Measurement Group
   Culver City, California

Alelia Munroe
   Consultant
   National Black Alcoholism and Addictions
      Council
   Orlando, Florida

Gail M. Nahwahquaw, B.S.
   Case Manager Consultant
   Consultant (Menominee)
   The HIV Center for Excellence
   Phoenix Indian Medical Center
   Phoenix, Arizona

Thomas Nicholson, Ph.D., M.P.H., M.A.Ed.
   Professor
   Department of Public Health
   Western Kentucky University
   Bowling Green, Kentucky

Kenneth L. Packer
   Health Education Consultant
   The Golden Skate
   Washingtonville, New York

Eileen Stark Pagan, M.S., R.N.C.
   Director of Nursing Services
   HELP/ Project Samaritan, Inc.
   Bronx, New York

Billy Pick, J.D., M.S.W.
   Program Manager
   AIDS Office
   San Francisco Department of Public Health
   San Francisco, California

Mel Pohl, M.D.
   Charter Hospital
   Las Vegas, Nevada

John F. Robertson, Ph.D.
   Executive Director
   Robertson Psychological and Consulting
      Services
   National Black Alcoholism and Addictions
      Council
   Utica, New York

Andrea Ronhovde, L.C.S.W.
   Director
   Alexandria Mental Health HIV/AIDS Project
   Alexandria Mental Health Center
   Alexandria, Virginia

Jeffrey H. Samet, M.D., M.A., M.P.H.
   Associate Professor of Medicine
   Boston University School of Medicine
   Boston, Massachusetts

Christine Smith, M.S.W.
   Senior Analyst
   ABT Associates
   Cambridge, Massachusetts

Mary Sowder, L.P.C., C.D.A.C.
   Vice President
   Texas HIV Connection
   Workers Assistance Program
   Austin, Texas

Ronald D. Stall, Ph.D., M.P.H.
   Center for AIDS Prevention Studies
   University of California at San Francisco
   San Francisco, California

Richard T. Suchinsky, M.D.
  Associate Chief for Addictive Disorders and
    Psychiatric Rehabilitation
  Mental Health and Behavioral Sciences
    Services
  Department of Veterans Affairs
  Washington, D.C.

David C. Thompson
  Public Health Advisor
  Division of Practice and Systems
    Development
  Center for Substance Abuse Treatment
  Rockville, Maryland

Mark E. Wallace, M.D.
  Psychiatrist
  New York City Human Resources
    Administration
  Office of Health and Mental Services
  New York, New York

Gloria Weissman
  Director
  Program Development Staff
  Division of Community Based Programs
  HIV/AIDS Bureau
  Health Resources and Services
    Administration
  Rockville, Maryland

Christopher J. Welsh, M.D.
  Clinical Assistant Professor
  Alcohol and Drug Abuse/Psychiatry
  Medical Director
  HIV/LAAM Program
  University of Maryland
  Baltimore, Maryland

Barbara C. Zeller, M.D.
  Medical Director
  HELP/Project Samaritan, Inc.
  Bronx, New York

Janet Zwick
  Director
  Division of Substance Abuse and Health
    Promotion
  Iowa Department of Public Health
  Des Moines, Iowa

GPO U.S. GOVERNMENT PRINTING OFFICE: 2009-349-358/43621